Dietary Polyphenols and Human Health

Dietary Polyphenols and Human Health

Editor

Anna Tresserra-Rimbau

MDPI • Basel • Beijing • Wuhan • Barcelona • Belgrade • Manchester • Tokyo • Cluj • Tianjin

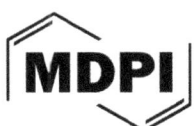

Editor
Anna Tresserra-Rimbau
University of Barcelona
Barcelona

Editorial Office
MDPI
St. Alban-Anlage 66
4052 Basel, Switzerland

This is a reprint of articles from the Special Issue published online in the open access journal *Nutrients* (ISSN 2072-6643) (available at: https://www.mdpi.com/journal/nutrients/special_issues/Dietary_Polyphenols_and_Human_Health).

For citation purposes, cite each article independently as indicated on the article page online and as indicated below:

LastName, A.A.; LastName, B.B.; LastName, C.C. Article Title. *Journal Name* **Year**, *Volume Number*, Page Range.

ISBN 978-3-03943-793-1 (Hbk)
ISBN 978-3-03943-794-8 (PDF)

Cover image courtesy of Oriol Pagès.

© 2020 by the authors. Articles in this book are Open Access and distributed under the Creative Commons Attribution (CC BY) license, which allows users to download, copy and build upon published articles, as long as the author and publisher are properly credited, which ensures maximum dissemination and a wider impact of our publications.

The book as a whole is distributed by MDPI under the terms and conditions of the Creative Commons license CC BY-NC-ND.

Contents

About the Editor vii

Anna Tresserra-Rimbau
Dietary Polyphenols and Human Health
Reprinted from: *Nutrients* **2020**, *12*, 2893, doi:10.3390/nu12092893 1

**Daniela Martini, Stefano Bernardi, Cristian Del Bo', Nicole Hidalgo Liberona,
Raul Zamora-Ros, Massimiliano Tucci, Antonio Cherubini, Marisa Porrini, Giorgio Gargari,
Raúl González-Domínguez, Gregorio Peron, Benjamin Kirkup, Paul A Kroon,
Cristina Andres-Lacueva, Simone Guglielmetti and Patrizia Riso**
Estimated Intakes of Nutrients and Polyphenols in Participants Completing the MaPLE Randomised Controlled Trial and Its Relevance for the Future Development of Dietary Guidelines for the Older Subjects
Reprinted from: *Nutrients* **2020**, *12*, 2458, doi:10.3390/nu12082458 5

**Meropi D. Kontogianni, Aswathy Vijayakumar, Ciara Rooney, Rebecca L. Noad,
Katherine M. Appleton, Danielle McCarthy, Michael Donnelly, Ian S. Young,
Michelle C. McKinley, Pascal P. McKeown and Jayne V. Woodside**
A High Polyphenol Diet Improves Psychological Well-Being: The Polyphenol Intervention Trial (PPhIT)
Reprinted from: *Nutrients* **2020**, *12*, 2445, doi:10.3390/nu12082445 23

**Emma L. Wightman, Philippa A. Jackson, Joanne Forster, Julie Khan, Julia C. Wiebe,
Nigel Gericke and David O. Kennedy**
Acute Effects of a Polyphenol-Rich Leaf Extract of *Mangifera indica* L. (Zynamite) on Cognitive Function in Healthy Adults: A Double-Blind, Placebo-Controlled Crossover Study
Reprinted from: *Nutrients* **2020**, *12*, 2194, doi:10.3390/nu12082194 39

Jing Sun, Hong Jiang, Weijing Wang, Xue Dong and Dongfeng Zhang
Associations of Urinary Phytoestrogen Concentrations with Sleep Disorders and Sleep Duration among Adults
Reprinted from: *Nutrients* **2020**, *12*, 2103, doi:10.3390/nu12072103 55

Nancy Saji, Nidhish Francis, Lachlan J. Schwarz, Christopher L. Blanchard and Abishek B. Santhakumar
Rice Bran Phenolic Extracts Modulate Insulin Secretion and Gene Expression Associated with β-Cell Function
Reprinted from: *Nutrients* **2020**, *12*, 1889, doi:10.3390/nu12061889 81

**Borkwei Ed Nignpense, Kenneth A Chinkwo, Christopher L Blanchard and
Abishek B Santhakumar**
Black Sorghum Phenolic Extract Modulates Platelet Activation and Platelet Microparticle Release
Reprinted from: *Nutrients* **2020**, *12*, 1760, doi:10.3390/nu12061760 95

Sara Castro-Barquero, Anna Tresserra-Rimbau, Facundo Vitelli-Storelli, Mónica Doménech, Jordi Salas-Salvadó, Vicente Martín-Sánchez, María Rubín-García, Pilar Buil-Cosiales, Dolores Corella, Montserrat Fitó, Dora Romaguera, Jesús Vioque, Ángel María Alonso-Gómez, Julia Wärnberg, José Alfredo Martínez, Luís Serra-Majem, Francisco José Tinahones, José Lapetra, Xavier Pintó, Josep Antonio Tur, Antonio Garcia-Rios, Laura García-Molina, Miguel Delgado-Rodriguez, Pilar Matía-Martín, Lidia Daimiel, Josep Vidal, Clotilde Vázquez, Montserrat Cofán, Andrea Romanos-Nanclares, Nerea Becerra-Tomas, Rocio Barragan, Olga Castañer, Jadwiga Konieczna, Sandra González-Palacios, Carolina Sorto-Sánchez, Jessica Pérez-López, María Angeles Zulet, Inmaculada Bautista-Castaño, Rosa Casas, Ana María Gómez-Perez, José Manuel Santos-Lozano, María Ángeles Rodríguez-Sanchez, Alicia Julibert, Nerea Martín-Calvo, Pablo Hernández-Alonso, José V Sorlí, Albert Sanllorente, Aina María Galmés-Panadés, Eugenio Cases-Pérez, Leire Goicolea-Güemez, **Miguel Ruiz-Canela, Nancy Babio, Álvaro Hernáez, Rosa María Lamuela-Raventós and Ramon Estruch**
Dietary Polyphenol Intake is Associated with HDL-Cholesterol and A Better Profile of Other Components of the Metabolic Syndrome: A PREDIMED-Plus Sub-Study
Reprinted from: *Nutrients* **2020**, *12*, 689, doi:10.3390/nu12030689 . . . . **107**

Inés Domínguez-López, María Yago-Aragón, Albert Salas-Huetos, Anna Tresserra-Rimbau and Sara Hurtado-Barroso
Effects of Dietary Phytoestrogens on Hormones throughout a Human Lifespan: A Review
Reprinted from: *Nutrients* **2020**, *12*, 2456, doi:10.3390/nu12082456 . . . . **125**

Viviana Sandoval, Hèctor Sanz-Lamora, Giselle Arias, Pedro F. Marrero, Diego Haro and Joana Relat
Metabolic Impact of Flavonoids Consumption in Obesity: From Central to Peripheral
Reprinted from: *Nutrients* **2020**, *12*, 2393, doi:10.3390/nu12082393 . . . . **151**

Estefanía Márquez Campos, Linda Jakobs and Marie-Christine Simon
Antidiabetic Effects of Flavan-3-ols and Their Microbial Metabolites
Reprinted from: *Nutrients* **2020**, *12*, 1592, doi:10.3390/nu12061592 . . . . **205**

About the Editor

Anna Tresserra-Rimbau is Serra-Hunter tenure teacher in the Department of Nutrition, Food Science and Gastronomy of the Faculty of Pharmacy and Food Science of the University of Barcelona. She is a member of the INSA-UB (Institute for Research on Nutrition and Food Safety) and the CIBEROBN consortium (Spanish Biomedical Research Centre in Physiopathology of Obesity and Nutrition). Her main research topic is the influence of polyphenols and polyphenol-rich foods on chronic diseases. She has participated in many different national and international projects, mainly human intervention studies such as the PREDIMED, the PREDIMEDplus, and the SI! Program.

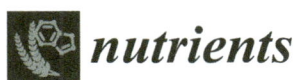

Editorial

Dietary Polyphenols and Human Health

Anna Tresserra-Rimbau [1,2]

1. Department of Nutrition, Food Science and Gastronomy, XaRTA, INSA, School of Pharmacy and Food Sciences, University of Barcelona, 08028 Barcelona, Spain; annatresserra@ub.edu
2. Centro de Investigación Biomédica en Red Fisiopatología de la Obesidad y la Nutrición (CIBEROBN), Instituto de Salud Carlos III, 28029 Madrid, Spain

Received: 18 September 2020; Accepted: 21 September 2020; Published: 22 September 2020

Plant-based foods are the main source of phytochemicals, including polyphenols, a large family of compounds with highly diverse chemical structures. The impact of polyphenols, ranging from simple gallic acid to the most complex proanthocyanidins, on different biological processes has been irrefutably demonstrated by numerous studies [1].

Multiple approaches, each with their strengths and weaknesses, have been used to investigate the effects of polyphenols, all making an important and complementary contribution to the field. In vitro and in vivo experimental models play a vital role in the elucidation of the mechanisms of action underlying the health benefits observed in human trials. However, their results cannot always be easily extrapolated to human beings, partly because of considerable interindividual variability and other external factors. For instance, potential effect-modulating variables, such as sex, age, smoking habits, body mass index, and hormone levels, need to be identified, as does the influence of other foods, nutrients and even culinary techniques [1,2]. Additionally, we should not forget the importance of gut microbiota and genetic polymorphisms, which lead to varied circulating metabolites with different biological activities and health impacts [3].

A more recent approach is the use of omics, an integration of disciplines such as metabolomics, genomics, epigenomics, and foodomics based on cutting-edge experimental techniques, including mass spectrometry. The comprehensive ultra-large data sets they generate allow the scientific community to answer new and complex questions [4].

Daily dietary intake of polyphenols is thought to be approximately 1 g, although this estimate is based on subjective food frequency questionnaires, in which participants tend to overestimate the consumption of healthier items. Moreover, despite the availability of useful and comprehensive databases on polyphenol content in food, the concentrations depend on a wide range of factors, including plant variety, ripeness, environmental conditions, cropping systems, cooking, and storage, all of which add to the complexity of calculating intake [5].

In this Special Issue on "Dietary Polyphenols and Human Health", a series of 10 papers are presented, including three literature reviews [6–8] and seven original research papers [9–15]. The described research contributes to filling some of the gaps in our knowledge about the beneficial effects of dietary polyphenols on chronic health conditions, notably cardiovascular disease, type 2 diabetes, neurological impairment, and also certain risk factors.

In their review, Sandoval et al. describe the molecular mechanisms and signaling pathways involved in the metabolic impact of each group of flavonoids on obesity and related disorders, focusing on the liver, white and brown adipose tissue and central nervous system [6]. Márquez-Campos et al. have collected and summarized the available literature on the antidiabetic effects of both parent flavan-3-ol compounds and their microbial metabolites. The role of microbiota is especially relevant, as flavan-3-ols are poorly absorbed and their metabolization and absorption largely depend on the activity of colonic bacteria [7]. In the third review, Domínguez-López et al. explore the effects of phytoestrogens on human hormone-dependent outcomes throughout the human lifespan, divided into stages of pregnancy, childhood, adulthood, and the pre- and post-menopause [8].

Individual phytoestrogens are also the subject of a cross-sectional study by Sun et al., who are interested specifically in their impact on sleep quality. The association between urinary phytoestrogens (enterolactone, enterodiol, daidzein, O-desmethylangolensin, equol, and genistein) and sleeping disorders and sleep duration was examined in adults from the National Health and Nutrition Examination Survey 2005–2010. Discrepant results were found, depending on the metabolites and the race and sex of the participants, revealing the need for further studies with prospective cohorts and clinical trials [9].

Two of the other papers report clinical trials on the effect of polyphenols on the brain. In a study on psychological well-being (the PPhIT study), Kontogianni et al. concluded that participants with a high polyphenol intake had fewer depressive symptoms and better general mental and physical health compared to those on a low-phenolic diet [10]. The crossover study on mood and cognitive function performed by Wightman et al., where healthy participants received a single dose of a polyphenol-rich extract obtained from mango leaves (<60% mangiferin), revealed no significant results for mood, but cognitive function was enhanced [11].

Taking on the challenge of assessing polyphenol intake, Martini et al. used food frequency questionnaires to compare the nutrients afforded by two different dietary patterns (polyphenol rich and control) in older participants of the MaPLE study. Their ultimate goal is to develop dietary guidelines to increase the intake of these bioactive compounds [12]. Castro-Barquero et al. also used food frequency questionnaires to make a detailed estimation of the polyphenol intake in high cardiovascular risk participants of the PREDIMEDplus study. Monitoring metabolic syndrome symptoms, they found that some phenolic groups were inversely associated with better values of blood pressure, fasting plasma glucose, HDL cholesterol, and triglycerides [13]. Interestingly, both MaPLE and the PREDIMEDplus studies gave similar values for polyphenol intake.

The final two publications shed light on the mechanism of action of polyphenols. Saji et al. explore how a rice bran phenolic extract could target metabolic pathways associated with Type 2 diabetes mellitus, concluding that it modulated the expression of genes involved in β-cell dysfunction and insulin secretion through different mechanisms [14]. Focusing on the pathogenesis of cardiovascular diseases, Nignpense et al. performed a clinical trial with healthy volunteers to evaluate the effect of ingesting a sorghum extract. Although oxidative stress-related endothelial dysfunction and platelet aggregation were not reduced, a beneficial impact on platelet activation and platelet microparticle release was observed [15].

The growth of publications on bioactive compounds in the last years reflects the considerable interest of the scientific community in the field, but a great deal of research still needs to be done. A better understanding of the health benefits of polyphenols and their mechanisms of action will lead to improved (and perhaps individualized) nutritional recommendations aimed at enhancing human health.

Funding: This research received no external funding.

Acknowledgments: A.T.-R. thanks all the authors for their contributions to this Special Issue, all the reviewers for evaluating the submitted articles, and the editorial staff of the journal *Nutrients*, especially C-W, for always being so kind and helpful.

Conflicts of Interest: The author declares no conflict of interest.

References

1. Tresserra-Rimbau, A.; Lamuela-Raventos, R.M.; Moreno, J.J. Polyphenols, food and pharma. Current knowledge and directions for future research. *Biochem. Pharmacol.* **2018**, *156*, 186–195. [CrossRef] [PubMed]
2. Landberg, R.; Manach, C.; Kerckhof, F.M.; Minihane, A.M.; Saleh, R.N.M.; De Roos, B.; Tomas-Barberan, F.; Morand, C.; Van de Wiele, T. Future prospects for dissecting inter-individual variability in the absorption, distribution and elimination of plant bioactives of relevance for cardiometabolic endpoints. *Eur. J. Nutr.* **2019**, *58*, 21–36. [CrossRef] [PubMed]
3. Rowland, I.; Gibson, G.; Heinken, A.; Scott, K.; Swann, J.; Thiele, I.; Tuohy, K. Gut microbiota functions: Metabolism of nutrients and other food components. *Eur. J. Nutr.* **2018**, *57*, 1–24. [CrossRef] [PubMed]
4. Ulaszewska, M.M.; Weinert, C.H.; Trimigno, A.; Portmann, R.; Andres Lacueva, C.; Badertscher, R.; Brennan, L.; Brunius, C.; Bub, A.; Capozzi, F.; et al. Nutrimetabolomics: An Integrative Action for Metabolomic Analyses in Human Nutritional Studies. *Mol. Nutr. Food Res.* **2019**, *63*, 1800384. [CrossRef]
5. Rothwell, J.A.; Perez-Jimenez, J.; Neveu, V.; Medina-Remón, A.; M'Hiri, N.; García-Lobato, P.; Manach, C.; Knox, C.; Eisner, R.; Wishart, D.S.; et al. Phenol-Explorer 3.0: A major update of the Phenol-Explorer database to incorporate data on the effects of food processing on polyphenol content. *Database* **2013**, *2013*. [CrossRef]
6. Sandoval, V.; Sanz-Lamora, H.; Arias, G.; Marrero, P.F.; Haro, D.; Relat, J. Metabolic impact of flavonoids consumption in obesity: From central to peripheral. *Nutrients* **2020**, *12*, 2393. [CrossRef] [PubMed]
7. Márquez Campos, E.; Jakobs, L.; Simon, M.C. Antidiabetic effects of flavan-3-ols and their microbial metabolites. *Nutrients* **2020**, *12*, 1562. [CrossRef] [PubMed]
8. Domínguez-López, I.; Yago-Aragón, M.; Salas-Huetos, A.; Tresserra-Rimbau, A.; Hurtado-Barroso, S. Effects of dietary phytoestrogens on hormones throughout a human lifespan: A review. *Nutrients* **2020**, *12*, 2456. [CrossRef] [PubMed]
9. Sun, J.; Jiang, H.; Wang, W.; Dong, X.; Zhang, D. Associations of urinary phytoestrogen concentrations with sleep disorders and sleep duration among adults. *Nutrients* **2020**, *12*, 2103. [CrossRef] [PubMed]
10. Kontogianni, M.D.; Vijayakumar, A.; Rooney, C.; Noad, R.L.; Appleton, K.M.; McCarthy, D.; Donnelly, M.; Young, I.S.; McKinley, M.C.; McKeown, P.P.; et al. A high polyphenol diet improves psychological well-being: The polyphenol intervention trial (pphit). *Nutrients* **2020**, *12*, 2445. [CrossRef] [PubMed]
11. Wightman, E.L.; Jackson, P.A.; Forster, J.; Khan, J.; Wiebe, J.C.; Gericke, N.; Kennedy, D.O. Acute effects of a polyphenol-rich leaf extract of mangifera indica l. (zynamite) on cognitive function in healthy adults: A double-blind, placebo-controlled crossover study. *Nutrients* **2020**, *12*, 2194. [CrossRef] [PubMed]
12. Martini, D.; Bernardi, S.; Del Bo', C.; Liberona, N.H.; Zamora-Ros, R.; Tucci, M.; Cherubini, A.; Porrini, M.; Gargari, G.; González-Domínguez, R.; et al. Estimated intakes of nutrients and polyphenols in participants completing the maple randomised controlled trial and its relevance for the future development of dietary guidelines for the older subjects. *Nutrients* **2020**, *12*, 2458. [CrossRef]
13. Castro-Barquero, S.; Tresserra-Rimbau, A.; Vitelli-Storelli, F.; Doménech, M.; Salas-Salvadó, J.; Martín-Sánchez, V.; Rubín-García, M.; Buil-Cosiales, P.; Corella, D.; Fitó, M.; et al. Dietary polyphenol intake is associated with HDL-cholesterol and a better profile of other components of the metabolic syndrome: A PREDIMED-plus sub-study. *Nutrients* **2020**, *12*, 689. [CrossRef] [PubMed]
14. Saji, N.; Francis, N.; Schwarz, L.J.; Blanchard, C.L.; Santhakumar, A.B. Rice bran phenolic extracts modulate insulin secretion and gene expression associated with β-cell function. *Nutrients* **2020**, *12*, 1889. [CrossRef]
15. Nignpense, B.E.; Chinkwo, K.A.; Blanchard, C.L.; Santhakumar, A.B. Black sorghum phenolic extract modulates platelet activation and platelet microparticle release. *Nutrients* **2020**, *12*, 1760. [CrossRef] [PubMed]

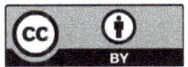

© 2020 by the author. Licensee MDPI, Basel, Switzerland. This article is an open access article distributed under the terms and conditions of the Creative Commons Attribution (CC BY) license (http://creativecommons.org/licenses/by/4.0/).

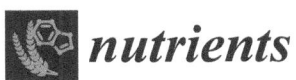

Article

Estimated Intakes of Nutrients and Polyphenols in Participants Completing the MaPLE Randomised Controlled Trial and Its Relevance for the Future Development of Dietary Guidelines for the Older Subjects

Daniela Martini [1,†], Stefano Bernardi [1,†], Cristian Del Bo' [1], Nicole Hidalgo Liberona [2,3], Raul Zamora-Ros [2,4], Massimiliano Tucci [1], Antonio Cherubini [5], Marisa Porrini [1], Giorgio Gargari [1], Raúl González-Domínguez [2,3], Gregorio Peron [2,3], Benjamin Kirkup [6], Paul A. Kroon [6], Cristina Andres-Lacueva [2,3], Simone Guglielmetti [1] and Patrizia Riso [1,*]

1. Department of Food, Environmental and Nutritional Sciences (DeFENS), Università degli Studi di Milano, 20133 Milan, Italy; daniela.martini@unimi.it (D.M.); stefano.bernardi@unimi.it (S.B.); cristian.delbo@unimi.it (C.D.B.); massimiliano.tucci@unimi.it (M.T.); marisa.porrini@unimi.it (M.P.); gargari.g@gmail.com (G.G.); simone.guglielmetti@unimi.it (S.G.)
2. Biomarkers and Nutrimetabolomics Laboratory, Department of Nutrition, Food Sciences and Gastronomy, XaRTA, INSA, Faculty of Pharmacy and Food Sciences, University of Barcelona. 08028 Barcelona, Spain; n.hidalgoliberona@ub.edu (N.H.L.); rzamora@idibell.cat (R.Z.-R.); raul.gonzalez@ub.edu (R.G.-D.); gregorio.peron@ub.edu (G.P.); candres@ub.edu (C.A.-L.)
3. CIBER de Fragilidad y Envejecimiento Saludable (CIBERfes), Instituto de Salud Carlos III, 08028 Barcelona, Spain
4. Unit of Nutrition and Cancer, Cancer Epidemiology Research Programme, Catalan Institute of Oncology (ICO), Bellvitge Biomedical Research Institute (IDIBELL), 08908 L'Hospitalet de Llobregat, Spain
5. Geriatria, Accettazione Geriatrica e Centro di ricerca per l'invecchiamento, IRCCS INRCA, 60127 Ancona, Italy; a.cherubini@inrca.it
6. Quadram Institute Bioscience, Norwich Research Park, Norwich NR4 7UG, UK; benjamin.kirkup@quadram.ac.uk (B.K.); paul.kroon@quadram.ac.uk (P.A.K.)
* Correspondence: patrizia.riso@unimi.it; Tel.: +39-02-503-16726
† Equally contributed as first author.

Received: 28 July 2020; Accepted: 13 August 2020; Published: 15 August 2020

Abstract: The evaluation of food intake in older subjects is crucial in order to be able to verify adherence to nutritional recommendations. In this context, estimation of the intake of specific dietary bioactives, such as polyphenols, although particularly challenging, is necessary to plan possible intervention strategies to increase their intake. The aims of the present study were to: (i) evaluate the nutritional composition of dietary menus provided in a residential care setting; (ii) estimate the actual intake of nutrients and polyphenols in a group of older subjects participating in the MaPLE study; and (iii) investigate the impact of an eight-week polyphenol-rich dietary pattern, compared to an eight-week control diet, on overall nutrient and polyphenol intake in older participants. The menus served to the participants provided ~770 mg per day of total polyphenols on average with small variations between seasons. The analysis of real consumption, measured using weighed food diaries, demonstrated a lower nutrient (~20%) and polyphenol intake (~15%) compared to that provided by the menus. The feasibility of dietary patterns that enable an increase in polyphenol intake with putative health benefits for age-related conditions is discussed, with a perspective to developing dietary guidelines for this target population.

Keywords: nursing home; residential care; aging; menu; flavonoids; phenolic acids

1. Introduction

It is well recognized that nutrition plays an important role in health status, with increasing evidence of associations between intake of specific dietary components and risk of many non-communicable diseases (NCDs), such as cardiovascular diseases (CVDs), type 2 diabetes, and some types of cancer. For instance, the Global Burden of Diseases has recently indicated that high intake of sodium, low intake of whole grains, and low intake of fruits are the leading dietary risk factors for deaths and disability-adjusted life-years (DALYs) worldwide [1]. These findings have been widely used to prepare national and international dietary guidelines aimed both at recommending the adequate intake of energy and nutrients for different targets of population and possibly at reducing the risk for the most common NCDs [2].

The ageing process affects the nutrient needs of older subjects, whose requirements for some nutrients may be reduced or increased with respect to younger adults. In this life-stage, a variety of factors such as sensory losses, chewing and swallowing problems, and medications may compromise dietary intake and lead to nutritional deficiencies and malnutrition, which has been contributing to the progression of many diseases and common syndromes in older people [3].

For this reason, specific recommendations have been proposed to meet the nutritional requirements of this target group; for instance, energy, protein and fibre intake should be individually adjusted by considering their nutritional status and physical condition and accounting for the presence of specific disease [4]. In addition to macronutrients, micronutrients also play a fundamental role in promoting health and preventing NCDs and their deficiencies are often common in aged people for a number of reasons including reduced food intake or lack of a varied diet, but they are also associated with the vicious cycle promoted by diseases and pharmacological treatments.

It is noteworthy that these factors may also affect the intake, absorption and/or metabolism of bioactive compounds such as polyphenols. In this regard, data on polyphenol intake in different older target groups are not univocal, possibly due to differences in geographical area considered, and in the individual characteristics in terms of health/disease status, and living conditions, as previously evidenced [5]. The interest in the assessment of polyphenol intake and the study of their potential impact on older subjects has been growing by considering several findings suggesting the protective role they can play against age-related diseases and in the promotion of healthy aging [6]. Regarding the changes on polyphenol intake with age, conflicting results have been reported so far, with some studies showing an increased intake [7,8] while others reporting no differences depending on age [9,10].

For the above-mentioned reasons, the nutritional assessment of older people represents a critical issue, which may be particularly true for those living in residential care settings where the prevalence of malnutrition has been reported to be extremely variable, ranging from 1.5 to 66.5% [11]. This represents a current clinical and public health concern at both the individual and population level [12,13]. Several methods have been developed for the assessment of energy and nutrient intake, including food-frequency questionnaires, food diaries and 24-h dietary recalls, all having pros and cons to be considered when choosing the best method to use in each specific context [14]. The estimation of micronutrients and bioactives like polyphenols is particularly challenging, mainly due to methodological issues, including the tool and the database used for the evaluation, as well as the type of polyphenol under consideration (e.g., total polyphenols versus single classes and subclasses of polyphenols) [5]. Being able to make accurate estimates of actual polyphenol intake is a fundamental requirement of developing a better understand of the role of these compounds and their relationship with health or disease conditions. In addition, this information is crucial to define potential polyphenol exploitation for the development of dietary strategies to prevent against age-associated diseases.

Based on these premises, the aim of this research was to evaluate the nutritional composition of nursing home dietary menus and to estimate the actual intake of nutrients and polyphenols in a group of older subjects living in a residential care setting. The assessments were performed as part of the MaPLE (Microbiome mAnipulation through Polyphenols for managing Leakiness in the Elderly) project, funded within the European Joint Programming Initiative "A Healthy Diet for a Healthy

Life" (JPI HDHL), with the aim to investigate benefits of a polyphenol-enriched diet on intestinal permeability in older subjects. An increased gut permeability, often associated with dysbiosis and inflammation, could play a role in the development of some age-related conditions. In this regard, it has been suggested that the intake of polyphenols may represent a promising strategy to improve intestinal permeability (IP) as demonstrated mainly in experimental studies suggesting the involvement of these bioactives in both direct and indirect modulatory mechanisms [15]. In this context, a more accurate estimation of the intake of polyphenols in a vulnerable target such as older subjects, in terms of amount, sources and distribution across the day and even in different seasons, can be of relevance. This could enable a better understanding of their potential benefits and the development of specific recommendations based on findings from dietary intervention studies.

2. Materials and Methods

2.1. Study Design and Population

The study design of the MaPLE randomized controlled trial (RCT) has been previously reported [16]. Briefly, the central hypothesis that this study sought to address was that a polyphenol-enriched dietary pattern would reduce IP and systemic inflammation and cause beneficial changes in various biomarkers of cardiometabolic health, and that this would be associated with changes in the gut microbiota in these older subjects. To this aim, volunteers were randomized to consume a polyphenol-rich diet (PR-diet) or a control diet (C-diet) for 8 weeks following a cross-over design separated by an 8-week wash-out. The development of the PR-diet and C-diet has been reported previously [16]. During the intervention, subjects were given three small portions of polyphenol-rich foods daily as substitutes for foods with lower polyphenol contents that were part of the C-diet (developed by analyzing the regular menus provided to the study participants and specifically assessing the nutrient and polyphenol composition). The characteristics and polyphenol content of the servings provided in the PR-diet for each product are reported in Table 1. The amount of polyphenols provided was more than double that deriving from the replaced products. Data shown include total polyphenol content (i.e., TPC) quantified by analysing products through the Folin–Ciocalteau method [17] and estimates of total polyphenols (i.e., TP). The estimation of TP was calculated as the sum of flavonoids, phenolic acids, lignans, stilbenes and other polyphenol classes expressed in mg (aglycone/100 g). The estimations were performed using an in-house ad hoc database of food composition on polyphenols, compiled from the USDA (fdc.nal.usda.gov/) for databases (for flavonoids, isoflavones and proanthocyanidins) and the Phenol-Explorer (PE; www.phenol-explorer.eu) database (for phenolic compounds lignans, stilbenes and other minor polyphenol classes) through a computer application developed that uses the relational database system. This methodology has been used and previously described [18–21]. Polyphenols were expressed as mg of aglycones per 100 g.

For the intervention study, all the participants were recruited from residents at Civitas Vitae, a large residential care setting (OIC Foundation including both nursing homes and independent residencies for older subjects, Padua, Italy) according to specific inclusion and exclusion criteria. Among inclusion criteria, subjects had to be aged 60 years and to have increased intestinal permeability evaluated by serum zonulin level as previously reported [16].

All the participants recruited into the study were self-sufficient and were in good cognitive health. The Ethics Committee of the Università degli Studi di Milano approved the study protocol (15/02/2016; ref.: 6/16/CE_15.02.16_Verbale_All-7). All the participants were provided with detailed information about their involvement in the study and gave their informed consent before beginning the intervention. The trial was registered in the ISRCTN Registry on 28 April 2017; ISRCTN10214981.

Table 1. Polyphenol content and composition of each serving of MaPLE products included in the dietary intervention, expressed as mg per serving.

	TPC	TP	Flavonoids	Phenolic Acids	Stilbenes	Lignans	Other
Blood orange juice	178	63.4	42.0	21.4	-	-	-
Blood orange fruit	178	34.8	23.1	11.8	-	-	-
Renetta apple	296	225.9	201.2	24.7	-	0.01	-
Renetta apple purée [+]	167	150.6	134.1	16.5	-	0.00	-
Whole blueberry [§]	291	259.5	165.1	94.5	-	-	-
Blueberry purée [✢]	259	199.0	163.6	35.4	-	0.0	0.02
Pomegranate juice	189	135.5	55.1	80.3	-	-	-
Green tea [*]	146	129.2	116.2	13.0	-	0.08	-
Cocoa powder [°]	234	92.2	90.5	1.7	-	0.00	0.01
Chocolate callets	337	167.8	165.4	2.4	0.01	-	-

[§] Frozen whole blueberry product was thawed and prepared before consumption; [✢] Blueberry purée was a ready-to-eat product; [°] Cocoa powder was dissolved in hot milk or water; [*] Green tea was prepared by solubilization of 200 mg of green tea extract in 200 mL of hot water; [+] Renetta apple purée was prepared in controlled conditions and stored at −18 °C until consumption. TPC, total polyphenol content by Folin–Ciocalteau assay; TP, total polyphenols determined by USDA and Phenol Explorer databases.

2.2. Nutritional and Polyphenol Composition of the Menus

To estimate the energy and nutrient composition of the planned meals regularly provided, the weekly menus during different seasons (summer, mid-season and winter) were evaluated (i.e., covering the whole intervention study). To this aim, Metadieta ® software (Me.te.da srl, S. Benedetto del Tronto, Italy) was used to include all the recipes and to estimate the nutritional composition of the different menus.

In addition, the TPC content of the menus was estimated by PE databases with the addition of our own data (characterized products in Table 1 used for the intervention) and other literature sources for those ingredients that were not available in those databases [22–24]. TP was instead estimated through the PE/USDA database, as also described in Section 2.1.

2.3. Evaluation of Actual Energy, Nutrient and Polyphenol Intake

During both intervention periods, weighed food records (WFR) were used to estimate food, energy, nutrient and polyphenol intake as reported in Section 2.2. In particular, up to six detailed daily diaries (recording the amount of foods provided and the amount actually consumed by weighing the leftovers) were analysed for each subject during the two intervention periods. In addition, one diary was filled in by participants at baseline and scheduled the day of blood drawings and sampling according to what was previously reported [16].

2.4. Statistical Analysis

Statistical analysis was conducted using the Statistical Package for Social Sciences software (IBM SPSS Statistics, Version 26.0, IBM corp., Chicago, IL, USA) and R statistical software (version 3.6.). One-way ANOVA was applied to analyse differences between the winter, mid-season and summer menus provided during the intervention in terms of nutrients and polyphenol composition. The nonparametric Wilcoxon–Mann–Whitney test with Benjamini–Hochberg correction pairing the data when possible was performed to ascertain differences at baseline between men and women in terms of actual intake and to verify the impact of treatment (PR vs. C-diet) and gender (men vs. women) on both nutrient and polyphenol intake in participants. The level of significance was set at $p \leq 0.05$. All results were expressed as mean ± standard deviation (SD).

3. Results

Fifty-one older subjects (22 men; 29 women; age ≥ 60 y) successfully completed the entire study, and the data reported here are for those 51 participants. Dropouts were not due to side effects of the dietary intervention itself.

3.1. Nutritional Composition of Menus

The nutritional composition of the nursing home menus provided during the intervention is reported in Table 2. The average estimated daily energy content of the summer menu was 140 kcal higher than for the winter menu. No differences were detected for the nutrients among seasonal menus, both when expressed as net quantity or as percentage of energy provided.

Table 2. Mean energy and nutrient composition of the nursing home menus across three seasons and overall mean composition.

Nutritional Factor	Winter Menu	Mid-Season Menu	Summer Menu	Mean Menu
Energy (kcal)	1889 ± 102 [a]	2012 ± 176 [a,b]	2028 ± 66 [b]	1976 ± 133
Total CHO (% of energy)	47.4 ± 3.2	46.4 ± 4.7	46.5 ± 3.0	46.8 ± 3.5
Simple CHO (% of energy)	20.6 ± 2.2	19.8 ± 0.6	20.3 ± 1.4	20.2 ± 1.5
Total protein (% of energy)	18.7 ± 2.5	20.0 ± 2.3	19.6 ± 2.7	19.4 ± 2.5
Animal protein (% of energy)	11.1 ± 2.8	13.4 ± 2.8	12.8 ± 2.5	12.4 ± 0.3
Plant protein (% of energy)	6.2 ± 0.9	6.2 ± 1.1	6.4 ± 0.8	6.3 ± 0.1
Total Lipids (% of energy)	34.1 ± 4.2	33.7 ± 4.1	34.0 ± 4.6	33.9 ± 4.1
SFA (% of energy)	8.7 ± 1.3	8.9 ± 2.0	8.6 ± 1.8	8.7 ± 1.6
MUFA (% of energy)	17.9 ± 3.3	16.9 ± 2.4	17.7 ± 2.2	17.5 ± 2.6
PUFA (% of energy)	3.7 ± 0.8	3.8 ± 0.7	3.9 ± 1.4	3.8 ± 1.0
ω-3 (% of energy)	0.7 ± 0.4	0.7 ± 0.4	0.7 ± 0.4	0.7 ± 0.4
ω-6 (% of energy)	3.0 ± 0.9	3.0 ± 0.8	3.2 ± 1.3	3.0 ± 1.0
Total Fibre (g/1000 Kcal)	12.2 ± 2.1	11.6 ± 2.4	12.3 ± 1.7	12.0 ± 2.0
Cholesterol (mg)	264 ± 91	358 ± 134	288 ± 123	303 ± 118
Total proteins (g)	88.1 ± 14.3	100.9 ± 19.6	98.8 ± 11.3	95.9 ± 15.7
Animal protein (g)	56.0 ± 13.8	68.3 ± 20.5	64.8 ± 10.9	63.0 ± 15.7
Plant protein (g)	30.6 ± 4.1	30.9 ± 4.2	32.6 ± 4.0	31.4 ± 4.0
Total lipids (g)	71.2 ± 7.8	75.3 ± 12.5	76.5 ± 12.3	74.3 ± 10.7
SFA (g)	18.3 ± 3.3	19.8 ± 4.6	19.4 ± 4.4	19.1 ± 4.0
MUFA (g)	37.3 ± 5.8	38.0 ± 7.1	40.1 ± 5.8	38.5 ± 6.0
PUFA (g)	7.7 ± 1.6	8.5 ± 2.1	8.7 ± 3.4	8.3 ± 2.4
Total ω-3 (g)	1.4 ± 0.8	1.5 ± 0.9	1.6 ± 0.9	1.5 ± 0.9
Total ω-6 (g)	6.2 ± 1.8	6.7 ± 2.1	7.1 ± 3.0	6.7 ± 3.0
Fibre (g/day)	22.9 ± 4.2	23.2 ± 4.4	24.8 ± 2.9	23.6 ± 3.8
Calcium (mg)	643 ± 254	666 ± 175	638 ± 112	649 ± 180
Iron (mg)	11.9 ± 2.0	14.2 ± 2.9	12.1 ± 1.0	12.7 ± 2.3
Vitamin B12 (mcg)	4.8 ± 2.2	5.3 ± 2.3	6.3 ± 5.1	5.5 ± 3.4
Vitamin C (mg)	225 ± 33	233 ± 28	242 ± 45	233 ± 35
Vitamin E (mg)	13.7 ± 1.9	15 ± 3.2	15.5 ± 2.4	14.8 ± 2.6
Vitamin B1 (mg)	1.4 ± 0.4	1.6 ± 0.4	1.5 ± 0.4	1.5 ± 0.4
Folates (mcg)	342 ± 78	377 ± 138	340 ± 70	353 ± 97
Vitamin B6 (mg)	2.3 ± 0.6	2.7 ± 0.7	2.5 ± 0.4	2.5 ± 0.6

Data represent the daily amounts with the units given in parentheses and are shown as mean ± standard deviation. Data have been calculated through the Metadieta ® software. Data with different letters in the same row are significantly different ($p < 0.05$). CHO, carbohydrates; SFA, saturated fatty acids; MUFA, monounsaturated fatty acids; PUFA, polyunsaturated fatty acids; ω-3, omega-3 fatty acids; ω-6, omega-6 fatty acids.

Regarding the polyphenol composition of the menu, as shown in Figure 1, no significant differences were observed among the different seasonal menus, which had an estimated mean TPC of about 770 mg/day.

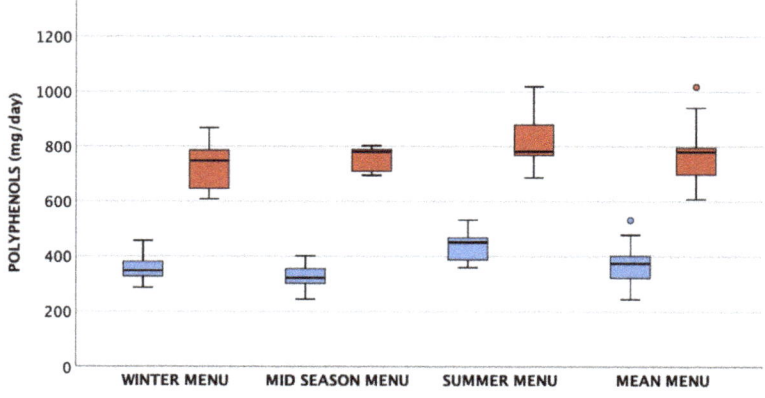

(A)

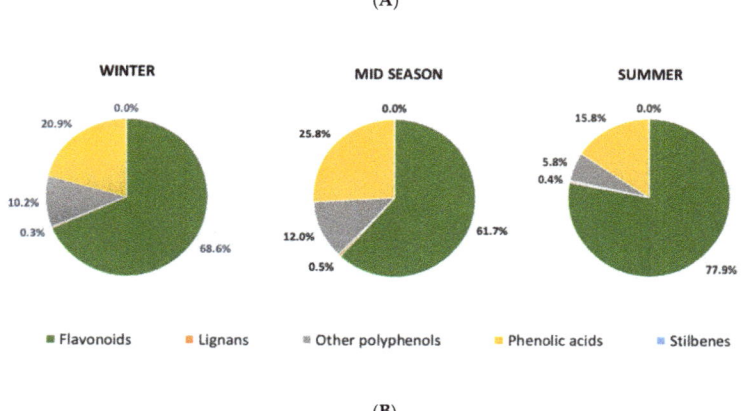

(B)

Figure 1. Box plot (panel **A**) showing polyphenol content in the seasonal menus, estimated through PE/USDA databases and other published data (TP in light blue) and by Folin–Ciocalteau data as reported in the PE database and other sources (TPC in red); percentage distribution of polyphenol classes (panel **B**) in the seasonal menus. Dots represent mild outliers that are more extreme than Q1 − 1.5 * IQR or Q3 + 1.5 * IQR but are not extreme data (where Q1=quartile 1; Q3=quartile 3; IQR=interquartile range).

3.2. Actual Energy, Nutrient and Polyphenol Intake at Baseline and during the Intervention

The actual energy, nutrient and polyphenol intake estimated at baseline for women, men and the whole group of participants is shown in Table 3. Overall, energy intakes, and accordingly nutrient intakes, were lower than calculated for the estimates based on the foods consumed from the menus, in keeping with the fact that not all the food was consumed for any particular meal. There were no significant differences between women and men for any of the dietary variables that were assessed at baseline. This was also confirmed by analysing the data obtained during the intervention study (Supplementary Materials Figure S1), except for simple carbohydrates in women and for total lipids and PUFA in men when comparing intake measured during the PR-diet and the C-diet ($p < 0.05$).

Finally, differences were observed in ω-6 fatty acids, iron and calcium intake following the PR-diet in both women and men.

Table 3. Daily mean energy, nutrient and polyphenol intake at baseline in the whole group of subjects, in women and men.

Variables	All ($n = 51$)	Women ($n = 29$)	Men ($n = 22$)	p-Value [†]
Energy (kcal)	1582 ± 108	1569 ± 110	1599 ± 105	0.318
Total CHO (% of energy)	50.0 ± 2.7	50.0 ± 2.7	49.8 ± 2.7	0.641
Simple CHO (% of energy)	20.4 ± 3.1	20.3 ± 3.3	20.5 ± 3.0	0.939
Proteins (% of energy)	17.8 ± 0.3	18.0 ± 0.8	17.7 ± 0.9	0.216
Animal proteins (% of energy)	12.1 ± 1.1	12.2 ± 1.0	11.8 ± 1.1	0.262
Plant proteins (% of energy)	5.7 ± 0.6	5.7 ± 0.6	5.7 ± 0.6	0.864
Total lipids (% of energy)	32.1 ± 2.3	31.9 ± 2.2	32.4 ± 2.5	0.441
SFA (% of energy)	8.6 ± 1.5	8.6 ± 1.4	8.7 ± 1.7	0.655
MUFA (% of energy)	16.3 ± 1.3	16.3 ± 1.1	16.4 ± 1.6	0.834
PUFA (% of energy)	3.2 ± 0.5	3.3 ± 0.6	3.2 ± 0.4	0.435
ω-3 (% of energy)	0.6 ± 0.2	0.6 ± 0.1	0.6 ± 0.2	0.753
ω-6 (% of energy)	2.5 ± 0.4	2.6 ± 0.5	2.5 ± 0.2	0.341
Total Fibre (g/1000 kcal)	11.2 ± 1.2	11.3 ± 1.1	11.1 ± 1.3	0.458
Cholesterol (mg)	207.7 ± 30.3	204.3 ± 29.9	212.2 ± 30.9	0.682
Total CHO (g)	210.7 ± 21.5	209.6 ± 22.8	212.2 ± 20.1	0.864
Simple CHO (g)	81.0 ± 15.2	80.8 ± 15.4	81.3 ± 15.2	0.954
Proteins (g)	70.3 ± 4.0	70.2 ± 4.0	70.4 ± 4.0	0.849
Animal proteins (g)	47.6 ± 3.9	47.9 ± 3.7	47.2 ± 4.2	0.536
Plant proteins (g)	22.4 ± 2.7	22.2 ± 2.7	22.7 ± 2.8	0.601
Total lipids (g)	56.2 ± 4.9	55.2 ± 3.8	57.5 ± 5.8	0.192
SFA (g)	15.2 ± 3.0	14.9 ± 2.7	15.5 ± 3.3	0.447
MUFA (g)	28.7 ± 2.4	28.3 ± 1.2	29.1 ± 3.4	0.575
PUFA (g)	5.7 ± 0.7	5.7 ± 0.7	5.7 ± 0.8	0.371
Total ω-3 (g)	1.1 ± 0.3	1.1 ± 0.1	1.1 ± 0.4	0.600
Total ω-6 (g)	4.5 ± 0.6	4.5 ± 0.6	4.4 ± 0.5	0.274
Fibre (g/day)	17.8 ± 2.4	17.8 ± 2.2	17.8 ± 2.6	0.932
Calcium (mg)	804 ± 135	808 ± 128	799 ± 147	0.761
Iron (mg)	9.4 ± 0.9	9.4 ± 0.7	9.4 ± 1.0	0.879
Vitamin B12 (μg)	4.2 ± 1.0	4.2 ± 0.4	4.3 ± 1.5	0.394
Vitamin C (mg)	111.8 ± 56.1	115.1 ± 45.2	107.4 ± 68.8	0.464
Vitamin E (mg)	11.4 ± 2.9	11.5 ± 1.3	11.2 ± 4.1	0.327
Vitamin B1 (mg)	0.8 ± 0.2	0.8 ± 0.1	0.7 ± 0.2	0.156
Folates (μg)	302 ± 73	311 ± 54	289 ± 93	0.536
Vitamin B6 (mg)	1.5 ± 0.3	1.5 ± 0.2	1.4 ± 0.3	0.588
Flavonoids (mg)	181.1 ± 137.5	174.4 ± 123.7	190.8 ± 157.8	0.984
Phenolic acids (mg)	130.9 ± 36.0	126.6 ± 28.6	137.1 ± 44.5	0.598
Stilbenes (mg)	0.04 ± 0.06	0.04 ± 0.06	0.04 ± 0.07	0.542
Lignans (mg)	0.8 ± 0.2	0.8 ± 0.2	0.8 ± 0.2	0.737
Other polyphenols (mg)	27.8 ± 4.3	28.0 ± 3.7	27.6 ± 5.0	0.723

All data are presented as mean ± standard deviation (SD); Data with $p < 0.05$ are significantly different. CHO, carbohydrates; SFA, saturated fatty acids; MUFA, monounsaturated fatty acids; PUFA, polyunsaturated fatty acids; ω-3, omega-3 fatty acids; ω-6, omega-6 fatty acids. [†] Comparison between women and men using Wilcoxon–Mann–Whitney test.

Regarding polyphenols, flavonoids and phenolic acids were the most consumed classes and were comparable between women and men.

3.3. Polyphenol Intake at Baseline and during Intervention

Figure 2 shows the polyphenol intake at baseline and in the two intervention periods. At baseline, the intake of TPC was 663.4 ± 147.5 mg/d and comparable between women (669.2 ± 160.1 mg/d) and men (655.2 ± 130.8 mg/d). The consumption of PR-products significantly ($p < 0.0001$) increased the intake of TPC by about 600 mg/d compared to the C-diet and was comparable in both men and women.

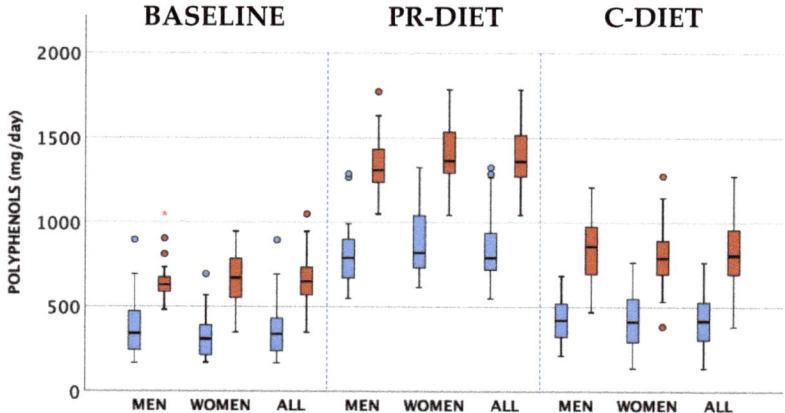

Figure 2. Polyphenol intake at baseline and in polyphenol (PR)-diet and control (C)-diet in the whole group of subjects and stratified by gender. The intake has been estimated using the PE and USDA databases and other published data (TP in light blue) and by Folin–Ciocalteau data as reported in the PE database and other sources (TPC in red). Dots represent mild outliers that are more extreme than Q1 − 1.5 * IQR or Q3 + 1.5 * IQR but are not extreme data. Asterisks are extreme data that are more extreme than Q1 − 3 * IQR or Q3 + 3 * IQR (where Q1=quartile 1; Q3=quartile 3; IQR=interquartile range).

Table 4 shows the contribution of different polyphenol classes to the total polyphenol intake during the PR and C-diet. Flavonoids were the main subclass increased in the PR-rich diet and accounted for 74.6%, followed by phenolic acids (23.3%), while lignans and other polyphenols accounted for the remainder. A treatment effect ($p < 0.0001$) for total flavonoids and phenolic acids was observed (Table 4), while a gender effect was observed for stilbenes showing a higher intake in men compared to women ($p = 0.033$).

Table 4. Intake of total polyphenols and classes (according to PE/USDA databases) during the PR-diet and the C-diet.

Title 1	Flavonoids	Phenolic Acids	Stilbenes	Lignans	Other Polyphenols
PR-diet					
All	634.3 ± 171.8	198.1 ± 52.2	0.2 ± 0.4	0.8 ± 0.3	16.4 ± 5.3
Men	594.6 ± 152.2	201.1 ± 74.3	0.4 ± 0.6	0.7 ± 0.3	16.7 ± 6.3
Women	662.1 ± 163.5	195.9 ± 42.0	0.1 ± 0.2	0.8 ± 0.3	16.2 ± 5.3
p value #	0.098	0.810	0.108	0.206	0.827
C-diet					
All	273.8 ± 119.8	128.2 ± 60.9	0.3 ± 0.5	0.9 ± 0.4	17.0 ± 5.4
Men	260.9 ± 109.6	128.8 ± 57.8	0.4 ± 0.4	0.9 ± 0.4	15.9 ± 5.7
Women	282.9 ± 125.6	127.8 ± 63.0	0.2 ± 0.5	0.9 ± 0.4	17.8 ± 4.9
p value #	0.453	0.271	0.033	0.745	0.271
p value †	<0.0001	<0.0001	0.386	0.303	0.164
p value ¥	<0.0001	0.001	0.575	0.068	0.807
p value §	<0.0001	<0.0001	0.348	0.060	0.331

All data are expressed as mean ± standard deviation (SD); PR, polyphenol-rich diet; C, control diet. † Comparison between PR-diet vs. C-diet in women. ¥ Comparison between PR-diet vs. C-diet in men. # Comparison between women and men in PR-diet and C-diet. § Comparison between PR-diet vs. C-diet in all subjects. Comparisons have been performed using the Wilcoxon–Mann–Whitney test.

Considering the total polyphenol (TP) contribution from the different meals, in the PR-diet, ~50% of polyphenol intake derives from snacks and the remaining ~50% from breakfast, lunch and dinner (Figure 3). In particular, there is a significant contribution to mid-morning and afternoon snacks from the intake of PR-products. Conversely, during the C-diet, only ~15% of the total polyphenols consumed were derived from snacks.

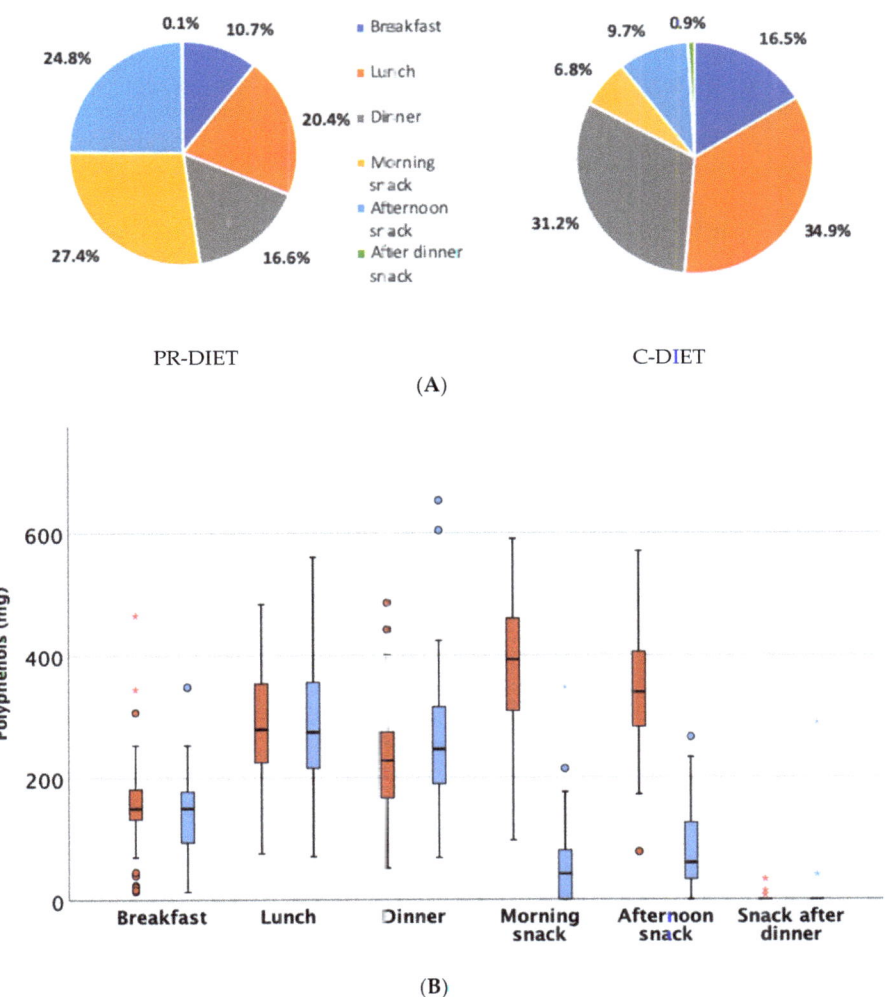

Figure 3. Total phenolic contribution from different meals during the polyphenol (PR)-diet and the control (C)-diet expressed as percentage (Panel **A**), or expressed as amount in mg during the PR-diet (in red) and the C-diet (in blue) as estimated through PE/USDA databases and other published data (Panel **B**). Dots represent mild outliers that are more extreme than Q1 − 1.5 * IQR or Q3 + 1.5 * IQR but are not extreme data. Asterisks are extreme data that are more extreme than Q1 − 3 * IQR or Q3 + 3 * IQR (where Q1=quartile 1; Q3=quartile 3; IQR=interquartile range).

Overall, through the analysis of the menu items provided to the volunteers and recorded in the WFRs during the two intervention periods and by considering the frequencies of consumption of the single ingredients, we estimated the main polyphenol sources contributing to the different meal times.

During the PR-diet, the main foods providing polyphenols at breakfast were fruit and fruit-derived products (e.g., orange, grape, orange juice, apricot jam, etc.), followed by barley coffee and minor contributions from coffee and tea. Polyphenol-rich products on the PR-rich diet were occasionally consumed at breakfast, where green tea, pomegranate juice, chocolate callets and blood orange juice were the most commonly consumed. For lunch and dinner, the main sources during the PR-diet were vegetables (e.g., chard, asparagus, broccoli, carrots), extra virgin olive oil, legumes and spices. A few participants occasionally consumed white wine in small portions (usually 1 glass), which also made a contribution to the polyphenol intake. PR-rich products were mainly consumed as mid-morning and mid-afternoon snacks, as reported in Figure 3. During the C-diet, we found similar foods providing polyphenols at breakfast, lunch and dinner compared to the PR-diet, except for the introduced PR-rich products. Major differences between the two treatments were largely due to the snack foods because only fruits and fruit-based products (i.e., juices), cakes (including sometime chocolate-based cakes) or yogurt were available during the C-diet, whereas a more extensive range of PR-foods were available as snacks on the PR-rich diet.

4. Discussion

The evaluation of the adequacy of diets in older subjects is of utmost importance not only to identify possible deviations from desirable nutritional targets but also to contribute to the development of new recommendations that address gaps in the current guidance. In this context, the MaPLE project has given us the unique opportunity to assess dietary intake in a well-controlled setting where it is also possible to analyse the daily menus provided to the residents, while considering all the recipes and ingredients used for the preparation of the meals. At the same time, long-term residences often have facilities enabling the measurement of food intake (e.g., by collecting multiple weighed food records) and this represents the best procedure to estimate actual consumption. Menu planning in residential care involves modifications of recipes during the year to take account of seasonal changes in ingredient availability and this may partially affect not only nutritional characteristics in terms of macro- and micro- nutrients but also food sources of bioactive compounds with potential impact on host metabolism and other functions.

In the present study, the evaluation of three different menus showed that overall they were comparable in terms of nutritional composition, and also that they were in line with the dietary recommendations for older subjects in Italy (i.e., Italian Reference Intake) [2], with some dissimilarities that are worth highlighting. In regards to total energy, menus provided suitable amounts for the target population, at least in consideration of the main Italian guidelines developed for dietary management in residential care [25]. Some studies carried out in nursing homes showed lower energy provided by menus [26,27], while others reported data higher or similar to our observation [28–30]. The distribution in macronutrients was consistent with the recommendations: carbohydrates accounted for ~47% of total energy intake on average (reference intake range: 45–60% energy (E)), although we found there was a higher intake of simple carbohydrate in comparison with the recommendations (20% E vs. < 15% E) due to the wide use of fruit juices and hot beverages with added sugars as has been commonly reported in this target population. Protein intake derived mainly from animal sources (about two-thirds) and was higher in comparison with the suggested dietary target (1.1 g/kg/day), while total lipid intake was within the reference intake range (20–35% E). Specifically, SFAs were in accordance with the national/international recommendation (<10% E), while total PUFAs were slightly lower than 5% E due to the low intake of ω-6 in favour of higher MUFAs, as can often be found in the Mediterranean areas. The amount of fibre provided by the menus was slightly lower than the suggested dietary target of 25 g per day defined by Italian and international guidelines [2,31]. Regarding micronutrients, iron contribution was adequate while, as also reported in the literature, calcium content in the three menus was lower than the population reference intake (PRI, 1200 mg for both women and men ≥ 60 years) [2]. However, it is worth noting that these data included only calcium derived from recipes and did not consider contributions from other sources such as water and supplements. Vitamin B1, B6 and B12 provided by menus were higher than reference values, while folates were slightly lower than the established population reference intake of 400 µg per day. With regard to antioxidants, vitamins E and C were both adequate, in particular vitamin C largely exceeded the PRI levels (i.e., 85 mg and 105 mg per day for women and men respectively). Overall, the results on the nutritional composition of the menus suggest that, although they are generally developed following specific guidelines, it is still possible to improve the content of critical nutrients such as fibre, specific micronutrients and bioactives, above all in institutionalised subjects as also reported in the literature [29,30].

Notably, actual food intake in older subjects can be significantly lower with respect to that provided by the menus. For these reasons, we also estimated the actual food consumption through the analysis of detailed and repeated weighed food records. Measured energy and nutrient intake were indeed lower than that provided through the menus (by about 20%), with no differences between women and men. In this regard, it is underlined that the subjects enrolled in the present study generally had a good nutritional status, evidenced also by their anthropometric characteristics (BMI = 26.8 ± 5.5 kg/m^2).

The energy intakes we have reported here (mean approximately 1580 kcal) were slightly lower than those found in the InCHIANTI study, performed on about 1200 free-living older subjects (>65 years) in Tuscany, in which mean energy intakes ranged from 1764 to 2260 kcal/d and from 1521 to 1793 kcal/d in men and women, respectively [32]. However, despite the higher energy intake, in the InCHIANTI study, a large group of subjects reported inadequate intakes of protein, calcium and other nutrients, which have been independently associated with frailty [33]. In our assessments, the lower food intake was associated with reduced protein intake (about 0.9 g/kg day on average), increasing the rate of inadequate intake above all in male subjects (about 22% with intake ≤ 0.71 g/kg per day and only 18% with intake ≥ 1.1 g/kg per day as defined by the suggested dietary target). The consumption of simple carbohydrates in older subjects was confirmed to be higher than the suggested values, while the fat intake appeared to be within the suggested intake range, although the amount of ω-6 fatty acids remained lower than recommended values, as did the intake of calcium, vitamins B1, B6 and folates. These results confirmed previous observations of a potential risk of long-term inadequate intake of nutrients that are fundamental for maintenance of functional and metabolic integrity in older subjects, and that these inadequate intakes are likely due to the actual food intake being significantly less than the amount of food provided to the care home residents in each meal (i.e., incomplete meal consumption is likely a major cause). Moreover, there is not only a problem related to overall food intake but also to specific classes of products that appear to be consumed in lower amounts with respect to others, for example justifying a low intake of fibre that has been found for most, if not all, the subjects under study. This is an underestimated consideration that should be a target for future multidisciplinary research that is able to finally implement guidelines for the achievement of nutritional targets through traditional or possibly alternative strategies.

A major focus in this study was polyphenols because these compounds have the potential to provide further specific benefits to the target population under study. It has been reported that there is a large variation in the polyphenol content of foods available in different periods of the year [34–36], and for this reason we specifically analysed recipes and ingredients used to develop seasonal menus and the results obtained showed a relatively comparable amount of these bioactive compounds (about 770 mg per day on average as TPC) among the different seasons. We could not find other data on the impact of seasonality on polyphenol content of dietary plans provided in long-term residences for older people, while more literature is available in free-living older subjects. In this regard, in the Blue Mountains Eye Study, a longitudinal study performed in Australia [35], the authors found that season did not affect the overall total flavonoid intake in a group of adult and older subjects; however, it was relatively higher in spring and lower in autumn in line with our results. Conversely, Tatsumi et al. [37] showed that total antioxidant intake in a Japanese population (39–77 years) was highest in winter and lowest in summer. The authors attributed this difference to the participants' selection of food (in particular fruits and vegetables) but also beverages across seasons.

In our study, the assessment of actual food consumption at baseline indicated a mean TPC intake of ~660 mg/d (i.e., evaluated by Folin–Ciocalteau through the PE database and specific literature), about 15% less than the amount estimated in the menus served to the study participants. Although a thorough comparison with other published data must be done cautiously because of the differences in the populations under study and the methods and databases used for estimating the intakes of total polyphenols and polyphenol classes, the overall actual intake estimated in the present study seems to be comparable with mean intake observed in the InChianti study [20], but lower with respect to others previously reported.

In fact, assessments in older subjects estimated polyphenol intakes from 333 mg/day up to 1492 mg/day, as reported previously [5]. For example, in the PREDIMED study evaluating a big cohort of Spanish older subjects aged 55–80 years, a mean polyphenol intake of 820 ± 323 mg/day expressed as glycosides was estimated through the PE database, by analysis of food consumption data obtained from FFQs [38]. With regard to the contribution of the classes, total flavonoid intake is generally the larger part of the intake, while data available in some studies suggest that up to 30–40% of the total polyphenol intake can be represented by phenolic acids [5]. Results from the EPIC cohort showed that older subjects tended to have increased intake of flavonoids, stilbenes, lignans, and other polyphenols with respect to younger individuals, while no differences were found for total polyphenol intake [7], and similar findings were reported by Karam and colleagues [8], also showing an impact of gender. In our study in a controlled setting, the data confirmed that the flavonoid subclass was the greatest contributor to total polyphenol intake followed by phenolic acids, while no differences were detected between men and women. Some studies have suggested a higher total and subclass polyphenol intake in females compared to males [8,10], above all when standardized by energy intake, and this may also be the reason for the lack of differences in our study. In addition, it is relevant that the overall lower availability of food alternatives for selection in controlled, with respect to a free-living condition, may have affected eating behaviour, increasing the comparability of the dietary intake.

With regard to polyphenol food sources, tea and coffee have been underlined as the main polyphenol contributors in northern European older subjects, while red wine, extra virgin olive oil and fruit are the main sources in Southern Europe [7,39]. In our evaluation, fruit and fruit juices, vegetable and extra virgin olive oil represent the main food categories providing polyphenols. In addition, we could not demonstrate a different selection of polyphenol sources depending on gender, despite some studies having reported a higher contribution from fruit and vegetables in females compared to males [8,34]. It is noteworthy that in the nursing home, the intake of coffee and wine was strongly limited, if not denied, to limit risks associated with caffeine and alcohol consumption and this may represent an important behavioural difference with respect to what may be observed in free-living older subjects.

The evaluation of habitual polyphenol intake in the older target group was a fundamental step in the process of developing a reliable and evidence based polyphenol rich dietary pattern to use for the intervention trial. In particular, the aim was to approximately double the habitual polyphenol intake of the nursing home residents when on the PR-rich diet in order to reach amounts in the highest quantile of intake identified in previous observational studies, where older subjects were included or specifically considered [7,21,40].

Indeed, the main objective of the MaPLE study was to investigate whether the increased intake of polyphenols might cause a reduction in intestinal permeability (IP) and inflammation associated with an improved intestinal microbial ecosystem, also affecting metabolic and functional activities in the older subjects [16]. In particular, the intervention was developed by replacing three portions per day of low polyphenol foods/beverages with specific products rich in polyphenols. The selection of the products was performed by considering different aspects: (i) the total amount of polyphenols provided, (ii) the contribution of the different polyphenol classes, (iii) the adequate portion of food able to provide a reliable high dose of polyphenols, and (iv) the possible food preparation in order to ensure polyphenol bioavailability. Additionally, foods selection was carried out by considering the characteristics of the target group and their specific needs in terms of acceptability and suitability in the context of residential care settings. Through the administration of the selected foods, we provided mainly flavonoids (approximately four times higher compared to the amount introduced through the C-diet) and phenolic acids. These bioactives have been suggested as potential modulators of critical factors and specific targets regulating IP, including the impact on microbiota composition and activities [15,41]. Overall, our results demonstrate that it is possible to obtain a significant increase in polyphenol intake in older subjects, through the use of small amounts of well-accepted polyphenol-rich food products. Moreover, it has been demonstrated that the intake is well tolerated and without undesirable effects. Participants appreciated the products and were interested in continuing with the dietary protocol after the end of the trial, suggesting that older people can change their diet if it does not dramatically modify their eating habits.

An interesting observation highlighted was that older subjects preferred the consumption of PR-products during the intervention as mid-morning and afternoon snacks. In fact, the protocol adopted did not fix the timing for the PR-food intake, but the products should have been consumed within the day according to preferences and/or habits. For this reason, our results give an important contribution to the development of dietary guidelines for this target population. At the same time, the analysis of the pattern of consumption of polyphenol-rich foods may also contribute to a better understanding of chronobiological aspects related to the effect of bioactive compounds. In this regard, it has been suggested that the inclusion of polyphenols within the meals may have an impact on related metabolic responses, e.g., through reduction of glucose and lipid levels, inflammation, oxidative stress, and blood pressure, associated with food intake [42–44]. Consuming most of the polyphenols outside of the main meals could also affect their bioavailability for direct absorption and their use as substrates for microbial transformation.

This work has several strengths mainly related to the well-controlled setting of the intervention, enabling both the evaluation of the nutrient and bioactive content of the menus and the actual intake during the whole intervention, ensuring high adherence to dietary instructions. Conversely, possible study limitations include the small sample size and the partial generalizability to free-living community dwelling older subjects. Finally, the limited food choices available in the main standard menus provided could have reduced the possibility of showing gender differences.

5. Conclusions and Perspectives

In conclusion, the assessments performed within the MaPLE project have further underlined the need for a careful revision of dietary menus addressed for older subjects not only to optimize the intake of essential nutrients, but also of bioactive compounds, such as polyphenols, in order to lower the risk of chronic diseases and improve specific metabolic and functional activities during aging. In this context, we have shown that there is a possibility to develop feasible and reliable polyphenol-rich dietary patterns that can be appreciated and consumed by the older population with excellent compliance, while assuring a significant increase in the intake of these bioactive compounds. Moreover, the products and preparations included in the dietary menu have been easily managed in the residential care setting and this is a practical aspect of relevance for the success of new recommendations.

Further studies are needed to: (i) improve tools available to better estimate polyphenol intake and enable comparison of different data in the literature, as previously reported [5]; and (ii) improve dietary recommendations by defining the amount of polyphenol needed in order to obtain, if confirmed, the postulated health benefits in the older subjects. This is not an easy task and imply a strong research effort that needs to consider the potential impact of these results for the development of evidence-based dietary guidelines for the management of age-related conditions.

Supplementary Materials: The following are available online at http://www.mdpi.com/2072-6643/12/8/2458/s1, Figure S1: comparison of percentage energy and nutrient intake during 8-week polyphenol-rich diet (PR-diet) and control diet (C-diet) in older women and men.

Author Contributions: P.R. and S.G. designed the trial and in collaboration with A.C., C.A.-L. and P.A.K. optimised the study protocol including the development of the polyphenol rich dietary pattern. D.M., S.B., C.D.B. and P.R. drafted the manuscript. S.B., M.T., supervised by M.P. and P.R., evaluated the nutritional composition of dietary plans and estimated the actual nutrient intake. N.H.L., R.Z.-R. and C.A.-L. estimated the actual dietary polyphenol intake in collaboration with R.G.-D. and G.P., D.M., C.D.B., B.K. and G.G. performed the statistical analysis. All authors have read and agreed to the published version of the manuscript.

Funding: This research was undertaken as part of the MAPLE project (Gut and blood microbiomics for studying the effect of a polyphenol-rich dietary pattern on intestinal permeability in the elderly), which was funded through the European Joint Programming Initiative "A Healthy Diet for a Healthy Life" (JPI-HDHL-http://www.healthydietforhealthylife.eu/) with national funding support provided by Mipaaf (Italy; D.M. 8245/7303/2016), MINECO (Spain, PCIN-2015-238) and the BBSRC (UK, BB/N023951/1). In addition, C.A.-L. thanks 2017SGR1546 from AGAUR, CIBERFES (co-funded by the FEDER Program from EU) and ICREA Academia award 2018.

Acknowledgments: C.D.B. is grateful for support granted by "Piano di sostegno alla ricerca- Linea 2, azione A-grant number "PSR2019-CDELB". P.R. and C.D.B. acknowledge the European Cooperation for Science and Technology (COST Action) CA16112 "NutRedOx: Personalized Nutrition in Aging Society: Redox Control of Major Age-related Diseases". P.R. thanks also Coordinated Research Center (CRC) "Innovation for Well-Being and Environment (I-WE). R.Z.-R. was supported by the "Miguel Servet" program (CP15/00100) from the Institute of Health Carlos III (Co-funded by the European Social Fund (ESF)-ESF investing in your future). PAK and BK are grateful for additional support from the BBSRC (UK) through an Institute Strategic Programme Grant ('Food Innovation and Health'; Grant No. BB/R012512/1) and its constituent project BBS/E/F/000PR10346 (Theme 3, Digestion and Fermentation in the Lower GI Tract) to Quadram Institute Bioscience. We are grateful to the valuable contribution and dedication of our older volunteers and to the nursing and medical staff working at OIC Foundation (Padua, Italy). We would like to specifically acknowledge Alberto Fantuzzo, Chiara Cavazzini, Lorella Pinton, Paolo Bergantin, Rosanna Ceccato, Pamela Soranzo, and Silvana Giraldini and Guido Masnata. We are also grateful to all the physicians (Michela Rigon, Lorena D'Aloise, Antonio Merlo, Elisabetta Bernardinello, Nadia Malacarne, Silvana Bortoli, Fabiola Talato, Agostino Corsini, Maria Licursi, Nicoletta Marcon, Angela Sansone), the nurses and other personnel at the residential care who were essential to complete the study successfully. Giulia Minto and Nicola Fassetta are acknowledged for their help during the evaluation of food intake. Finally, the authors are grateful to Barry Callebaut, Indena, Melinda, Oranfrizer, Roberts Berrie, Zuegg for their kind contribution of products used for the intervention.

Conflicts of Interest: The authors declare no conflict of interest. The funders had no role in the design of the study; in the collection, analyses, or interpretation of data; in the writing of the manuscript, or in the decision to publish the results.

References

1. Afshin, A.; Sur, P.J.; Fay, K.A.; Cornaby, L.; Ferrara, G.; Salama, J.S.; Mullany, E.C.; Abate, K.H.; Abbafati, C.; Abebe, Z.; et al. Health effects of dietary risks in 195 countries, 1990–2017: A systematic analysis for the Global Burden of Disease Study 2017. *Lancet* **2019**, *393*, 1958–1972. [CrossRef]
2. SINU. *LARN—Livelli di Assunzione di Riferimento di Nutrienti ed Energia—IV Revisione*; SICS: Milan, Italy, 2014; ISBN 9788890685224.
3. Amarya, S.; Singh, K.; Sabharwal, M. Changes during aging and their association with malnutrition. *J. Clin. Gerontol. Geriatr.* **2015**, *6*, 78–84. [CrossRef]
4. Volkert, D.; Beck, A.M.; Cederholm, T.; Cruz-Jentoft, A.; Goisser, S.; Hooper, L.; Kiesswetter, E.; Maggio, M.; Raynaud-Simon, A.; Sieber, C.C.; et al. ESPEN guideline on clinical nutrition and hydration in geriatrics. *Clin. Nutr.* **2019**, *38*, 10–47. [CrossRef] [PubMed]
5. Del Bo', C.; Bernardi, S.; Marino, M.; Porrini, M.; Tucci, M.; Guglielmetti, S.; Cherubini, A.; Carrieri, B.; Kirkup, B.; Kroon, P.; et al. Systematic Review on Polyphenol Intake and Health Outcomes: Is there Sufficient Evidence to Define a Health-Promoting Polyphenol-Rich Dietary Pattern? *Nutrients* **2019**, *11*, 1355.
6. Cherniack, E.P. *Polyphenols and Aging*; Malavolta, M., Mocchegiani, E., Eds.; Elsevier Inc.: London, UK, 2016; ISBN 9780128018163.
7. Zamora-Ros, R.; Knaze, V.; Rothwell, J.A.; Hémon, B.; Moskal, A.; Overvad, K.; Tjønneland, A.; Kyrø, C.; Fagherazzi, G.; Boutron-Ruault, M.-C.; et al. Dietary polyphenol intake in Europe: The European Prospective Investigation into Cancer and Nutrition (EPIC) study. *Eur. J. Nutr.* **2016**, *55*, 1359–1375. [CrossRef] [PubMed]

8. Karam, J.; Bibiloni, M.M.; Tur, J.A. Polyphenol estimated intake and dietary sources among older adults from Mallorca Island. *PLoS ONE* **2018**, *13*, e0191573. [CrossRef] [PubMed]
9. Miranda, A.M.; Steluti, J.; Fisberg, R.M.; Marchioni, D.M. Dietary intake and food contributors of polyphenols in adults and elderly adults of Sao Paulo: A population-based study. *Br. J. Nutr.* **2016**, *115*, 1061–1070. [CrossRef]
10. Ziauddeen, N.; Rosi, A.; Del Rio, D.; Amoutzopoulos, B.; Nicholson, S.; Page, P.; Scazzina, F.; Brighenti, F.; Ray, S.; Mena, P. Dietary intake of (poly)phenols in children and adults: Cross-sectional analysis of UK National Diet and Nutrition Survey Rolling Programme (2008–2014). *Eur. J. Nutr.* **2019**, *58*, 3183–3198. [CrossRef]
11. Bell, C.L.; Lee, A.S.W.; Tamura, B.K. Malnutrition in the nursing home. *Curr. Opin. Clin. Nutr. Metab. Care* **2015**, *18*, 17–23. [CrossRef]
12. Serrano-Urrea, R.; Garcia-Meseguer, M.J. Malnutrition in an Elderly Population without Cognitive Impairment Living in Nursing Homes in Spain: Study of Prevalence Using the Mini Nutritional Assessment Test. *Gerontology* **2013**, *59*, 490–498. [CrossRef]
13. Vandewoude, M.F.J.; van Wijngaarden, J.P.; De Maesschalck, L.; Luiking, Y.C.; Van Gossum, A. The prevalence and health burden of malnutrition in Belgian older people in the community or residing in nursing homes: Results of the NutriAction II study. *Aging Clin. Exp. Res.* **2019**, *31*, 175–183. [CrossRef] [PubMed]
14. FAO. *Dietary Assessment. A Resource Guide to Method Selection and Application in Low Resource Settings*; Elsevier: Rome, Italy, 2018; ISBN 9780120883936.
15. Bernardi, S.; Del Bo', C.; Marino, M.; Gargari, G.; Cherubini, A.; Andrés-Lacueva, C.; Hidalgo-Liberona, N.; Peron, G.; González-Dominguez, R.; Kroon, P.; et al. Polyphenols and Intestinal Permeability: Rationale and Future Perspectives. *J. Agric. Food Chem.* **2020**, *68*, 1816–1829. [CrossRef] [PubMed]
16. Guglielmetti, S.; Bernardi, S.; Del Bo', C.; Cherubini, A.; Porrini, M.; Gargari, G.; Hidalgo-Liberona, N.; Gonzalez-Dominguez, R.; Peron, G.; Zamora-Ros, R.; et al. Effect of a polyphenol-rich dietary pattern on intestinal permeability and gut and blood microbiomics in older subjects: Study protocol of the MaPLE randomised controlled trial. *BMC Geriatr.* **2020**, *20*, 77. [CrossRef] [PubMed]
17. Singleton, V.L.; Rossi, J.A. Colorimetry of total phenolics with phosphomolybdic-phosphotungstic acid reagents. *Am. J. Enol. Vitic.* **1965**, *16*, 144–158.
18. Zamora-Ros, R.; Rabassa, M.; Cherubini, A.; Urpi-Sarda, M.; Llorach, R.; Bandinelli, S.; Ferrucci, L.; Andres-Lacueva, C. Comparison of 24-h volume and creatinine-corrected total urinary polyphenol as a biomarker of total dietary polyphenols in the Invecchiare InCHIANTI study. *Anal. Chim. Acta* **2011**, *704*, 110–115. [CrossRef]
19. Zamora-Ros, R.; Rabassa, M.; Cherubini, A.; Urpí-Sardà, M.; Bandinelli, S.; Ferrucci, L.; Andres-Lacueva, C. High Concentrations of a Urinary Biomarker of Polyphenol Intake Are Associated with Decreased Mortality in Older Adults. *J. Nutr.* **2013**, *143*, 1445–1450. [CrossRef]
20. Rabassa, M.; Zamora-Ros, R.; Andres-Lacueva, C.; Urpi-Sarda, M.; Bandinelli, S.; Ferrucci, L.; Cherubini, A. Association between both total baseline urinary and dietary polyphenols and substantial physical performance decline risk in older adults: A 9-year follow-up of the InCHIANTI study. *J. Nutr. Health Aging* **2016**, *20*, 478–484. [CrossRef]
21. Rabassa, M.; Cherubini, A.; Zamora-Ros, R.; Urpi-Sarda, M.; Bandinelli, S.; Ferrucci, L.; Andres-Lacueva, C. Low Levels of a Urinary Biomarker of Dietary Polyphenol Are Associated with Substantial Cognitive Decline over a 3-Year Period in Older Adults: The Invecchiare in Chianti Study. *J. Am. Geriatr. Soc.* **2015**, *63*, 938–946. [CrossRef]
22. Nibir, Y.M.; Sumit, A.F.; Akhand, A.A.; Ahsan, N.; Hossain, M.S. Comparative assessment of total polyphenols, antioxidant and antimicrobial activity of different tea varieties of Bangladesh. *Asian Pac. J. Trop. Biomed.* **2017**, *7*, 352–357. [CrossRef]
23. Vrhovsek, U.; Rigo, A.; Tonon, D.; Mattivi, F. Quantitation of Polyphenols in Different Apple Varieties. *J. Agric. Food Chem.* **2004**, *52*, 6532–6538. [CrossRef]
24. Cleverdon, R.; Elhalaby, Y.; McAlpine, M.; Gittings, W.; Ward, W. Total Polyphenol Content and Antioxidant Capacity of Tea Bags: Comparison of Black, Green, Red Rooibos, Chamomile and Peppermint over Different Steep Times. *Beverages* **2018**, *4*, 15. [CrossRef]

25. Ministero della Salute. *Linee di Indirizzo Nazionale per la Ristorazione Ospedaliera e Assistenziale*; Ministero della salute: Rome, Italy, 2011.
26. Trang, S.; Fraser, J.; Wilkinson, L.; Steckham, K.; Oliphant, H.; Fletcher, H.; Tzianetas, R.; Arcand, J. A Multi-Center Assessment of Nutrient Levels and Foods Provided by Hospital Patient Menus. *Nutrients* **2015**, *7*, 9256–9264. [CrossRef]
27. Thibault, R.; Chikhi, M.; Clerc, A.; Darmon, P.; Chopard, P.; Genton, L.; Kossovsky, M.P.; Pichard, C. Assessment of food intake in hospitalised patients: A 10-year comparative study of a prospective hospital survey. *Clin. Nutr.* **2011**, *30*, 289–296. [CrossRef] [PubMed]
28. Coulston, A.M.; Mandelbaum, D.; Reaven, G.M. Dietary management of nursing home residents with non-insulin-dependent diabetes mellitus. *Am. J. Clin. Nutr.* **1990**, *51*, 67–71. [CrossRef] [PubMed]
29. Rodríguez Rejón, A.I.; Ruiz López, M.D.; Malafarina, V.; Puerta, A.; Zuñiga, A.; Artacho, R. Menus offered in long-term care homes: Quality of meal service and nutritional analysis. *Nutr. Hosp.* **2017**, *34*, 584. [CrossRef] [PubMed]
30. Vucea, V.; Keller, H.H.; Morrison, J.M.; Duncan, A.M.; Duizer, L.M.; Carrier, N.; Lengyel, C.O.; Slaughter, S.E. Nutritional quality of regular and pureed menus in Canadian long term care homes: An analysis of the Making the Most of Mealtimes (M3) project. *BMC Nutr.* **2017**, *3*, 80. [CrossRef]
31. World Health Organization. *Food Based Dietary Guidelines in the WHO European Region*; WHO Regional Office for Europe: Copenhagen, Denmark, 2003.
32. Bartali, B.; Salvini, S.; Turrini, A.; Lauretani, F.; Russo, C.R.; Corsi, A.M.; Bandinelli, S.; D'Amicis, A.; Palli, D.; Guralnik, J.M.; et al. Age and Disability Affect Dietary Intake. *J. Nutr.* **2003**, *133*, 2868–2873. [CrossRef]
33. Bartali, B.; Frongillo, E.A.; Bandinelli, S.; Lauretani, F.; Semba, R.D.; Fried, L.P.; Ferrucci, L. Low Nutrient Intake Is an Essential Component of Frailty in Older Persons. *J. Gerontol. Ser. A Biol. Sci. Med. Sci.* **2006**, *61*, 589–593. [CrossRef]
34. Taguchi, C.; Kishimoto, Y.; Takeuchi, I.; Tanaka, M.; Iwashima, T.; Fukushima, Y.; Kondo, K. Estimated Dietary Polyphenol Intake and Its Seasonal Variations among Japanese University Students. *J. Nutr. Sci. Vitaminol. (Tokyo)* **2019**, *65*, 192–195. [CrossRef]
35. Kent, K.; Charlton, K.E.; Lee, S.; Mond, J.; Russell, J.; Mitchell, P.; Flood, V.M. Dietary flavonoid intake in older adults: How many days of dietary assessment are required and what is the impact of seasonality? *Nutr. J.* **2018**, *17*, 7. [CrossRef]
36. Taguchi, C.; Fukushima, Y.; Kishimoto, Y.; Saita, E.; Suzuki-Sugihara, N.; Yoshida, D.; Kondo, K. Polyphenol Intake from Beverages in Japan over an 18-Year Period (1996–2013): Trends by Year, Age, Gender and Season. *J. Nutr. Sci. Vitaminol. (Tokyo)* **2015**, *61*, 338–344. [CrossRef] [PubMed]
37. Tatsumi, Y.; Ishihara, J.; Morimoto, A.; Ohno, Y.; Watanabe, S. Seasonal differences in total antioxidant capacity intake from foods consumed by a Japanese population. *Eur. J. Clin. Nutr.* **2014**, *68*, 799–803. [CrossRef] [PubMed]
38. Tresserra-Rimbau, A.; Medina-Remón, A.; Pérez-Jiménez, J.; Martínez-González, M.A.; Covas, M.I.; Corella, D.; Salas-Salvadó, J.; Gómez-Gracia, E.; Lapetra, J.; Arós, F.; et al. Dietary intake and major food sources of polyphenols in a Spanish population at high cardiovascular risk: The PREDIMED study. *Nutr. Metab. Cardiovasc. Dis.* **2013**, *23*, 953–959. [CrossRef] [PubMed]
39. Grosso, G.; Stepaniak, U.; Topor-Mądry, R.; Szafraniec, K.; Pająk, A. Estimated dietary intake and major food sources of polyphenols in the Polish arm of the HAPIEE study. *Nutrition* **2014**, *30*, 1398–1403. [CrossRef]
40. Tresserra-Rimbau, A.; Guasch-Ferré, M.; Salas-Salvadó, J.; Toledo, E.; Corella, D.; Castañer, O.; Guo, X.; Gómez-Gracia, E.; Lapetra, J.; Arós, F.; et al. Intake of Total Polyphenols and Some Classes of Polyphenols Is Inversely Associated with Diabetes in Elderly People at High Cardiovascular Disease Risk. *J. Nutr.* **2015**, *146*, 767–777.
41. Peron, G.; Hidalgo-Liberona, N.; González-Domínguez, R.; Garcia-Aloy, M.; Guglielmetti, S.; Bernardi, S.; Kirkup, B.; Kroon, P.A.; Cherubini, A.; Riso, P.; et al. Exploring the Molecular Pathways Behind the Effects of Nutrients and Dietary Polyphenols on Gut Microbiota and Intestinal Permeability: A Perspective on the Potential of Metabolomics and Future Clinical Applications. *J. Agric. Food Chem.* **2020**, *68*, 1780–1789. [CrossRef]
42. Amiot, M.J.; Riva, C.; Vinet, A. Effects of dietary polyphenols on metabolic syndrome features in humans: A systematic review. *Obes. Rev.* **2016**, *17*, 573–586. [CrossRef]

43. Cao, H.; Ou, J.; Chen, L.; Zhang, Y.; Szkudelski, T.; Delmas, D.; Daglia, M.; Xiao, J. Dietary polyphenols and type 2 diabetes: Human Study and Clinical Trial. *Crit. Rev. Food Sci. Nutr.* **2019**, *59*, 3371–3379. [CrossRef]
44. Kim, Y.; Keogh, J.; Clifton, P. Polyphenols and Glycemic Control. *Nutrients* **2016**, *8*, 17. [CrossRef]

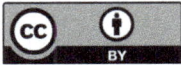

© 2020 by the authors. Licensee MDPI, Basel, Switzerland. This article is an open access article distributed under the terms and conditions of the Creative Commons Attribution (CC BY) license (http://creativecommons.org/licenses/by/4.0/).

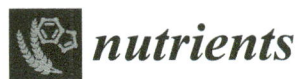

Article

A High Polyphenol Diet Improves Psychological Well-Being: The Polyphenol Intervention Trial (PPhIT)

Meropi D. Kontogianni [1], Aswathy Vijayakumar [2], Ciara Rooney [2], Rebecca L. Noad [2,3], Katherine M. Appleton [4], Danielle McCarthy [5], Michael Donnelly [2], Ian S. Young [2,5], Michelle C. McKinley [2,5], Pascal P. McKeown [2,3] and Jayne V. Woodside [2,5,*]

1. Department of Nutrition and Dietetics, Harokopio University, Eleftheriou Venizelou 70, 17671 Kallithea, Greece; mkont@hua.gr
2. Centre for Public Health, Queen's University Belfast, Belfast BT12 6BA, UK; a.vijayakumar@qub.ac.uk (A.V.); crooney34@hotmail.com (C.R.); rebeccanoad@gmail.com (R.L.N.); michael.donnelly@qub.ac.uk (M.D.); I.Young@qub.ac.uk (I.S.Y.); m.mckinley@qub.ac.uk (M.C.M.); P.P.McKeown@qub.ac.uk (P.P.M.)
3. Cardiology Department, Belfast Health and Social Care Trust, Belfast BT9 7AB, UK
4. Department of Psychology, Bournemouth University, Bournemouth BH12 5BB, UK; k.appleton@bournemouth.ac.uk
5. Institute for Global Food Security, Queen's University Belfast, Belfast BT9 5DL, UK; D.McCarthy@qub.ac.uk
* Correspondence: j.woodside@qub.ac.uk

Received: 29 May 2020; Accepted: 12 August 2020; Published: 14 August 2020

Abstract: Mental ill health is currently one of the leading causes of disease burden worldwide. A growing body of data has emerged supporting the role of diet, especially polyphenols, which have anxiolytic and antidepressant-like properties. The aim of the present study was to assess the effect of a high polyphenol diet (HPD) compared to a low polyphenol diet (LPD) on aspects of psychological well-being in the Polyphenol Intervention Trial (PPhIT). Ninety-nine mildly hypertensive participants aged 40–65 years were enrolled in a four-week LPD washout period and then randomised to either an LPD or an HPD for eight weeks. Both at baseline and the end of intervention, participants' lifestyle and psychological well-being were assessed. The participants in the HPD group reported a decrease in depressive symptoms, as assessed by the Beck Depression Inventory-II, and an improvement in physical component and mental health component scores as assessed with 36-Item Short Form Survey. No differences in anxiety, stress, self-esteem or body image perception were observed. In summary, the study findings suggest that the adoption of a polyphenol-rich diet could potentially lead to beneficial effects including a reduction in depressive symptoms and improvements in general mental health status and physical health in hypertensive participants.

Keywords: polyphenols; fruits; berries; vegetables; dark chocolate; psychological well-being; depression; physical health; mental health

1. Introduction

Mental ill health, manifesting itself in a wide range of conditions such as depression, anxiety and stress [1], represents one of the leading causes of burden of disease worldwide, also substantially increasing the risk of cardiovascular disease, diabetes and cancer [2–4] and adversely affecting quality of life (QoL), relationships and the ability to work [5]. Northern Ireland has the highest prevalence of mental illness within the UK, and psychiatric morbidity is 25% higher than in the UK [6].

Thus, research is required in order to establish inexpensive and effective techniques to reduce the incidence of mental health problems and to improve the psychological well-being of the population. Alongside genetic and biological factors, researchers have increasingly begun to examine the role of lifestyle factors, including dietary intake, in the promotion of psychological well-being and the prevention of mental illness [7,8]. Studies that have explored potential associations between nutrient intake (namely carbohydrates, B vitamins and antioxidants such as vitamins C, E and polyphenols) or foods rich in these nutrients (e.g., fruits, vegetables, legumes, coffee, chocolate) and psychological well-being have produced conflicting results [9–12].

Polyphenols, in particular, have gained increasing attention from health researchers in recent years due to their biological properties, as well as their abundance within the human diet [13]. A growing number of epidemiological studies support a role for polyphenols in the prevention of chronic non-communicable diseases such as cardiovascular disease (CVD) [14], cancer [15] and neurodegenerative diseases [14,16]. Furthermore, animal studies have demonstrated the ability of polyphenols to improve cognitive performance and memory [17,18] and, more recently, these results have been replicated in human studies [19,20]. Regarding mental health, a growing body of data from animal and human studies has emerged supporting the role of a variety of dietary polyphenols in affecting behaviour and mood through anxiolytic and antidepressant-like properties, mediated through multiple molecular and cellular pathways [21]. Moreover, given that recent studies have demonstrated the pathophysiological role of oxidative stress and inflammation in the onset and progression of depression, polyphenols have been examined both in vitro and in vivo as a potential antidepressant treatment, although randomised controlled trials are still scarce in the field [22,23]. The richest sources of polyphenols in the human diet include fruits (e.g., berries, grapes, apples and plums), vegetables (e.g., cabbage, eggplant, onions, peppers), plant-derived beverages including tea, coffee, red wine and fruit juices (e.g., apple juice), seeds, nuts and chocolate (particularly dark chocolate) [24,25]. In terms of a food-based approach, several of the above-mentioned foods have been studied both in observational and intervention studies for potential effects on outcomes related to mental well-being, mood, psychological distress and life satisfaction [26], although, potentially due in part to the great variation in study design, results are not consistent. Studying diet on a dietary pattern level will be beneficial in allowing potential complicated or cumulative intercorrelations, interactions and synergies to be revealed, given that different polyphenols may have different effects on outcomes of mental health [27–29].

The aim of the present study was to assess the effect of a polyphenol-rich dietary pattern (comprising fruits, including berries; vegetables and dark chocolate) in comparison to a control diet (low fruits and vegetables, <2 portions/day, and no dark chocolate) on aspects of psychological well-being and mental health status including mood, QoL, body image perception and self-esteem as secondary outcomes measured within the Polyphenol Intervention Trial (PPhIT) [30].

2. Materials and Methods

2.1. Setting and Study Population

PPhIT was a randomised, controlled, parallel-group, single-blinded dietary intervention trial, primarily designed to test whether increasing overall polyphenol dietary intake would affect microvascular function and a range of other markers of CVD risk, such as systolic blood pressure and lipid profile, in patients with hypertension. All participants underwent a full assessment at baseline (week 0) (described below); then, they entered a washout period, during which they consumed a low polyphenol diet, and afterwards were randomised to either a low polyphenol diet (LPD) or a high polyphenol diet (HPD) group for 8 weeks (Figure 1). A full assessment was repeated for all the participants at the end of the 8-week intervention (week 12), while at the end of the washout period (week 4), participants also underwent a dietary intake assessment, anthropometric measurements and blood and urine sample collection.

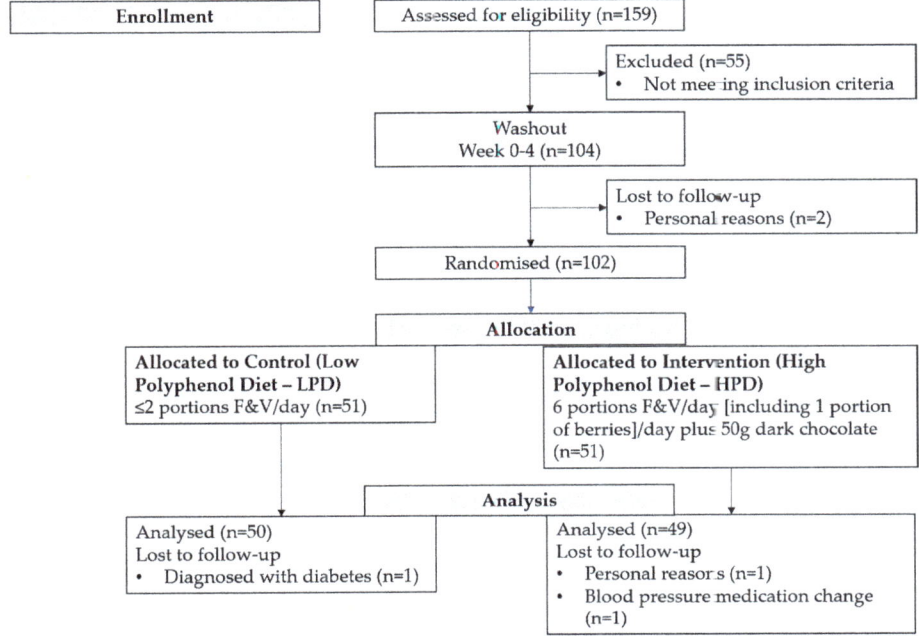

Figure 1. CONSORT diagram summarizing flow of participants through the study.

Participants aged 40–65 years, with documented grade I (140–159/90–99 mmHg) or grade II (160–179/100–109 mmHg) hypertension, were eligible. Participants with diabetes mellitus, acute coronary syndrome or transient ischaemic attack within three months, pregnancy or lactation, fasting triglyceride concentration >4 mmol/L, alcohol consumption (>28 units/week for men and >21 units/week for women), oral anticoagulant therapy or antioxidant supplements, dietary restrictions that would limit ability to comply with the study diets, body mass index >35 kg/m^2 or with an impalpable brachial artery were excluded from the study. Recruitment for PPhIT began in February 2011 and was completed by January 2013. All participants were informed about the aims and procedures of the study and gave their written consent. The study had ethical approval from the Office of Research Ethics Committee Northern Ireland (ref 10/NIR03/39) and was registered at ClinicalTrials.gov (ref NCT01319786). Details of the primary aim of the study, population, design, recruitment procedures and main findings have been published elsewhere [30]. Below, we provide some additional details on selected aspects of the evaluation that pertain to the analyses reported in this manuscript.

2.2. Dietary Intervention

The intervention commenced with a four-week "washout period" for all participants, during which they were asked to consume two portions or less of fruits and vegetables (F&V) per day and to exclude berries and dark chocolate (LPD). At the end of this period, subjects were randomised to either continue with the above LPD for a further 8-week "intervention period" or to consume an HPD of six portions of F&V (including one portion of berries per day) and 50 g of dark chocolate per day (Figure 1). A portion of fruit and vegetables was quantitatively defined using household measures as outlined by UK guidelines (https://www.nhs.uk/live-well/eat-well/5-a-day-portion-sizes/), i.e., 1 apple, 1 orange, half a grapefruit or one glass (150 mL) fruit juice, 3 tablespoons of vegetables [31]. All participants in the HPD had a self-selected weekly delivery of F&V and dark chocolate (Lindt® 70% cocoa) free of charge to their homes from a local supermarket and were provided with written material regarding

F&V portion sizes, recipes and sample diet plans. In addition, each participant, regardless of dietary allocation, was also contacted by telephone at weekly intervals to provide support and encouragement and to discuss potential barriers encountered in relation to achieving the dietary goals.

Dietary intake and compliance with the intervention were assessed through 4-day food diaries completed on four occasions: on the four days leading up to the week 0 visit (baseline measurement), on the four days leading up to the week 4 visit (washout period measurement), at week 8 (intervention measurement) and on the four days leading up to the final week 12 visit (a second intervention period measurement). Circulating blood and urine levels of a panel of nutritional biomarkers, with detailed methodology given below, were also used to assess compliance. Self-reported F&V, berries and dark chocolate consumed per day (as recorded in the food diaries) were extracted and entered into a Microsoft Excel spreadsheet. The spreadsheet contained pre-determined formulae which transformed the actual amounts of F&V and berries consumed into "portions" according to the "5-a-day" message.

2.3. Other Lifestyle Parameters

A "lifestyle and medical" questionnaire was used at week 0 to record participant demographic, lifestyle and medical information. The questionnaire had 16 items in total and assessed several aspects including vitamin and mineral supplement usage, smoking and alcohol habits, history of education, current occupational status, current medication, history of steroid use and, for females, use of hormone replacement therapy and details of menstrual cycle. Information regarding changes in medication use, smoking and alcohol patterns, as well as infections/illnesses were also recorded throughout the study.

Participants' physical activity levels were recorded at weeks 0, 4 and 12 to ensure that habitual activity levels were not altered for the duration of the study. The Recent Physical Activity Questionnaire (RPAQ), designed by the Medical Research Council (MRC Epidemiology Unit, Cambridge, UK), was used to measure physical activity. The questionnaire assesses physical activity within the preceding four weeks based on three primary areas: activity at home, activity at work (including travel to and from work) and recreational activities. The RPAQ has been shown to be a valid instrument for calculating total energy expenditure, physical activity energy expenditure and physical activity in healthy adults [32]. In terms of analysis, physical activity as recorded in the questionnaire was converted to total metabolic equivalent of task (MET) hours per day of sedentary, light, moderate and vigorous activity.

2.4. Anthropometric, Clinical and Biochemical Assessments

Participants attended the Royal Victoria Hospital (Belfast, Northern Ireland, UK) for assessments on three occasions throughout the study: baseline (week 0), washout period (week 4) and intervention (week 12). Body weight of participants was measured to the nearest 100 g and height to the nearest 0.5 cm. Body mass index (BMI) was calculated as weight (kg) divided by height squared (m^2). Waist circumference (WC) and hip circumference (HC) were tape-measured to the nearest 0.1 cm. Blood pressure (BP) was measured using an Omron M5-1 automatic BP monitor (Omron Healthcare, Hoofddorp, The Netherlands). Three consecutive readings were recorded, and a mean BP was calculated from the 2nd and 3rd readings. To measure the primary endpoint of PPhIT (microvascular function), venous occlusion plethysmography was conducted on participants by determining forearm blood flow during incremental intra-arterial infusions of acetylcholine and sodium nitroprusside, as previously described [30]. Blood samples were also collected. Fasting serum lipid profiles (total cholesterol, high density lipoprotein (HDL) and triglycerides) were assessed using standard enzymatic colorimetric assays on an automated Cobas® 8000 Modular system biochemical analyser (Roche Diagnostics Ltd., West Sussex, UK). Low-density lipoprotein (LDL) cholesterol was calculated using a standard Friedewald formula [33]. Blood and urine markers of micronutrient status were assessed at weeks 0 and 12 to objectively measure compliance to the intervention diet. Plasma vitamin C was measured on a FLUOstar Optima plate reader (BMG Labtech, Ortenberg, Germany), adapted from the method of Vuilleumier and Keck [34]. Serum concentrations of six carotenoids (α-carotene, β-carotene, β-cryptoxanthin, lutein, lycopene and zeaxanthin) were measured by reverse phase high performance liquid chromatography (HPLC), as described by Craft [35]. Urine collected from the volunteers between evening meal and midnight the evening before each study visit was analysed, including an enzymatic hydrolysis step, to quantify total epicatechin content, using an Agilent Technologies 1100 series HPLC (Agilent Technologies, Stockport, UK) directly linked to a Waters Micromass Quattro Ultima Platinum API triple quadrupole mass spectrometer (Waters, Dublin, Ireland).

2.5. Psychological Well-Being, Self-Esteem and Body Image

Aspects of psychological well-being and mental health status were evaluated through several scales and questionnaires that were completed at weeks 0 and 12. The decision to use these questionnaires only twice was made for three reasons: (i) the study wished to investigate the effect of the intervention diet in comparison to normal psychological well-being, rather than psychological well-being under the controlled conditions of the washout period; (ii) to reduce participants' burden at week 4 visits, which were already long (2.5 h) in duration due to vascular function and dietary assessments; (iii) distributing the surveys at three time points may have been disadvantageous in terms of allowing participants to become familiar with their format, which may have influenced responses. All questionnaires are commonly used for assessing various aspects of mental health and psychological well-being in the general population.

The Positive and Negative Affect Schedule (PANAS) was used for evaluating subjective mood. The questionnaire measures two distinctive dimensions: positive affect (PA) and negative affect (NA) [36]. PA is associated with pleasurable engagement with the environment, including feelings of enthusiasm and alertness as well as feeling active. NA refers to unpleasurable engagement with the environment, comprising feelings of anger, contempt, disgust, guilt, fear and nervousness. Whilst related, PA and NA represent two distinct and independent dimensions of mood. Participants were asked to respond to 10 items representing PA and 10 items representing NA on a five-point scale. Higher scores represent higher positive and negative affect, respectively. This was the only questionnaire assessing psychological well-being that was also completed at week 4, in order to monitor psychological well-being at the end of the washout period.

Depressive symptomology was assessed with the Beck Depression Inventory-II (BDI-II), a 21-item, self-report questionnaire developed by Beck and colleagues [37]. Each item on the BDI-II has four statements which relate to the severity of a particular depressive symptom, and respondents are asked to choose the one statement which best describes how they have been feeling in the preceding two weeks. Higher scores indicate higher levels of depression (scores 0–13 = minimal; 14–19 = mild; 20–28 = moderate; 29–63 = severe). The shorter version (21 items) of the Depression Anxiety Stress Scale (DASS-21) was also completed to measure depression, anxiety and stress [38]. The DASS-21 questionnaire was introduced nine months into the recruitment of the participants. DASS-21 has seven items per subscale and asks participants to rate the extent to which they experienced each emotional state the preceding week using a four-point Likert scale (0 = Did not apply to me at all, 3 = Applied to me very much or most of the time). Higher scores are indicative of higher levels of depression, anxiety and stress.

The Rosenberg Self-Esteem Scale was used as a global measure of self-esteem [39,40]. The questionnaire consists of a ten-item Likert scale, completed using a four-point scale from strongly agree to strongly disagree. Scores can range from 0 to 30, with higher scores indicating higher self-esteem. Finally, body image satisfaction was assessed through the Multidimensional Body Self-Relations Questionnaire—Appearance Scales (MSRQ-AS), a 34-item validated measure of body image perception for use in general populations (www.body-images.com) [41]. This version contains five subscales: appearance evaluation (satisfaction with ones looks), appearance orientation (levels of investment in one's appearance), overweight preoccupation (weight anxiety, vigilance, dieting etc), self-classified weight (how one perceives and labels one's weight) and body area satisfaction (satisfaction with areas of body). The questionnaire contains a series of statements and asks participants to indicate the extent to which each statement applies to them personally, with higher scores generally indicating greater body image satisfaction.

2.6. Mental and Physical Health

Mental and physical health were assessed with the RAND Medical Outcomes Study 36-item Short Form Health Survey (SF-36) [42,43]. A total of 36 questions are included in the RAND SF-36 survey and eight key areas are explored in the SF-36 including physical functioning, role limitations due to physical problems, pain, general health, energy/fatigue, social functioning, role limitations due to emotional problems and emotional well-being. The raw data were recoded using the RAND SF-36 scoring instructions available online. Additionally, the eight areas were combined to obtain the scoring for physical and mental health components. As the eight different components consist of different numbers of questions, the normal scores were transformed to T-scores, as described by Hays et al. 1993 [44] and Hays et al. 1995 [45]. Physical functioning, role limitations due to physical problems, pain and general health were combined to obtain the physical health component and role limitations due to emotional problems, energy/fatigue, emotional well-being and social functioning were combined to obtain the mental health component.

2.7. Statistical Analyses

The sample size calculation was based on the PPhIT primary outcome, namely microvascular function. According to this, detection of a 33% difference between groups in microvascular function, measured by forearm blood flow responses to an endothelium-dependent vasodilator, with 90% power, using a 2-tailed test at the 5% significance level, would require 50 participants per group. The current analysis reports secondary outcomes, for which power calculations were not performed.

Results are expressed as mean ± standard deviation for normally distributed continuous variables and as medians and interquartile ranges for continuous skewed variables. Categorical variables are presented as absolute (*n*) and relative frequencies (%). The normality of variables was checked through the Shapiro–Wilk test and graphically through histograms. Concentration measures of micronutrients were logarithmically transformed and were summarised as geometric median and interquartile range. The principal analysis for each outcome variable was a between-group comparison of change using independent sample t tests or Mann–Whitney U test for continuous parametric and non-parametric variables, respectively, and chi-squared test for categorical variables. Within-group comparisons were performed using paired sample t tests or Wilcoxon signed-rank test for parametric and non-parametric continuous variables, respectively. Statistical significance was set at $p \leq 0.05$. All statistical methods were conducted using PASW Statistics 18 for Windows (SPSS Inc., Chicago, IL, USA).

3. Results

3.1. General Results

Ninety-nine participants completed the PPhIT study, including 53 (53.5%) males. Participants had a mean age of 54.9 ± 6.9 years, with ages ranging from 40 to 65 years. The majority (52%) of the sample were obese (BMI ≥ 30 kg/m^2). In total, 12.1% were current smokers, and 43.4% stated that they had smoked in the past. Baseline characteristics according to dietary group (LPD versus HPD) are shown in Table 1. Overall, the groups were similar upon entering the study, with no statistically significant differences in anthropometric, lifestyle and basic clinical characteristics.

Table 1. Baseline (week 0) participant characteristics according to the Polyphenol Intervention Trial (PPhIT) study group allocation.

	Low Polyphenol ($n_{max} = 50$)	High Polyphenol ($n_{max} = 49$)	Between-Group Comparison p-Value *
Age (years)	55.6 ± 6.8	54.0 ± 7.0	0.25
Sex (males, n (%))	30 (60.0)	23 (46.9)	0.23
Education (years)	13.9 (12.0, 16.8)	13.6 (13.8, 15.8)	0.57
Body mass index (kg/m^2)	29.9 (26.9, 34.6)	31.15 (27.7, 33.5)	0.29
Waist circumference (cm)			
Male	106.5 (98.0, 116.3)	105.0 (98.0, 116.0)	0.86
Female	94.0 (85.3, 108.8)	96.0 (89.5, 108.5)	0.56
Current smoker n (%)	5 (10.0)	7 (14.3)	0.55
Use of antidepressants n (%)	7 (14.0)	8 (16.3)	0.79
Systolic blood pressure (mmHg)	143.7 ± 6.6	143.6 ± 8.0	0.95
Diastolic blood pressure (mmHg)	86.9 ± 3.3	85.9 ± 7.1	0.55
Total cholesterol (mmol/L)	5.3 ± 1.2	5.7 ± 1.2	0.10
HDL (mmol/L)	1.4 ± 0.3	1.3 ± 0.4	0.58
LDL (mmol/L)	4.3 ± 1.3	4.6 ± 1.2	0.18
Triglycerides (mmol/L)	1.7 (1.6, 2.1)	1.6 (1.5, 2.0)	0.46

HDL—high-density lipoprotein; LDL—low-density lipoprotein. Continuous variables are summarised as mean ± SD or medians and interquartile ranges. Categorical variables are summarised as n (%). * Between-group comparisons were made using independent sample t-tests ($p < 0.05$) or Mann–Whitney U test for continuous variables and chi-squared tests ($p < 0.05$) for categorical variables.

During the washout period, no changes were recorded in participants' physical activity habits, weight status, smoking habits, medication use or clinical condition compared to baseline in both HPD and LPD groups (data not shown). Additionally, mood evaluation according to PANAS questionnaire did not record any change between baseline and end of washout period (both $p > 0.05$) (data not shown). F&V intake per day declined significantly during washout, from 2.67 portions at week 0 to 1.38 portions at week 4 within the overall sample ($p < 0.001$), and significant reductions in blood levels of vitamin C ($p < 0.001$) and β-cryptoxanthin ($p = 0.05$), but not in any of the other carotenoids measured, were also recorded (data not shown).

Dietary intake of food groups and micronutrients, as well as weight status and physical activity levels both at baseline and at the end of the intervention period, are presented in Table 2, per intervention group. At baseline, there was no significant difference in intake of F&V, berries and dark chocolate and concentration of micronutrients between the LPD and HPD group. By the end of the intervention, there was a significant increase in intake of F&V, berries and dark chocolate in the HPD group, and the differences in change in intake between the two groups were statistically significant. Furthermore, there was a significant increase in the concentration of biomarkers, plasma vitamin C, serum lutein, β-cryptoxanthin, α-carotene and lycopene and urinary epicatechin over the course of the intervention in the HPD group, and the differences in the change in the concentration between the LPD and HPD group were statistically significant. These results indicate good compliance with the intervention diet, with significant between-group differences in change in all biomarkers measured except β-carotene. No differences were recorded in change in physical activity and weight status between the two intervention groups during the intervention.

Table 2. Baseline (week 0) and end of intervention (week 12) dietary intake, plasma, serum and urine micronutrient biomarkers, physical activity and weight status characteristics according to the Polyphenol Intervention Trial (PPhIT) study group allocation.

	Low Polyphenol Diet (n_{max} = 50)				High Polyphenol Diet (n_{max} = 49)				
	Week 0 [1]	Week 12	Median Change (IQR) [3]	Within Group (p Value) [4]	Week 0 [1]	Week 12	Median Change (IQR) [3]	Within Group (p Value) [4]	Between Group (p value) [5]
Dietary intake									
Fruits and vegetables intake (portions/day)	2.68 ± 1.68	1.24 ± 0.56	−1.44 (−1.87, −0.95)	<0.001	2.64 ± 1.70	6.73 ± 2.07	4.09 (3.45, 4.73)	<0.001	<0.001
	Week 0 [1]	Week 12	Median Change (IQR) [3]	Within Group (p value) [4]	Week 0 [1]	Week 12	Median Change (IQR) [3]	Within Group (p value) [4]	Between Group (p value) [5]
Berries (portions/day)	0 (0.00, 0.00)	0 (0.00, 0.00)	0 (0.00, 0.00)	0.69	0 (0.00, 0.00)	1 (0.80, 1.25)	1 (0.75, 1.17)	<0.001	<0.001
Dark chocolate (grams/day)	0 (0.00, 0.00)	0 (0.00, 0.00)	0 (0.00, 0.00)	0.18	0 (0.00, 0.00)	50 (37.50, 50.00)	50 (37.5, 50.0)	<0.001	<0.001
Micronutrient biomarkers									
Vitamin C (μmol/l) [6]	44.3 (28.70, 61.90)	34.2 (13.40, 49.50)	−7.60 (−26.50, 0.85)	<0.001	46.4 (31.70, 65.00)	55.7 (43.10, 68.20)	4.83 (−8.68, 20.75)	0.1	<0.001
Total carotenoids (μmol/l) [6]	1.09 (0.88, 1.43)	1.09 (0.72, 1.35)	−0.01 (−0.03, 0.01)	0.01	1.17 (0.96, 1.48)	1.33 (1.06, 1.66)	0.12 (−0.12, 0.40)	0.07	<0.001
Lutein (μmol/l) [6]	0.15 (0.12, 0.22)	0.14 (0.11, 0.20)	−0.01 (−0.03, 0.01)	0.08	0.14 (0.11, 0.20)	0.20 (0.15, 0.26)	0.04 (0.01, 0.07)	<0.001	<0.001
Zeaxanthin (μmol/l) [6]	0.04 (0.03, 0.05)	0.03 (0.03, 0.05)	−0.00 (−0.01, 0.01)	0.3	0.04 (0.03, 0.05)	0.04 (0.04, 0.06)	0 (−0.00, 0.01)	0.01	0.01
β-cryptoxanthin (μmol/l) [6]	0.06 (0.04, 0.07)	0.05 (0.03, 0.08)	−0.01 (−0.02, 0.01)	0.049	0.06 (0.04, 0.09)	0.07 (0.05, 0.09)	0.01 (−0.01, 0.03)	0.03	<0.001
α-carotene (μmol/l) [6]	0.12 (0.09, 0.15)	0.1 (0.08, 0.15)	−0.01 (−0.04, 0.01)	0.06	0.13 (0.11, 0.18)	0.15 (0.11, 0.20)	0.01 (−0.02, 0.03)	0.17	0.02
β-carotene (μmol/l) [6]	0.23 (0.16, 0.34)	0.22 (0.13, 0.32)	−0.01 (−0.09, 0.03)	0.07	0.27 (0.19, 0.44)	0.3 (0.21, 0.41)	−0.00 (−0.06, 0.08)	0.79	0.14
Lycopene (μmol/l) [6]	0.49 (0.38, 0.66)	0.47 (0.33, 0.58)	−0.04 (−0.19, 0.09)	0.07	0.5 (0.39, 0.61)	0.56 (0.40, 0.68)	0.05 (−0.14, 0.21)	0.31	0.048
Epicatechin (nmol/mg crt/L) [6]	0.43 (0.17, 1.10)	0.55 (0.26, 1.00)	0.04 (−0.24, 0.32)	0.37	0.64 (0.25, 0.97)	1.73 (0.51, 4.20)	0.89 (0.10, 3.57)	<0.001	<0.001
	Week 0 [1]	Week 12	Mean Change (95% CI) [2]	Within Group (p value) [4]	Week 0 [1]	Week 12	Mean Change (95% CI) [2]	Within Group (p value) [4]	Between Group (p value) [5]
Physical activity (MET hours/day)									
Sedentary activities	8.9 ± 4.7	8.6 ± 4.6	−0.3 (−1.0, 0.4)	0.6	8.4 ± 4.7	8.2 ± 4.8	−0.2 (−1.0, 0.7)	0.72	0.77
Moderate intensity	3.7 ± 5.6	2.6 ± 4.7	−1.1 (−2.3, 0.2)	0.1	3.9 ± 5.4	3.0 ± 5.4	−0.9 (−2.0, 0.2)	0.049	0.78
Vigorous intensity	1.1 ± 4.5	0.2 ± 0.5	−1.0 (−2.2, 0.3)	0.33	0.3 ± 1.6	0.1 ± 0.5	−0.2 (−0.6, 0.3)	0.89	0.63
Weight (kg)	87.2 ± 19.1	87.0 ± 19.1	−0.15 (−0.7, 0.4)	0.56	88.0 ± 20.1	88.2 ± 20.4	0.20 (−0.22, 6.2)	0.35	0.29

MET – metabolic equivalent of task. Data are presented as mean ± SD or medians and interquartile ranges (IQR). [1] There were no significant between-group differences in baseline values; [2] mean change was calculated as week 12- week 0 and is presented as mean change (95% CI); [3] median change was calculated as week 12- week 0 and is presented as median change (IQR); [4] within-group comparisons were performed using paired sample t tests and Wilcoxon signed-rank test ($p < 0.05$); [5] between-group comparisons were made using independent sample t-tests and Mann–Whitney U test ($p < 0.05$); [6] all variables are logarithmically transformed and summarised as geometric medians (IQ range) and change as geometric median change (IQR).

3.2. Changes in Aspects of Psychological Well-Being

Changes in measures of psychological well-being between baseline and intervention are illustrated in Table 3. There were no significant differences in scores of BDI-II, DASS-21 or PANAS between the LPD and HPD groups at baseline. There was a significant between-group difference ($p = 0.01$) in change in depressive symptoms as assessed with BDI-II, but no other significant effects were found between groups with regards to depression, anxiety or stress measured using the DASS-21 or positive and negative affect measured with PANAS. Regarding within-group changes, a borderline significant ($p = 0.05$) result was detected for a reduction in stress measured by DASS-21 within the HPD group, as well as an improvement in subjective mood (positive affect) ($p = 0.03$) measured by PANAS.

3.3. Changes in Self-Esteem and Body Image Perception

There were no significant differences in self-esteem or body image perception scores between the LPD and HPD groups at baseline. As shown in Table 3, there were also no significant differences between the HPD and LPD in self-esteem or body image perception scores at the end of the intervention.

3.4. Changes in Health-Related Quality of Life

There were no significant differences between groups at baseline with regards to health-related quality of life measured using the SF-36. There were statistically significant between-group differences in change in different component scores (general health ($p = 0.03$) and energy/fatigue ($p = 0.02$)) and the overall summary scores for the physical health component ($p = 0.04$) and mental health component ($p = 0.01$), with more positive changes demonstrated in the HPD group. In the HPD group, there were also within-group improvements in role limitations due to physical health ($p = 0.04$), general health ($p = 0.00$), energy/fatigue ($p = <0.001$), emotional well-being ($p = <0.001$) and social functioning ($p = 0.02$)

Table 3. Changes in mood, self-esteem, body image and quality of life indicators according to the Polyphenol Intervention Trial (PPhIT) study group allocation.

	Low Polyphenol Diet (n_{max} = 50)				High Polyphenol Diet (n_{max} = 49)				Between Group Change (p Value)[4]
	Week 0[1]	Week 12	Median Change (IQR)[2]	Within Group Change (p Value)[3]	Week 0[1]	Week 12	Median Change (IQR)[2]	Within Group Change (p Value)[3]	
BDI-II *	6.0 (2.0, 12.5)	7.0 (2.0, 11.0)	0.2 (−1.5, 1.9)	0.98	6.0 (3.0, 12.0)	2.0 (0.0, 6.0)	−3.4 (−5.4, −1.5)	<0.001	0.01
DASS-21 **									
Depression[5]	2.0 (0.0, 12.0)	6.0 (0.0, 10.5)	0 (−2.0, 6.0)	0.29	2.0 (0.0, 10.0)	0.0 (0.0, 6.0)	0 (−2.0, 0.0)	0.53	0.56
Anxiety[5]	4.0 (2.0, 9.0)	2.0 (0.0, 8.0)	0 (−3.0, 3.0)	0.86	4.0 (0.0, 10.0)	2.0 (0.0, 6.0)	0.0 (−2.0, 0.0)	0.16	0.8
Stress[5]	7.0 (2.0, 12.5)	8.0 (0.0, 16.0)	0 (−2.0, 4.0)	0.76	6.0 (2.0, 14.0)	4.0 (0.0, 10.0)	−2.0 (−6.0, 2.0)	0.05	0.14
PANAS ***									
Positive affect	29.9 (8.3)	30.4 (9.8)	0.5 (−1.5, 2.5)	0.63	33.0 (6.8)	35.2 (7.4)	2.2 (0.3, 4.1)	0.03	0.21
Negative affect	11.0 (10.0, 13.0)	11.0 (10.0, 13.0)	0.0 (−1.5, 1.5)	0.56	12.0 (10.0, 15.0)	10.0 (10.0, 14.0)	0.0 (−1.0, 0.5)	0.68	0.99
Rosenberg Self-Esteem Score †	26.0 (25.0, 28.0)	26.0 (25.0, 28.0)	0.0 (−2.0, 2.0)	0.74	26.0 (25.0, 27.0)	27.0 (24.0, 27.0)	0.0 (−2.0, 2.0)	0.68	0.53
MBSRQ-AS ††									
Appearance Evaluation	2.9 (2.4, 3.5)	3.0 (2.4, 3.6)	0.0 (−0.3, 0.4)	0.27	3.0 (2.5, 3.4)	3.1 (2.7, 3.6)	0.1 (−0.3, 0.4)	0.15	0.76
Appearance Orientation	3.0 (2.5, 3.7)	3.0 (2.5, 3.7)	0.0 (−0.3, 0.2)	0.35	3.2 (2.8, 3.5)	3.3 (2.9, 3.8)	0.2 (−0.2, 0.4)	0.16	0.1
Body areas Satisfaction	3.0 (2.7, 3.4)	3.3 (2.4, 3.7)	0.2 (−0.1, 0.4)	0.03	3.1 (2.7, 3.6)	3.3 (2.8, 3.8)	0.2 (−0.1, 0.3)	0.02	0.71
Overweight Preoccupation	2.3 (1.8, 2.8)	2.4 (1.8, 2.8)	0.0 (−0.3, 0.5)	0.87	2.5 (1.8, 3.2)	2.6 (1.8, 3.2)	0.0 (−0.5, 0.3)	0.45	0.72
Self-classified Weight[1]	4.0 (3.4, 4.0)	4.0 (3.0, 4.0)	0.0 (0.0, 0.0)	0.08	4.0 (3.5, 4.0)	4.0 (3.5, 4.0)	0.0 (0.0, 0.0)	0.43	0.5
SF-36 †††									
Physical Functioning	90 (75.0, 97.5)	90 (81.3, 100.0)	0 (0.0, 10.0)	0.07	95 (80.0, 100.0)	95 (85.0, 100.0)	0 (−5.0, 10.0)	0.15	0.44
Role limitations—physical health	100 (37.5, 100.0)	100 (37.5, 100.0)	0 (0.0, 25.0)	0.45	100 (75.0, 100.0)	100 (100.0, 100.0)	0.0 (0.0, 0.0)	<0.001	0.61
Pain	80 (47.5, 100.0)	80 (46.3, 100.0)	0 (−10.0, 10.0)	0.64	90 (60.0, 90.0)	90 (70.0, 100.0)	0 (−10.0, 22.5)	0.2	0.51
General health	65 (45.0, 75.0)	60 (50.0, 75.0)	0 (−10.0, 10.0)	0.47	65 (50.0, 75.0)	75 (65.0, 85.0)	10 (−5.0, 20.0)	<0.001	0.03
Physical health component	210.5 (168.5, 223.1)	200.9 (172.9, 217.2)	−6.4 (−17.0, 4.2)	0.09	213.2 (189.6, 225.1)	216.6 (201.4, 225.3)	2.2 (−8.1, 15.4)	0.2	0.04
Role limitations—emotional health	100 (100.0, 100.0)	100 (100.0, 100.0)	0.0 (0.0, 0.0)	0.99	100 (100.0, 100.0)	100 (100.0, 100.0)	0.0 (0.0, 0.0)	0.1	0.85
Energy/fatigue	55 (40.0, 72.5)	60 (45.0, 70.0)	5 (−5.0, 10.0)	0.39	60 (50.0, 80.0)	70 (60.0, 80.0)	5 (0.0, 20.0)	<0.001	0.02
Emotional well-being	76 (64.0, 84.0)	80 (62.0, 86.0)	0 (−8.0, 8.0)	0.73	80 (60.0, 88.0)	84 (72.0, 92.0)	4 (0.0, 16.0)	0	0.01
Social functioning	100 (75.0, 100.0)	100 (75.0, 100.0)	0 (−6.3, 0.0)	0.97	100 (75.0, 100.0)	100 (100.0, 100.0)	0 (0.0, 25.0)	0.02	0.08
Mental health component	209.1 (176.8, 222.3)	197.9 (175.0, 217.2)	−4.0 (−26.6, 8.1)	0.04	208 (181.4, 226.0)	218.3 (201.4, 226.8)	1.9 (−6.9, 19.1)	0.09	0.01

Data are presented as mean ± SD or medians and interquartile ranges (IQR). [1] There were no significant between-group differences in baseline values; [2] median change was calculated as week 12- week 0 and is presented as median change (IQR); [3] within-group comparisons were performed using paired sample t test or Wilcoxon signed-rank test ($p < 0.05$); [4] between-group comparisons were made using Mann–Whitney U test for continuous variables ($p < 0.05$); [5] n = 57 (LPD (n = 27), HPD (n = 30)); * BDI-II: Beck Depression Inventory Second Edition. Scores 0–13 = minimal depression, 14–19 = mild depression, 20–28 = moderate depression, 29–63 = severe depression; ** DASS-21; Depression Anxiety and Stress Scale 21 items. Depression score 0–9 = normal, Anxiety score 0–7 = normal, Stress score 0–14 = normal; *** PANAS; Positive and Negative Affect Scale. Higher score indicates higher positive and negative affect; † Rosenberg Self-Esteem Score; scores range from 0 to 30. Higher scores are indicative of higher self-esteem; †† MBSRQ-AS; Multi-Dimensional Body-Self Relations Questionnaire—Appearance Scales. Higher scores indicative of higher body image satisfaction; ††† Mental and physical health assessed using the RAND 36-Item Short Form Survey (SF-36). Physical functioning scores: "low" = limited a lot in performing all physical activities including bathing or dressing, "high" = performs all types of physical activities including the most vigorous without limitations due to health; Role limitations due to physical problems: "low" = problems with work or other daily activities as a result of physical health, "high" = no problems with work or other daily activities as a result of physical health, past 4 weeks; Pain: "high" = very severe and extremely limiting pain, "low" = no pain or limitations due to pain, past 4 weeks; General health perceptions: "high" = believes personal health is poor and likely to get worse, "low" = believes personal health is excellent. Physical health component = sum of physical functioning, role limitations—physical health, pain and general health. Role limitations due to emotional problems: "high" = problems with work or other daily activities as a result of emotional problems, "low" = no problems with work or other daily activities as a result of emotional problems, past 4 weeks; Energy/fatigue: "low" = feels tired and worn out all of the time, "low" = feels full of pep and energy all of the time, past 4 weeks; Emotional well-being: "high" = feelings of nervousness and depression all of the time, "low" = feels peaceful, happy and calm all of the time, past 4 weeks; Social functioning: "low" = extreme and frequent interference with normal social activities due to physical and emotional problems, "high" = performs normal social activities without interference due to physical or emotional problems, past 4 weeks. Mental health component = sum of role limitations—emotional health, energy/fatigue, emotional well-being and social functioning.

4. Discussion

Given the high prevalence of mental health problems and the potential effect of dietary patterns on their onset and/or treatment, the aim of the present study was to assess the effect of a polyphenol-rich dietary pattern (comprising fruits, including berries; vegetables and dark chocolate) on aspects of psychological well-being or mental health status, including mood, self-esteem and body image perception, as secondary outcomes of the PPhIT study. Despite some heterogeneity, the study findings suggest that the adoption of such a polyphenol-rich diet could potentially lead to beneficial effects on certain outcomes including depressed mood and physical and mental health in hypertensive participants.

There was a significant difference in change in depressive symptoms assessed with BDI-II between the HPD group and the LPD group, indicating a positive effect of the HPD, which is in agreement with a number of other observational studies focusing on the same outcome measure and polyphenol-rich foods. In the HPD group, a 66.6% reduction in BDI-II score was observed after the intervention. Button et al. 2015, using data from three randomised controlled trials (RCT) with a sample of $n = 1039$, identified that a 17.5% reduction in score was necessary to observe minimally clinically important differences [46]. Oliveria et al. (2019) found a negative association between depressive symptoms measured by BDI and high intake of polyphenol food items [47]. In the Finnish general population ($n = 2011$), daily intake of tea was associated with reduced risk of depressive symptoms defined by BDI scores [48]. Similarly, in the Mediterranean healthy eating, lifestyle and aging (MEAL) study ($n = 1572$), the dietary intake of phenolic acid, flavanones and anthocyanin were negatively associated with depressive symptoms measured using the Center for Epidemiologic Studies Depression Scale (CES-D-10) [49]. The positive effects observed in the present study may be attributable to other nutrients found in F&V, berries and dark chocolate which may work independently or synergistically to influence health outcomes. Brody (2002) found that vitamin C intake over a 14 day period led to a moderate reduction in depressive symptoms amongst 42 healthy young adults [50]. In our study, there was a significant difference in plasma vitamin C status between the LPD and HPD group. Similarly, there were significant increases in serum carotenoids, lutein, zeaxanthin, β-cryptoxanthin and urinary epicatechin within the HPD group, and some studies have suggested a link between these nutrients and improvements in psychological well-being including depression [51]. The antidepressant effects of polyphenols may be associated with both their antioxidant and anti-inflammatory properties, whereby there is a reduction in free radicals and cytokine dysregulation [12]. Lua and Wong (2012) found that the consumption of 50 g dark chocolate (70% cocoa) for three days was associated with significant improvement in depressed mood [52].

The primary outcome of the PPhIT study was to identify whether high consumption of F&V, berries and dark chocolate could improve microvascular function in hypertensive subjects [30]. High intake of polyphenol, specifically including F&V, berries and dark chocolate in diet, resulted in significant improvements in endothelium-dependent (acetylcholine) vasodilator [30]. Depression is often observed among individuals with vascular diseases such as hypertension, peripheral vascular disease and coronary artery disease, known as "vascular depression hypothesis" [53]. Studies have reported morphological changes in vascular structure and altered expression of endothelial cell molecules such as nitric oxide in patients with depression [53]. In the current study, the improvements in endothelium-dependent vasodilatation might have also resulted in improvements in depressed mood.

In light of the findings from the BDI-II, it is interesting that no notable effects of the polyphenol-rich diet were observed on depressed mood measured using the DASS-21 questionnaire in this study. The DASS-21 questionnaire was introduced as an amendment to PPhIT, given concerns that BDI-II is used to screen for depression in normal populations or to assess severity of depression in clinical populations, and therefore it was thought possible by the research team that the tool may not have been sensitive enough to pick up changes due to diet. Page et al. (2007) showed that DASS-21 has good psychometric properties and is moderately sensitive to changes that result from the treatment [54]. However, this resulted in a considerably smaller sample size for the analysis of the

DASS-21 questionnaire ($n = 57$) compared to BDI-II, which may have had implications in terms of the associated power available to detect differences between the two diet groups. The DASS-21 also showed no statistically significant differences in change between groups with regards to stress or anxiety. Furthermore, for both measures, scores on all scales at the start of the study are low, and negative affect scores for the PANAS are also low. These low scores are unsurprising in a volunteer sample for a study intended to improve health but may also have limited our chances of finding effects. Further study in groups with higher levels of poor psychological health, e.g., those with diagnoses of depression or anxiety, may be of value.

In the present study, significant improvements in quality of life between the HPD group and the LPD group measured using the SF-36 health survey questionnaire were found. There were statistically significant improvements in both physical and mental health components in the HPD group when compared with the LPD group. Data showing the effect of dietary interventions and especially of polyphenols/antioxidants on quality of life parameters are sparse and mainly limited to patients with chronic diseases such as multiple sclerosis, chronic fatigue syndrome and depression. Steptoe et al. (2004) found that a higher intake of fruits and vegetables through behavioural and nutrition education counselling was positively associated with physical health status but not mental health status measured using SF-36 among adults in a low-income neighbourhood [55]. A sub-study of the DASH trial also found that adhering to a fruit and vegetable-rich diet was associated with improved perception of quality of life [56]. It is important to acknowledge that while the self-reported improvements in physical and mental health scores observed within the current sample may be attributed to the foods consumed, they may also be wholly or partly influenced by taking part in the intervention and increased positivity that may come from making positive dietary changes. As pointed out in the study by Plaisted et al. (1999), improvements in QoL might be attributable to participants' awareness that they are consuming a healthy diet, which could have contributed to improved self-ratings of general health and mental health component [56]. In addition, given that depressive symptoms were improved in the HPD group, the improvements in mental health component may simply mirror these findings.

It is important to consider the results of this study in light of a number of methodological limitations. Firstly, as the primary purpose of PPhIT was to test the effect of a polyphenol-rich dietary pattern on microvascular and platelet function, the outcomes discussed here are secondary endpoints. Hence, as mentioned previously, it is possible that the study may not have been adequately powered to detect differences between the dietary groups, which may account for some of the null findings demonstrated. Secondly, the study sample comprised mildly hypertensive participants, which limits the generalisability of these results to the wider population. Furthermore, it is possible that selection bias exists within the current sample, given that the volunteers for this study were on the whole well-educated, and, as is the case with most clinical trials, are likely to have been more motivated with regard to improving their health than the general population. The participants in the HPD group were provided with the key intervention foods on a weekly basis, whereas the LPD group received no food provision as their diet was to remain unchanged. This may have increased the likely compliance of the HPD group with the intervention. Another limitation of this study was the use of self-report measures to measure psychological outcomes. Self-report measures can be disadvantageous in that they can be affected by forms of bias, including response, recall and social desirability bias, which can lead to inaccurate responses and conclusions [57]. However, given the subjective nature of psychological well-being, self-reporting is the most suitable method of obtaining information on individuals' personal experiences and emotions. The current study employed validated and previously used measures to collect information on individuals' personal experiences and emotions [58,59]. Additionally, it must be noted that the questionnaires described in this study were distributed at week 0 (baseline) and week 12 (intervention). It is possible that the washout period (week 0 to week 4) could have potentially affected people's psychological well-being and thus it may have been useful to additionally measure the endpoints at week 4. However, the decision to distribute the questionnaires at week 0 and week 12 was made for three main reasons: (i) to reduce participant burden at week 4 visits, which were already long

(2.5 h) in duration due to vascular function assessment and the dissemination of dietary advice; (ii) the study wished to investigate the effect of the intervention diet in comparison to normal psychological status, rather than psychological states under controlled conditions, which would have limited the applicability of the results; (iii) distributing the outcome measures at three time points may have been disadvantageous in terms of allowing participants to become familiar with their format, which may have induced response bias. Another limitation common to most studies analysing self-reported questionnaire data is the number of variables assessed, which may have increased the chance of type one errors (identification of the false positive) associated with hypothesis testing.

In contrast, one of the most obvious strengths of this study is its RCT study design. However, as the randomisation according to the groups only occurred at week 4, the presentation of week 0 data based on the allocated groups is rather artificial, and this must be considered a limitation. As further strengths, the study implemented a variety of techniques to encourage and monitor compliance. As a result of such efforts, participants were demonstrated to have good compliance with both diets, which was assessed both subjectively and objectively. Furthermore, the study had good retention of participants, with a less than 5% ($n = 5$) drop out level, all of which were due to reasons unrelated to the study.

5. Conclusions

In conclusion, the results from the present RCT trial showed heterogeneous findings regarding the effect of a polyphenol-rich dietary pattern on aspects of psychological well-being, with positive effects demonstrated on depressive symptoms and both the physical and mental health status components of the SF-36 quality of life measure. Further studies with psychological well-being impacts as primary endpoints, with appropriate study design and sample sizes, are needed in order to confirm the benefits of a polyphenol-rich dietary pattern on these outcomes.

Author Contributions: Conceptualization, C.R., R.L.N., K.M.A., I.S.Y., M.C.M., P.P.M. and J.V.W.; formal analysis, M.D.K., A.V., C.R., D.M. and J.V.W.; investigation, C.R. and R.L.N.; writing—original draft, M.D.K., A.V., C.R. and J.V.W.; writing—review and editing, M.D.K., A.V., C.R., R.L.N., K.M.A., D.M., M.D., I.S.Y., M.C.M., P.P.M. and J.V.W. All authors have read and agreed to the published version of the manuscript.

Funding: This study was funded by a Northern Ireland Health and Social Care Research and Development doctoral fellowship award (ref: EAT/4195/09) and Northern Ireland Chest Heart and Stroke scientific research grant (ref: 2010_17).

Acknowledgments: We acknowledge Margaret Cupples and the Northern Ireland Clinical Research Network (Primary Care) for their assistance with participant recruitment, Lesley Hamill for conducting the epicatechin analysis and Sarah Gilchrist for performing vitamin C and carotenoid analysis. We also thank all of the participants in the study for their time, interest, cooperation and contribution to the research.

Conflicts of Interest: The authors declare no conflict of interest. The funders had no role in the design of the study; in the collection, analyses, or interpretation of data; in the writing of the manuscript, and in the decision to publish the results.

References

1. The World Health Organization. The World Health Report 2001—Mental Health: New Understanding, New Hope. 2001. Available online: https://www.who.int/whr/2001/en/ (accessed on 10 December 2019).
2. The World Health Organization. The Global Burden of Disease: 2004 Update. 2004. Available online: https://www.who.int/healthinfo/global_burden_disease/2004_report_update/en/ (accessed on 10 December 2019).
3. Correll, C.U.; Solmi, M.; Veronese, N.; Bortolato, B.; Rosson, S.; Santonastaso, P.; Thapa-Chhetri, N.; Fornaro, M.; Gallicchio, D.; Collantoni, E. Prevalence, incidence and mortality from cardiovascular disease in patients with pooled and specific severe mental illness: A large-scale meta-analysis of 3,211,768 patients and 113,383,368 controls. *World Psychiatry* **2017**, *15*, 163–180. [CrossRef] [PubMed]
4. Lawrence, D.; Hancock, K.J.; Kisely, S. Cancer and mental illness. In *Comorbidity of Mental and Physical Disorders*; Karger Publishers: Basel, Switzerland, 2015; Volume 179, pp. 88–98.

5. Vigo, D.; Thornicroft, G.; Atun, R. Estimating the true global burden of mental illness. *Lancet Psychiatry* **2016**, *3*, 171–178. [CrossRef]
6. O'Neill, S.; Rooney, N. Mental health in Northern Ireland: An urgent situation. *Lancet Psychiatry* **2018**, *5*, 965–966. [CrossRef]
7. Ljungberg, T.; Bondza, E.; Lethin, C. Evidence of the importance of dietary habits regarding depressive symptoms and depression. *Int. J. Environ. Res. Public Health* **2020**, *17*, 1616. [CrossRef] [PubMed]
8. Velten, J.; Bieda, A.; Scholten, S.; Wannemüller, A.; Margraf, J. Lifestyle choices and mental health: A longitudinal survey with German and Chinese students. *BMC Public Health* **2018**, *18*, 632. [CrossRef] [PubMed]
9. Lim, S.Y.; Kim, E.J.; Kim, A.; Lee, H.J.; Choi, H.J.; Yang, S.J. Nutritional factors affecting mental health. *Clin. Nutr. Res.* **2016**, *5*, 143–152. [CrossRef]
10. Saghafian, F.; Malmir, H.; Saneei, P.; Milajerdi, A.; Larijani, B.; Esmaillzadeh, A. Fruit and vegetable consumption and risk of depression: Accumulative evidence from an updated systematic review and meta-analysis of epidemiological studies. *Br. J. Nutr.* **2018**, *119*, 1087–1101. [CrossRef]
11. Jacka, F.N.; O'Neil, A.; Opie, R.; Itsiopoulos, C.; Cotton, S.; Mohebbi, M.; Castle, D.; Dash, S.; Mihalopoulos, C.; Chatterton, M.L. A randomised controlled trial of dietary improvement for adults with major depression (the 'SMILES' trial). *BMC Med.* **2017**, *15*, 23. [CrossRef]
12. Smith, D.F. Benefits of flavanol-rich cocoa-derived products for mental well-being: A review. *J. Funct. Foods* **2013**, *5*, 10–15. [CrossRef]
13. Cory, H.; Passarelli, S.; Szeto, J.; Tamez, M.; Mattei, J. The role of polyphenols in human health and food systems: A mini-review. *Front. Nutr.* **2018**, *5*, 87. [CrossRef]
14. Potì, F.; Santi, D.; Spaggiari, G.; Zimetti, F.; Zanotti, I. Polyphenol health effects on cardiovascular and neurodegenerative disorders: A review and meta-analysis. *Int. J. Mol. Sci.* **2019**, *20*, 351. [CrossRef] [PubMed]
15. Rothwell, J.A.; Knaze, V.; Zamora-Ros, R. Polyphenols: Dietary assessment and role in the prevention of cancers. *Curr. Opin. Clin. Nutr. Metab. Care* **2017**, *20*, 512–521. [CrossRef] [PubMed]
16. Renaud, J.; Martinoli, M. Considerations for the use of polyphenols as therapies in neurodegenerative diseases. *Int. J. Mol. Sci.* **2019**, *20*, 1883. [CrossRef] [PubMed]
17. Carey, A.N.; Miller, M.G.; Fisher, D.R.; Bielinski, D.F.; Gilman, C.K.; Poulose, S.M.; Shukitt-Hale, B. Dietary supplementation with the polyphenol-rich açaí pulps (Euterpe oleracea Mart. and Euterpe precatoria Mart.) improves cognition in aged rats and attenuates inflammatory signaling in BV-2 microglial cells. *Nutr. Neurosci.* **2017**, *20*, 238–245. [CrossRef] [PubMed]
18. Bensalem, J.; Dudonné, S.; Gaudout, D.; Servant, L.; Calon, F.; Desjardins, Y.; Layé, S.; Lafenetre, P.; Pallet, V. Polyphenol-rich extract from grape and blueberry attenuates cognitive decline and improves neuronal function in aged mice. *J. Nutr. Sci.* **2018**, *7*, e19. [CrossRef]
19. Travica, N.; D'Cunha, N.M.; Naumovski, N.; Kent, K.; Mellor, D.D.; Firth, J.; Georgousopoulou, E.N.; Dean, O.M.; Loughman, A.; Jacka, F. The effect of blueberry interventions on cognitive performance and mood: A systematic review of randomized controlled trials. *Brain Behav. Immun.* **2020**, *85*, 96–105. [CrossRef]
20. Philip, P.; Sagaspe, P.; Taillard, J.; Mandon, C.; Constans, J.; Pourtau, L.; Pouchieu, C.; Angelino, D.; Mena, P.; Martini, D. Acute intake of a grape and blueberry polyphenol-rich extract ameliorates cognitive performance in healthy young adults during a sustained cognitive effort. *Antioxidants* **2019**, *8*, 650. [CrossRef]
21. Vauzour, D. Polyphenols and brain health. *OCL* **2017**, *24*, A202. [CrossRef]
22. Nabavi, S.M.; Daglia, M.; Braidy, N.; Nabavi, S.F. Natural products, micronutrients, and nutraceuticals for the treatment of depression: A short review. *Nutr. Neurosci.* **2017**, *20*, 180–194. [CrossRef]
23. Sureda, A.; Tejada, S. Polyphenols and depression: From chemistry to medicine. *Curr. Pharm. Biotechnol.* **2015**, *16*, 259–264. [CrossRef]
24. Bhagwat, S.; Haytowitz, D.B.; Holden, J.M. *USDA Database for the Flavonoid Content of Selected Foods, Release 3*; US Department of Agriculture: Washington, DC, USA, 2011.
25. Rizzoli, R.; Stevenson, J.C.; Bauer, J.M.; van Loon, L.J.; Walrand, S.; Kanis, J.A.; Cooper, C.; Brandi, M.L.; Diez-Perez, A.; Reginster, J.Y.; et al. The role of dietary protein and vitamin D in maintaining musculoskeletal health in postmenopausal women: A consensus statement from the European society for clinical and economic aspects of osteoporosis and osteoarthritis (ESCEO). *Maturitas* **2014**, *79*, 122–132. [CrossRef]

26. Rooney, C.; McKinley, M.C.; Woodside, J.V. The potential role of fruit and vegetables in aspects of psychological well-being: A review of the literature and future directions. *Proc. Nutr. Soc.* **2013**, *72*, 420–432. [CrossRef] [PubMed]
27. Jesus, M.; Silva, T.; Cagigal, C.; Martins, V.; Silva, C. Dietary patterns: A New therapeutic approach for depression? *Curr. Pharm. Biotechnol.* **2019**, *20*, 123–129. [CrossRef] [PubMed]
28. Li, Y.; Lv, M.; Wei, Y.; Sun, L.; Zhang, J.; Zhang, H.; Li, B. Dietary patterns and depression risk: A meta-analysis. *Psychiatry Res.* **2017**, *253*, 373–382. [CrossRef] [PubMed]
29. Jacka, F.N.; Cherbuin, N.; Anstey, K.J.; Butterworth, P. Does reverse causality explain the relationship between diet and depression? *J. Affect. Disord.* **2015**, *175*, 248–250. [CrossRef] [PubMed]
30. Noad, R.L.; Rooney, C.; McCall, D.; Young, I.S.; McCance, D.; McKinley, M.C.; Woodside, J.V.; McKeown, P.P. Beneficial effect of a polyphenol-rich diet on cardiovascular risk: A randomised control trial. *Heart* **2016**, *102*, 1371–1379. [CrossRef] [PubMed]
31. The National Health Service (NHS). 5 A Day Portion Sizes. 2018. Available online: https://www.nhs.uk/live-well/eat-well/5-a-day-portion-sizes/ (accessed on 2 May 2020).
32. Besson, H.; Brage, S.; Jakes, R.W.; Ekelund, U.; Wareham, N.J. Estimating physical activity energy expenditure, sedentary time, and physical activity intensity by self-report in adults. *Am. J. Clin. Nutr.* **2010**, *91*, 106–114. [CrossRef]
33. Friedewald, W.T.; Levy, R.I.; Fredrickson, D.S. Estimation of the concentration of low-density lipoprotein cholesterol in plasma, without use of the preparative ultracentrifuge. *Clin. Chem.* **1972**, *18*, 499–502. [CrossRef]
34. Vuilleumier, J.; Keck, E. Fluorometric assay of vitamin C in biological materials using a centrifugal analyser with fluorescence attachment. *J. Micronutr. Anal.* **1989**, *5*, 25–34.
35. Craft, N.E. Carotenoid reversed-phase high-performance liquid chromatography methods: Reference compendium. *Methods Enzymol.* **1992**, *213*, 185–205.
36. Watson, D.; Clark, L.A.; Tellegen, A. Development and validation of brief measures of positive and negative affect: The PANAS scales. *J. Pers. Soc. Psychol.* **1988**, *54*, 1063–1070. [CrossRef]
37. Beck, A.T.; Steer, R.A.; Brown, G.K. Beck depression inventory-II. *Psychol. Corp* **1996**, *78*, 490–498.
38. Antony, M.M.; Bieling, P.J.; Cox, B.J.; Enns, M.W.; Swinson, R.P. Psychometric properties of the 42-item and 21-item versions of the depression anxiety stress scales in clinical groups and a community sample. *Psychol. Assess.* **1998**, *10*, 176–181. [CrossRef]
39. Rosenberg, M. *Society and the Adolescent Self-Image*; Princeton University Press: Princeton, NJ, USA, 2015.
40. Alessandri, G.; Vecchione, M.; Eisenberg, N.; Łaguna, M. On the factor structure of the rosenberg (1965) general self-esteem scale. *Psychol. Assess.* **2015**, *27*, 621–635. [CrossRef] [PubMed]
41. Cash, T.F. *MBSRQ Users™ Manual*; Old Dominion University Press: Norfolk, VA, USA, 2000.
42. Ware Jr, J.E.; Sherbourne, C.D. The MOS 36-item short-form health survey (SF-36): I. Conceptual framework and item selection. *Med. Care* **1992**, *30*, 473–483. [CrossRef]
43. McHorney, C.A.; Ware Jr, J.E.; Raczek, A.E. The MOS 36-item short-form health survey (SF-36): II. Psychometric and clinical tests of validity in measuring physical and mental health constructs. *Med. Care* **1993**, *31*, 247–263. [CrossRef] [PubMed]
44. Hays, R.D.; Sherbourne, C.D.; Mazel, R.M. The rand 36 item health survey 1.0. *Health Econ.* **1993**, *2*, 217–227. [CrossRef] [PubMed]
45. Hays, R.D.; Sherbourne, C.D.; Mazel, R.M. *User's Manual for the Medical Outcomes Study (Mos) Core Measures of Health-Related Quality of Life*; Rand Corporation: Santa Monica, CA, USA, 1995.
46. Button, K.; Kounali, D.; Thomas, L.; Wiles, N.; Peters, T.; Welton, N.; Ades, A.; Lewis, G. Minimal clinically important difference on the beck depression inventory-II according to the patient's perspective. *Psychol. Med.* **2015**, *45*, 3269–3279. [CrossRef] [PubMed]
47. Oliveira, N.G.d.; Teixeira, I.T.; Theodoro, H.; Branco, C.S. Dietary total antioxidant capacity as a preventive factor against depression in climacteric women. *Dement. Neuropsychol.* **2019**, *13*, 305–311. [CrossRef]
48. Hintikka, J.; Tolmunen, T.; Honkalampi, K.; Haatainen, K.; Koivumaa-Honkanen, H.; Tanskanen, A.; Viinamäki, H. Daily tea drinking is associated with a low level of depressive symptoms in the finnish general population. *Eur. J. Epidemiol.* **2005**, *20*, 359–363. [CrossRef]

49. Godos, J.; Castellano, S.; Ray, S.; Grosso, G.; Galvano, F. Dietary polyphenol intake and depression: Results from the mediterranean healthy eating, lifestyle and aging (meal) study. *Molecules* **2018**, *23*, 999. [CrossRef] [PubMed]
50. Brody, S. High-dose ascorbic acid increases intercourse frequency and improves mood: A randomized controlled clinical trial. *Biol. Psychiatry* **2002**, *52*, 371–374. [CrossRef]
51. Payne, M.E.; Steck, S.E.; George, R.R.; Steffens, D.C. Fruit, Vegetable, and antioxidant intakes are lower in older adults with depression. *J. Acad. Nutr. Diet.* **2012**, *112*, 2022–2027. [CrossRef] [PubMed]
52. Lua, P.; Wong, S. Dark chocolate consumption on anxiety, depression and health-related quality of life of patients with cancer: A randomised clinical investigation. *Malays. J. Psychiatry* **2012**, *21*, 1–11.
53. Baruah, J.; Vasudevan, A. The vessels shaping mental health or illness. *Open Neurol. J.* **2019**, *13*, 1–9. [CrossRef] [PubMed]
54. Page, A.C.; Hooke, G.R.; Morrison, D.L. Psychometric properties of the depression anxiety stress scales (DASS) in depressed clinical samples. *Br. J. Clin. Psychol.* **2007**, *46*, 283–297. [CrossRef] [PubMed]
55. Steptoe, A.; Perkins-Porras, L.; Hilton, S.; Rink, E.; Cappuccio, F.P. Quality of life and self-rated health in relation to changes in fruit and vegetable intake and in plasma vitamins C and E in a randomised trial of behavioural and nutritional education counselling. *Br. J. Nutr.* **2004**, *92*, 177–184. [CrossRef]
56. Plaisted, C.S.; Lin, P.H.; Ard, J.D.; McClure, M.L.; Svetkey, L.P. The effects of dietary patterns on quality of life: A substudy of the dietary approaches to stop hypertension trial. *J. Am. Diet. Assoc.* **1999**, *99*, S84–S89. [CrossRef]
57. Van de Mortel, T.F. Faking it: Social desirability response bias in self-report research. *Aust. J. Adv. Nurs.* **2008**, *25*, 40–48.
58. García-Batista, Z.E.; Guerra-Peña, K.; Cano-Vindel, A.; Herrera-Martínez, S.X.; Medrano, L.A. Validity and reliability of the beck depression inventory (BDI-II) in general and hospital population of dominican republic. *PLoS ONE* **2018**, *13*, e0199750. [CrossRef]
59. Osman, A.; Wong, J.L.; Bagge, C.L.; Freedenthal, S.; Gutierrez, P.M.; Lozano, G. The depression anxiety stress scales-21 (DASS-21): Further examination of dimensions, scale reliability, and correlates. *J. Clin. Psychol.* **2012**, *68*, 1322–1338. [CrossRef] [PubMed]

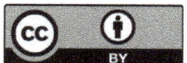

© 2020 by the authors. Licensee MDPI, Basel, Switzerland. This article is an open access article distributed under the terms and conditions of the Creative Commons Attribution (CC BY) license (http://creativecommons.org/licenses/by/4.0/).

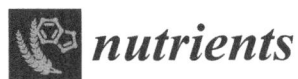

Article

Acute Effects of a Polyphenol-Rich Leaf Extract of *Mangifera indica* L. (Zynamite) on Cognitive Function in Healthy Adults: A Double-Blind, Placebo-Controlled Crossover Study

Emma L. Wightman [1,2], Philippa A. Jackson [2], Joanne Forster [2], Julie Khan [2], Julia C. Wiebe [3], Nigel Gericke [3,4] and David O. Kennedy [2,*]

[1] NUTRAN, Northumbria University, Newcastle-upon-Tyne NE1 8ST, UK; emma.l.wightman@northumbria.ac.uk
[2] Brain, Performance and Nutrition Research Centre, Northumbria University, Newcastle-upon-Tyne NE1 8ST, UK; philippa.jackson@northumbria.ac.uk (P.A.J.); jo.forster@northumbria.ac.uk (J.F.); julie.khan@northumbria.ac.uk (J.K.)
[3] Nektium Pharma, Agüimes, 35118 Las Palmas de Gran Canaria, Spain; jwiebe@nektium.com (J.C.W.); n.gericke@nektium.com (N.G.)
[4] Department of Botany and Plant Biotechnology, University of Johannesburg, Auckland Park 2006, Johannesburg 2092, South Africa
* Correspondence: david.kennedy@northumbria.ac.uk

Received: 17 June 2020; Accepted: 21 July 2020; Published: 23 July 2020

Abstract: Extracts made from the leaves of the mango food plant (*Mangifera indica* L., Anacardiaceae) have a long history of medicinal usage, most likely due to particularly high levels of the polyphenol mangiferin. In rodent models, oral mangiferin protects cognitive function and brain tissue from a number of challenges and modulates cerebro-electrical activity. Recent evidence has confirmed the latter effect in healthy humans following a mangiferin-rich mango leaf extract using quantitative electroencephalography (EEG). The current study therefore investigated the effects of a single dose of mango leaf extract, standardised to contain >60% mangiferin (Zynamite®), on cognitive function and mood. This study adopted a double-blind, placebo-controlled cross-over design in which 70 healthy young adults (18 to 45 years) received 300 mg mango leaf extract and a matched placebo, on separate occasions, separated by at least 7 days. On each occasion, cognitive/mood assessments were undertaken pre-dose and at 30 min, 3 h and 5 h post-dose using the Computerised Mental Performance Assessment System (COMPASS) assessment battery and the Profile of Mood States (POMS). The results showed that a single dose of 300 mg mango leaf extract significantly improved performance accuracy across the tasks in the battery, with domain-specific effects seen in terms of enhanced performance on an 'Accuracy of Attention' factor and an 'Episodic Memory' factor. Performance was also improved across all three tasks (Rapid Visual Information Processing, Serial 3s and Serial 7s subtraction tasks) that make up the Cognitive Demand Battery sub-section of the assessment. All of these cognitive benefits were seen across the post-dose assessments (30 min, 3 h, 5 h). There were no interpretable treatment related effects on mood. These results provide the first demonstration of cognition enhancement following consumption of mango leaf extract and add to previous research showing that polyphenols and polyphenol rich extracts can improve brain function.

Keywords: cognition; attention; memory; brain; polyphenols; mangiferin; mango leaf extract

1. Introduction

The roots, leaves, fruit and bark of the food plant *Mangifera indica* (mango) have a long history of therapeutic use within traditional medicinal systems for a wide range of conditions. For example, extracts, teas and infusions made from mango leaves have been used for the treatment of diabetes, malaria, diseases of the digestive system, lungs, and kidneys, and as a topical treatment for wounds and burns [1]. The bioactivity of mango leaf extracts may be due to particularly high levels [2] of xanthones. This group of polyphenols are found in a restricted group of plant species [3], including members of the *Hypericum* genus that provide us with a number of medicinal herbal extracts [4], but they are rarely consumed in the diet, with only a few exceptions other than mango itself (e.g., [5]). The predominant member of this structural group in mango leaf is mangiferin, a xanthone glucoside that has been shown to have potential anti-inflammatory, antioxidant, immunomodulatory, neuroprotective, antiproliferative, antidiabetic, DNA protective, and hypoglycaemic properties [6–10].

Whilst structurally distinct from the flavonoids and other polyphenols that are ubiquitous in plant derived foods, mangiferin [8,11–14] likely owes its beneficial bioactivity to some similar mechanisms of action as found in the wider polyphenol group class [15], including interactions with, and modulation of, diverse components of a wide range of mammalian cellular signal transduction pathways. These pathways, in turn, control gene transcription and a plethora of cellular responses, including cell proliferation, apoptosis, and the synthesis of growth factors, and vasodilatory and inflammatory molecules. In the central nervous system, specific additional interactions attributed to polyphenols include direct neurotransmitter and neurotrophin receptor and signalling pathway interactions, and increased synthesis of neurotrophins and vasodilatory molecules, which, in turn, foster angiogenesis/neurogenesis [15–20]. These mechanisms potentially underlie the observation of consistent beneficial cardiovascular effects from meta-analyses of multiple intervention studies [21–23], and demonstrations of improved cognitive function [24–28], following diverse polyphenols.

In line with these mechanistic cellular effects, rodent studies have demonstrated that a single administration of mangiferin can improve memory in uncompromised rats [29] and that either single doses or extended supplementation with mangiferin can attenuate the memory deficits or depressive/anxiety behaviours associated with a range of brain insults and challenges. This includes the cholinergic antagonist scopolamine [30], sleep deprivation [31], the injection of lipopolysaccharides [32] and aluminium chloride-induced neurotoxicity in mice [9]. Consistent ex vivo evidence focussing on the hippocampus also shows that mangiferin can protect rodent neuronal tissue from the increase in inflammatory cytokines [9,30–32] and the decrease in neurotrophins such as brain-derived neurotrophic factor (BDNF) [9,31], associated with multifarious brain insults. Similarly, mangiferin has been shown to protect the rodent brain from lead-induced structural damage and decrease oxidative stress via interactions within the Nrf2 signalling pathways in rats [10].

A number of recent studies have assessed the potential efficacy of a mango leaf extract standardized to a minimum of 60% mangiferin (Zynamite®). In terms of physical performance, several of these studies have assessed the ergogenic effects in humans of both acute [33–36] and longer-term supplementation [34] with this mango leaf extract combined with the polyphenols luteolin or quercetin. This research has demonstrated an improved performance during high intensity exercise [33–35], increased brain oxygenation [33,34], maximal aerobic capacity [33], increased muscle oxygen extraction [34,35] and the attenuation of muscle damage and improvements in the time course of decreased muscle performance [37].

With regard to brain function, in rats, oral administration of mango leaf extract attenuated electroencephalography (EEG) power measured via implanted electrodes (frontal cortex, hippocampus, striatum, reticular formation) across the spectra and brain regions under investigation, with the most striking findings in the alpha and beta wavebands. These effects were synergistically increased by the co-administration of caffeine. A concomitant ex vivo study also demonstrated that 7 days supplementation with the mango leaf extract lead to increased hippocampal pyramidal cell excitability [38]. In a subsequent multi-disciplinary series of studies [39], both the ex vivo hippocampal excitability and the attenuation of EEG spectral power across brain regions in rats were confirmed both for mango leaf extract and mangiferin, confirming this polyphenol as the likely active component of the extract. In two subsequent pilot studies (also reported in [39]), both involving 16 healthy young humans, quantitative EEG was employed at rest and during cognitive task performance 90- and 60-min post-dose respectively. In the first study, in comparison to control, mango leaf extract resulted in modest reductions in 'eyes open' power in delta and theta power, and a more pronounced increase in power during cognitive task performance, with significant increases in all wavebands across scalp electrodes interrogating the association cortex. These results were supported by more modest EEG changes in the second study, but no evidence of a synergistic relationship with caffeine. Cognitive task performance and mood were not significantly modulated by mango leaf extract.

The extant literature demonstrating functional benefits following polyphenol consumption, and the previous rodent and pilot human studies assessing the effects of mangiferin and mango leaf extract described above, suggest that a mango leaf extract with high levels of the polyphenol mangiferin may exert beneficial effects on human brain function, including the enhancement of cognitive function. The current exploratory, double-blind, placebo-controlled, balanced crossover study therefore assessed the effects of a single dose of mango leaf extract (Zynamite®) on cognitive function and psychological state 30 min, 3 h and 5 h post-dose in a large sample of healthy adults.

2. Methods

2.1. Design

This study adopted a randomised, double-blind, placebo-controlled, balanced crossover design, in which the acute effects of a single dose of 300 mg mango leaf extract and placebo were assessed on cognitive function and psychological state/mood at 30 min, 3 h and 5 h post-dose. All study procedures were reviewed and approved by Northumbria University's Department of Psychology Ethics Committee (Ref: 17741) and were conducted according to the principles of the Declaration of Helsinki. The trial was pre-registered at ClinicalTrials.gov (NCT04299217).

2.2. Participants

The required sample size for the study (N = 72) was calculated (GPower 3.0) on the basis of delivering adequate power (0.8) to detect a small effect size (f = 0.1). The power to detect the anticipated medium effect size (f = 0.25) exceeded 0.95.

A total of 75 participants were randomised. Three participants subsequently withdrew from the study after completing one testing visit. Two participants were removed from the dataset during blind data review due to a persistent inability to achieve performance criteria across tasks.

The final per-protocol analysis sample therefore comprised 70 participants (F 37/M 33; mean age 26.9 years, range 18–45 years; 5 vegetarians and 1 vegan). All participants self-reported that they were healthy and free from any relevant medical condition or disease, including psychiatric and neurodevelopmental disorders; that they were not taking any prescription or illicit drugs, food supplements or nicotine containing products; that they were not pregnant, lactating or seeking to become pregnant. Participants were also excluded if they consumed >500 mg caffeine per day (>6 × 150 mL cups of filter coffee), had high blood pressure (>systolic 159 mm Hg or diastolic 99 mm Hg) or had a body mass index outside of the range 18.5–35 kg/m^2. Participant dispositions are shown in Figure 1.

The final number of participants' data points (excluding missing data and data points removed during blind data review) included in the analysis of data from each individual outcome are shown in the relevant tables.

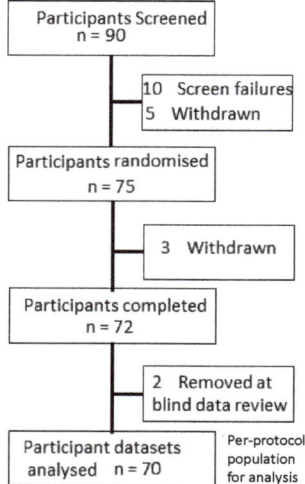

Figure 1. Participant disposition.

2.3. Treatments

Zynamite® mango leaf extract is comprised of components within the following ranges: mangiferin—60–65%; homomangiferin—3–5%; isomangiferin—up to 1%; leaf polysaccharides—6–20%; hydrolysable and non-hydrolysable tannins—up to 1%; fibre, minerals, moisture—6 to 15%. Details of the manufacturing process are provided elsewhere [39].

Participants were randomly allocated to receive 300 mg mango leaf extract or placebo (maltodextrin) in methylcellulose capsules of identical appearance, during each of their two assessment days. Testing days were separated by a minimum of 7 days to ensure washout. The order in which participants received the two interventions was counterbalanced across the group via random allocation to a counterbalancing schedule. Individual treatments were delivered to the trial facility in individual sealed plastic envelopes, labelled with the participants' randomisation numbers and visit (1 or 2) according to the computer-generated double-blind randomisation schedule.

There were no significant adverse events that could be linked to administration of the treatments and no significant difference in the incidence of minor adverse events (e.g., mild headache) between the placebo and mango leaf extract treatments.

2.4. Psychological Measures

2.4.1. Cognitive Tasks

All of computerised cognitive/mood assessments were identical, and were carried out via laptop computers and response boxes using the Computerised Mental Performance Assessment System (COMPASS, Northumbria University, Newcastle upon Tyne, UK). This software platform incorporates the presentation of classic and custom computerised cognitive tasks, with fully randomised parallel versions of each task delivered at each assessment for each individual. A similar selection of tasks has previously been shown to be sensitive to diverse nutritional interventions [40–43]. Within the 60-min assessment the participants also completed a 30-min component known as the Cognitive Demand Battery (CDB), which comprises the prolonged repetition of a series of demanding tasks that assess working memory, executive function and attention. The objective of this battery is to assess the impact of treatment on speed/accuracy and mental fatigue during continuous performance of cognitively demanding tasks. The CDB has also been shown to be sensitive to modulation by a wide range of nutritional interventions [43–46]. The individual tasks making up the cognitive assessment (including the CDB) are shown in Figure 2 and described in more detail in the online Supplementary Materials (Section I).

Figure 2 also shows the contribution of individual tasks to the principal performance measures, which were derived by averaging the data (either msec for speed, or % correct/maximum score for accuracy) from individual tasks into the following global performance outcomes: 'Speed of Performance' and 'Accuracy of Performance'; and the following cognitive domain factor scores 'Speed of Attention', 'Accuracy of Attention', 'Speed of Memory', 'Working Memory', and 'Episodic Memory'. The derivation of the global scores and cognitive factors are described in more detail in the online Supplementary Materials (Section II). These global measures and cognitive domain factors have been shown to be sensitive to nutritional manipulations previously [40–42].

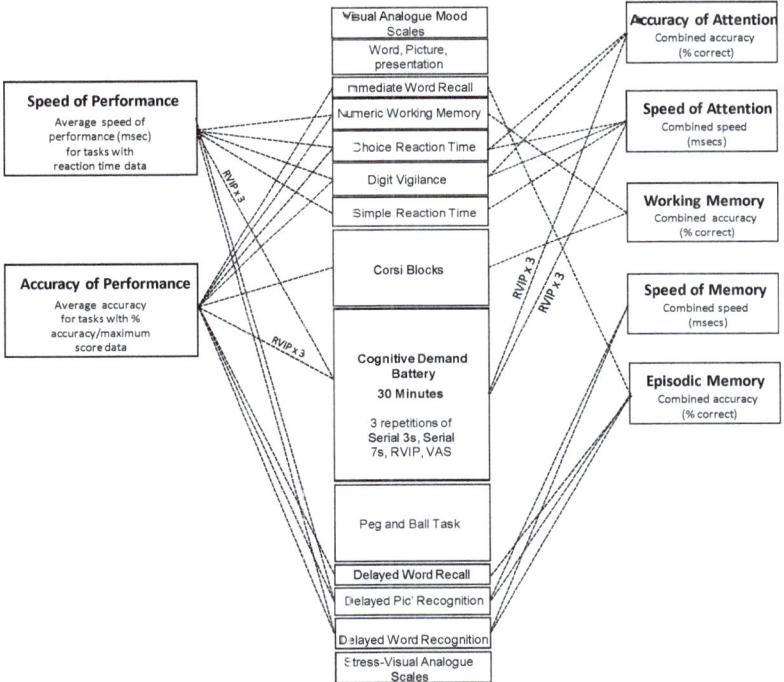

Figure 2. Cognitive assessments. The running order of tasks and their contribution to the cognitive factors (to the right) and global performance measures (to the left) derived from the overall battery. The same assessment was completed at the pre-treatment baseline and at 30 min, 3 h and 5 h post-dose on each assessment day. The selection of tasks took a total of 60 min to complete, with the Cognitive Demand Battery comprising 30 min of this. The individual tasks are described in more detail in the supplementary online materials (Section I). Rapid Visual Information Processing task (RVIP). Visual analogue scale (VAS).

2.4.2. Mood and Psychological State

Before each cognitive assessment, participants completed the Profile of Mood States (POMS-2) Adult Short Form [47]. As part of the COMPASS battery, and before the cognitive tasks, participants completed the Visual Analogue Mood Scales (VAMS), a set of 18 visual analogue scales anchored by pairs of antonymic mood/state adjectives (e.g., Alert–Inattentive; Lethargic–Energetic). Participants rated where they would position themselves between the adjectives anchoring each line according to how they felt at that moment. The individual item scores were combined to give an average (% along the line) score on three factors that had previously been derived by factor analysis:

'Alertness', 'Tranquillity' and 'Stress'. After the cognitive tasks participants also completed a further four stress visual analogue scales (S-VAS) that required them to rate their current psychological state between 'not at all' and 'extremely' with regard to their levels of stress, anxiety, calmness and relaxation. These were combined into two scores 'stress/anxiety' and 'calm/relaxed' with a higher score (average % along the line) representing more of the descriptor.

2.5. Procedure

Participants were required to attend the Brain, Performance and Nutrition Research Centre (Northumbria University) for three visits. The first visit comprised a screening and training session where, once written informed consent had been obtained, participants were screened according to the inclusion/exclusion criteria. Eligible participants then provided lifestyle and demographic data and their height, weight, waist to hip ratio and blood pressure were measured. They completed a short training session in which they practiced the cognitive tasks. Practice took the form of three repetitions of shortened versions of the COMPASS cognitive tasks, followed by the completion of the full-length, 60-min battery twice. During and at the end of the practice session, participants' performance was checked against standard minimum performance criteria and additional guidance was provided as necessary. At the end of this visit, participants were briefed as to what to expect on testing visits and were provided with pre-testing instructions.

Within four weeks of the screening visit, participants returned to the laboratory for their first testing visit at an agreed time in the morning that remained consistent across all testing visits. A maximum of 5 participants were tested on any day, and all participants were visually isolated in individual testing booths. Participants arrived at the laboratory having refrained from alcohol for 24 h, caffeine overnight and having consumed a simple breakfast of cereal and/or toast at home no later than an hour before arrival. Once participants arrived at the lab, they were not permitted to eat any food (aside from food items provided by the study staff) or drink (except for water) or chew gum. Continued compliance with the inclusion/exclusion criteria was assessed. This was followed by completion of the POMS and a 60-min computerised cognitive and mood assessment (COMPASS—including the 30-min Cognitive Demand Battery (CDB), Visual analogue mood scales (VAMS) and stress visual analogue scales (S-VAS)—see Figure 2.). Cognitive tasks were completed with the participants visually isolated from each other. After the first cognitive/mood assessment, participants consumed their treatment for the day and completed cognitive/mood assessments, identical to the above, commencing at 30 min, 3 h and 5 h post-dose. An additional, brief, 5-min assessment investigating the participants' response to a laboratory stressor, plus pre/post-dose blood sampling for half of the participants (for quantification of neurotrophins and catecholamines), took place after the pre-treatment and 30-min post-dose cognitive/mood assessments (For methodology see [48]), the results of this theoretically distinct investigation are to be reported elsewhere). All participants were scheduled to return to the laboratory 7 days later, with a maximum allowable leeway of an additional 7 days should exceptional circumstances arise in the meantime. This second testing day was identical to the previous day, with the exception that participants consumed a different treatment on each of the two days. The timelines of the testing day are presented in Figure 3.

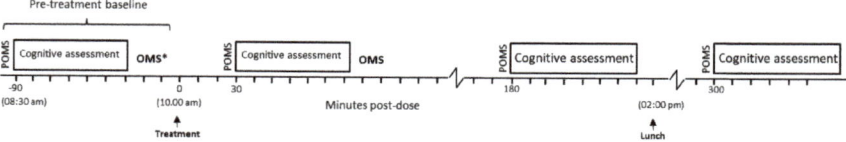

Figure 3. The timelines of the testing day for individual participants, showing the core cognitive assessment schedule. Profile of Mood States (POMS), 5 min Observed Multi-Tasking Stressor (*OMS) (methodology and results to be reported elsewhere).

Participants were provided with a standardised lunch (comprising a cheese sandwich on white bread, crisps and a custard pot) between the 180 and 300 min post-dose assessments and were given the option of a snack (hot decaffeinated tea or coffee and digestive biscuits) after completion of the stressor following the 30-min post-dose assessment. No alternative drinks, snacks or lunches were permitted.

2.6. Analysis

The study statistical analysis plan was formulated before the completion of data collection. Given the exploratory nature of the study, and the lack of any relevant human data, a small sub-set of primary outcomes was not pre-defined. Given the study intervention and objectives, a per protocol analysis was deemed the most appropriate.

All outcomes were analysed using SPSS (version 24.0, IBM corp., Armonk, NY, USA). During blind data review a number of participants' individual task datasets were removed due to technical or performance issues (for details of the issues and number of datasets involved see supplementary online materials). Prior to the primary analysis of the effects of treatment, pre-dose baseline differences between treatment were investigated by one-way (treatment group [placebo v mango leaf extract]) paired t tests, or in the case of the Cognitive Demand Battery (CDB) two-way (treatment x repetition) ANOVA. There were no significant differences between treatment groups at baseline.

For all cognitive and mood measures, the primary analysis of post-dose data was by Linear Mixed Models (LMM) using the MIXED procedure in SPSS (version 22.0, IBM corp.) with pre-dose baseline data for each outcome included as a covariate. For all LMM analyses, the 'compound symmetry' covariance structure provided the best fit, with the exception of 'mental fatigue' from the CDB for which an autoregressive covariance structure (AR1) was more appropriate.

For the cognitive outcomes derived from the COMPASS battery and the mood outcomes, terms were fitted for treatment (placebo/mango leaf extract) and assessment (30 min, 3 h, 5 h) and their interaction. For the CDB measures an additional 'repetition' term was added along with the appropriate interactions. Given that the treatment orders were balanced across the sample, or exactly or nearly balanced with regard to the participants contributing to each outcome (and given that treatment carry-over effects were highly unlikely), treatment order was not included as a factor in the analysis.

In order to establish the time course of any effects, pre-defined planned comparisons were conducted between treatments at each assessment time point (30 min, 3 h, 5 h) with a Bonferroni adjustment for the number of comparisons undertaken per outcome (i.e., 3). Only those planned comparisons conducted on data from outcomes that evinced a significant treatment related main or interaction effect are reported below.

3. Results

3.1. Cognitive Task Global and Factor Outcomes

The global outcomes and cognitive factors derived from the COMPASS battery showed that mango leaf extract resulted in significantly improved accuracy of performance across tasks and throughout the testing day (i.e., at 30 min, 3 h and 5 h post-dose). See Figure 4 below. There was a main effect of treatment on the global Accuracy of Performance measure (representing data from the eleven tasks that return % accuracy/maximum score data) ($F (1, 335) = 22.8$, $p < 0.001$). Reference to the planned comparisons at each assessment showed that this effect was evident throughout the post-dose testing period (30 min $p = 0.03$, 3 h $p = 0.02$, 5 h $p = 0.009$). There were also significant main effects in terms of improved accuracy following mango leaf extract on the Accuracy of Attention factor ($F (1, 315) = 16.697$, $p < 0.001$) and the Episodic Memory factor ($F (1, 345) = 6.94$, $p = 0.009$). With regard to the time course of these effects, whilst the Bonferroni adjusted comparisons of Episodic Memory scores did not reach significance during the individual assessments, Accuracy of Attention was improved at both the 3 h ($p = 0.048$) and 5 h ($p = 0.01$) post-dose assessments. Data (plus F score and p) for the cognitive outcomes derived from the COMPASS battery are presented in the online Supplementary Materials (Table S1.).

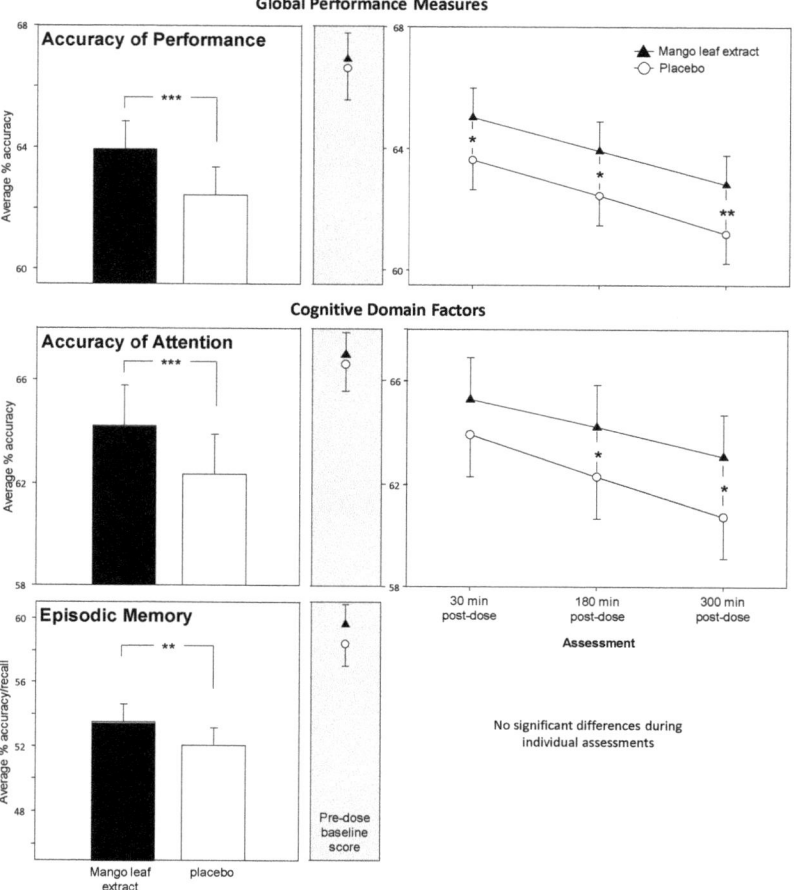

Figure 4. The effects of mango leaf extract on the global outcome measures and factor scores derived from the Computerised Mental Performance Assessment System (COMPASS) cognitive tasks. Left-hand panels show the main effect of treatment averaged across assessments; middle panels show the pre-dose baseline scores; right-hand panels show time course data from each post-dose assessment for those measures that saw significant effects on the planned comparisons (Bonferroni). The global Accuracy of Performance measure represents averaged data from the eleven tasks from the battery that return % accuracy/maximum score data: Accuracy of Attention represents averaged % accuracy data from the five attention tasks; and Episodic Memory represents averaged % accuracy/recall across the four long-term memory tasks. *, $p < 0.05$; **, $p < 0.01$, ***, $p < 0.001$ versus placebo. Number of participants contributing to the measure: Accuracy of Performance, $n = 68$, Episodic Memory, $n = 70$, Accuracy of Attention, $n = 64$.

3.2. Cognitive Demand Battery (CDB)

In keeping with the improved accuracy seen across the COMPASS task factors, performance in all three CDB tasks was improved across the testing day following mango leaf extract. See Figure 5. The Rapid Visual Information Processing task (RVIP) was improved across assessments in terms of

% of targets accurately detected (F (1, 1071) = 23.186, $p < 0.001$) with planned comparisons showing that these effects were apparent at the 30 min ($p = 0.047$) and 5 h ($p = 0.001$) assessments, with a trend towards the same effect at 3 h post-dose ($p = 0.059$). Performance was also improved on both the Serial 3s task (F (1, 1156) = 10.9, $p < 0.001$) and Serial 7s task (F (1, 1156) = 9.642, $p = 0.002$) in terms of number of correct subtractions across the testing day. Comparisons at each assessment showed that while the differences between groups did not reach significance during any individual assessment for the Serial 7s task, Serial 3s performance was enhanced at the 3 h assessment ($p = 0.014$), with a trend towards the same at 30 min post-dose ($p = 0.088$). There was no effect on ratings of mental fatigue during completion of the battery. Data (plus F score and p) for the CDB outcomes are presented in the online Supplementary Materials (Table S2.).

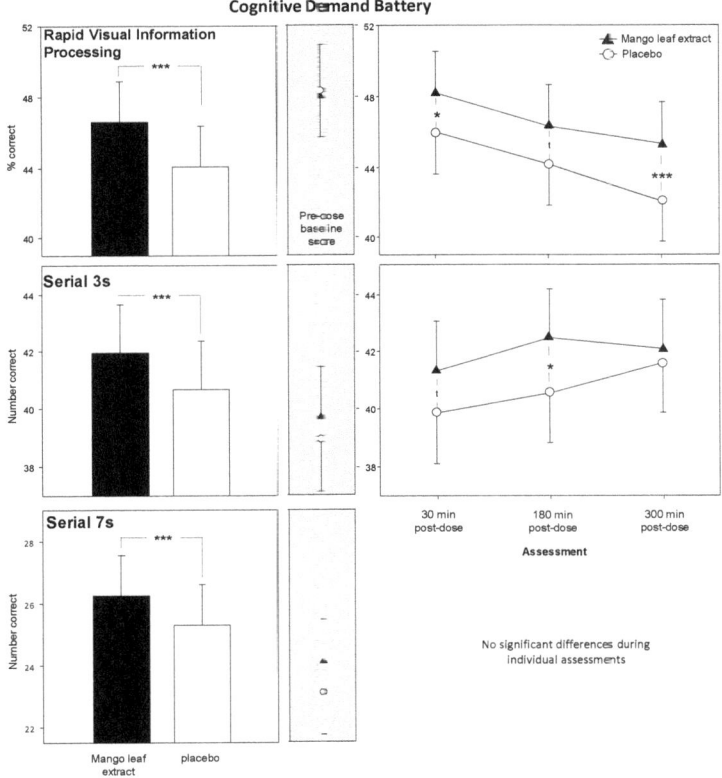

Figure 5. The effects of mango leaf extract on the Cognitive Demand Battery outcomes. Each task was repeated three times per assessment (total Cognitive Demand Battery (CDB) completion time, 30 min per assessment). Left-hand panels show the main effect of treatment averaged across assessments/repetitions; middle panels show the pre-dose baseline scores averaged across the three repetitions; right-hand panels show time course data from each post-dose assessment (averaged across the three repetitions per assessment) for those measures that saw significant effects on the planned comparisons (Bonferroni) of mango leaf extract versus placebo. t, $p < 0.1$; *, $p < 0.05$; ***; $p < 0.001$ in comparison to placebo. Number of participants contributing to the measure: RVIP, $n = 64$, Serial 3s/7s, $n = 69$.

3.3. Mood and Psychological State

There were no effects of treatment on any mood parameter (VAMS, S-VAS, POMS), with the exception of reduced calm/relaxed ratings on the S-VAS following mango leaf extract across testing assessments (F (1, 345) = 5.44, p = 0.02). See Figure 6. There were no significant differences on the comparisons made at each assessment for this outcome. Data from the POMS, VAMS and S-VAS data are presented in the online Supplementary Materials (Table S3.).

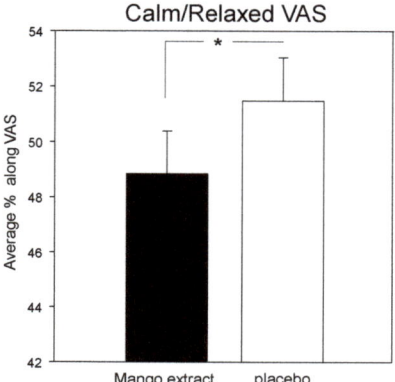

Figure 6. The effects of mango leaf extract on the calm/relaxed stress visual analogue scales (S-VAS) measure. There were no significant differences on the planned comparisons of data from each assessment. *, $p < 0.05$ in comparison to placebo.

4. Discussion

In the current study a single dose of mango leaf extract (Zynamite®) lead to significant, broad improvements in performance across a battery of cognitive tasks throughout the 6 h following consumption. There were no interpretable benefits found for any measure of mood/psychological state.

Cognitive improvements were seen on the global Accuracy of Performance measure, which comprised averaged % accuracy or % maximum score data from 11 computerised tasks. It was also seen more specifically in the cognitive sub-factors 'Accuracy of Attention', representing the overall % accuracy whilst performing the five attention tasks (excludes simple reaction time) within the battery and 'Episodic Memory', which represents the % recall or accuracy of the four long-term memory tasks. Performance benefits were also seen across all three of the tasks that make up the 30-min Cognitive Demand Battery, with improved RVIP accuracy and increased numbers of correct subtractions generated by participants on both the Serial 3s and Serial 7s tasks. These cognitive effects, taken as a whole, were evident as main effects across the post-dose testing day, which comprised 60 min assessments starting at 30 min, 3 h and 5 h post-dose, without any clear pattern of augmentation or attenuation over time. There were no benefits seen in terms of increased speed of task performance on the timed tasks, or indeed on the mood and psychological state measures.

Clearly, one question raised by these results is whether the effects seen here represent a truly global improvement in accuracy across cognitive domains, or whether they simply reflect the consequences of improved attention. Certainly, attention and episodic memory are inter-related, with enhanced attention leading to improved encoding and retrieval of information. It has been suggested that episodic memory processes are themselves, to an extent, 'acts of attention' [49]. As the attention and episodic memory tasks comprised the majority of the tasks that contributed to the global accuracy measure, it is possible that the improvements to the latter are simply a reflection of broad improvements to attention. However, the improvements in Serial 3s and Serial 7s subtraction task performance would be more difficult to accommodate solely within an attention framework. Whilst both subtraction tasks have attentional components, they draw more heavily on both working memory and executive function, particularly the more difficult Serial 7s, which requires greater executive resources in order to carry out the more complex manipulation of numbers [24]. Enhanced performance on these tasks, alongside improved accuracy across the tasks, therefore, seems to confirm that the benefits of mango leaf extract were seen broadly across cognitive domains.

The results also suggest that the modulation of cerebro-electrical activity (measured using EEG) seen in healthy adults following a single dose of Zynamite mango leaf extract [39] is most likely indicative of a benefit to brain function. The cognitive benefits seen here are broadly in line with previous demonstrations of improved cognitive function following both acute [24–26] and chronic administration [27,28] of polyphenol rich extracts. Several polyphenol studies also employed the Cognitive Demand Battery used here (but at a single post-dose time point), with demonstrations of improved performance across all three tasks following cocoa-flavanols [24], improved Serial 3s performance following fruit flavanols [50], but no benefits following resveratrol [51]. Of note, the global performance measures derived from the cognitive tasks utilised here have proved sensitive to the acute and chronic administration of a Nepalese pepper extract [42] and acute administration of a green oat extract to middle-aged adults [41]. However, both of these interventions contain other potentially bioactive phytochemicals alongside polyphenols, and in both cases global speed of performance was enhanced, rather than the improved global accuracy seen in the current study.

Previous research has demonstrated similarities in EEG cerebro-electrical response following both mango leaf extract and caffeine in rodents [38], but somewhat different responses to these two individual treatments in humans [39]. The cognitive effects of caffeine comprise modest but consistent improvements that are restricted to the performance of tasks measuring attention, with no reliable effect on other cognitive domains including long-term (episodic) memory [52–55]. Similarly, the duration of the effects seen following mango leaf extract do not follow the time course of caffeine's effects, which would become apparent by 30 min post-dose and would be expected to attenuate by 6 h post-dose. It is therefore notable that the pattern of cognitive benefits seen in the present study following the mango leaf extract are broader and longer lasting than those that would be expected after caffeine.

In terms of mechanism of action, a recent study investigating receptor binding and brain relevant enzyme inhibition found that mangiferin only significantly inhibited catechol-O-methyl transferase (COMT), the enzyme responsible for the degradation of catecholamine neurotransmitters [39]. Several other polyphenols that also feature a catechol moiety, including flavanols and oleacein, have also been shown to inhibit COMT [56,57]. COMT's catabolic pathway is most prevalent in brain tissue with low concentrations of catecholamine reuptake transporters, and therefore COMT inhibition predominantly affects dopaminergic function in the prefrontal cortex and hippocampus [58], potentially leading to improved working memory, selective attention, and executive function [59]. Clearly, the benefits seen in the current study correspond with these cognitive domains. However, whilst there is some evidence that COMT inhibitors may modulate these aspects of cognitive function, the overall pattern is for their effects to be bidirectionally moderated by COMT genotype (val158met polymorphism) [59–61]. COMT inhibition per se is therefore unlikely to be the primary mechanism underpinning the straightforward cognitive benefits seen here across a sample of mixed COMT genotypes.

Other potential 'direct' brain-relevant mechanisms of action previously established for mangiferin include acetylcholinesterase (AChE) inhibition [30,62] or other potential cholinergic mechanisms of action [63]. Increased acetylcholine activity would be expected to have a beneficial, inter-related effect on both focussed attention and memory consolidation/retrieval [64] and, therefore, could encompass many of the effects seen in the current study. However, it is equally likely that the effects seen here may be related to 'indirect' interactions within mammalian cellular signal transduction pathways, a property that mangiferin shares with other polyphenols [8,11–14]. These interactions potentially drive downstream modulation of neuroinflammation, neurotransmission, neurotrophin receptor and signalling pathway interactions, and increased synthesis of neurotrophins and vasodilatory molecules, leading to increased angiogenesis/neurogenesis and local cerebral blood flow [15–19]. These indirect cellular interactions may underlie the consistent demonstrations in humans of increased cerebral blood-flow [51,65–69] and peripherally measured brain-derived neurotrophic factor [26] seen following diverse polyphenols. Again, potentially diffuse beneficial effects within the brain could be conceived as potentially leading to broad benefits to cognitive function across domains, as seen here.

Clearly, a strength of the current study is that it represents the first concerted investigation of the effects of mangiferin, or indeed any xanthone glycoside, on human cognitive function. Conversely, this was, by its nature, an exploratory study, and the absence of pre-defined primary outcomes, due to a lack of previous data to guide their formulation, could be considered a limitation. Certainly the absence of primary endpoints allows a greater freedom for the interpretation of the results than will be enjoyed in future research, and it is hoped that the results of the current study will be useful in terms of directing the research questions and outcomes addressed by more studies involving this compound.

It should also be acknowledged that the results herein relate to a molecule, or group of molecules (xanthones) that are unlikely to be encountered in meaningful quantities in the typical diet, and therefore the results can only realistically be extrapolated to supplementation with mangiferin-rich extracts. Whilst the results tell us little about the benefits of polyphenols consumed as part of the everyday diet it might be noteworthy that the dose of 300 mg employed here contained an amount of polyphenols that is achievable through the consumption of polyphenol rich foods.

In conclusion, a single dose of mango leaf extract (Zynamite®) with high levels of the polyphenol mangiferin, lead to broad improvements in cognitive function that were seen across assessments spanning from 30 min to 6 h post-dose. These benefits were seen most strikingly in terms of participants' improved attention and long-term memory task performance and in their extended performance of cognitively demanding tasks, including those requiring executive function resources.

Supplementary Materials: The following are available online at http://www.mdpi.com/2072-6643/12/8/2194/s1. Section I: Individual COMPASS and CDB cognitive task descriptions. Section II: Derivation of the global outcome measures and cognitive domain factors, including notes on lost data. Section III: Table S1. (data from global measures and cognitive factors), Table S2. (data from Cognitive Demand Battery), Table S3. (data from the mood measures).

Author Contributions: D.O.K., E.L.W., P.A.J., J.C.W., N.G. formulated the research question and overall methodology. All of the authors (D.O.K., E.L.W., P.A.J., J.F., J.K., J.C.W., N.G.) were actively involved in the practical planning of the research described herein. J.F and J.K. supervised the collection of the data. D.O.K. analysed the data and E.L.W. and D.O.K. compiled the first draft of the paper. All authors contributed to and reviewed the subsequent drafts and final publication. All authors have read and agreed to the published version of the manuscript.

Funding: The study was sponsored by Nektium Pharma.

Acknowledgments: The following people were involved in the day to day running of the study and/or data collection: Amy Ferguson, Jennifer Webster, Fiona Dodd, Michael Patan, Ellen Smith, Rian Elcoate, Jessica Greener, Lucy Keeler, Charlotte Kenney, Faye Williams, Evan Davies, Leah Smith, Veronika Rysinova.

Conflicts of Interest: Nektium Pharma produced the Mangifera indica extract and sponsored the study. J.C.W. is employed by Nektium Pharma, and N.G. works as a consultant for Nektium Pharma. However, neither J.C.W., N.G. nor any other representative of Nektium Pharma had any role in the running of the study, or the analysis, or the interpretation of the data. None of the other authors have a conflict of interest.

References

1. Ediriweera, M.K.; Tennekoon, K.H.; Samarakoon, S.R. A review on ethnopharmacological applications, pharmacological activities, and bioactive compounds of Mangifera indica (mango). *Evid. Based Complement. Alternat. Med.* **2017**, *2017*. [CrossRef] [PubMed]
2. Tayana, N.; Inthakusol, W.; Duangdee, N.; Chewchinda, S.; Pandith, H.; Kongkiatpaiboon, S. Mangiferin content in different parts of mango tree (*Mangifera indica* L.) in Thailand. *Songklanakarin J. Sci. Technol.* **2019**, *41*. [CrossRef]
3. Vieira, L.; Kijjoa, A. Naturally-occurring xanthones: Recent developments. *Curr. Med. Chem.* **2005**, *12*, 2413–2446. [CrossRef] [PubMed]
4. Kitanov, G.M.; Nedialkov, P.T. Mangiferin and isomangiferin in some Hypericum species. *Biochem. Syst. Ecol.* **1998**, *26*, 647–653. [CrossRef]

5. Chitchumroonchokchai, C.; Riedl, K.M.; Suksumrarn, S.; Clinton, S.K.; Kinghorn, A.D.; Failla, M.L. Xanthones in mangosteen juice are absorbed and partially conjugated by healthy adults. *J. Nutr.* **2012**, *142*, 675–680. [CrossRef]
6. Khare, P.; Shanker, K. Mangiferin: A review of sources and interventions for biological activities. *Biofactors* **2016**, *42*, 504–514.
7. Sekar, V.; Chakraborty, S.; Mani, S.; Sali, V.; Vasanthi, H. Mangiferin from Mangifera indica fruits reduces post-prandial glucose level by inhibiting α-glucosidase and α-amylase activity. *S. Afr. J. Bot.* **2019**, *120*, 129–134. [CrossRef]
8. Gold-Smith, F.; Fernandez, A.; Bishop, K. Mangiferin and cancer: Mechanisms of action. *Nutrients* **2016**, *8*, 396. [CrossRef]
9. Kasbe, P.; Jangra, A.; Lahkar, M. Mangiferin ameliorates aluminium chloride-induced cognitive dysfunction via alleviation of hippocampal oxido-nitrosative stress, proinflammatory cytokines and acetylcholinesterase level. *J. Trace Elem. Med. Biol.* **2015**, *31*, 107–112. [CrossRef]
10. Li, H.-W.; Lan, T.-J.; Yun, C.-X.; Du, Z.-C.; Luo, X.-f.; Hao, E.-W.; Deng, J.-G. Mangiferin exerts neuroprotective activity against lead-induced toxicity and oxidative stress via Nrf2 pathway. *Chin. Herb. Med.* **2020**, *12*, 36–46. [CrossRef]
11. Yang, S.; Kuang, G.; Zhang, L.; Wu, S.; Zhao, Z.; Wang, B.; Yin, X.; Gong, X.; Wan, J. Mangiferin Attenuates LPS/D-GalN-Induced Acute Liver Injury by Promoting HO-1 in Kupffer Cells. *Front. Immunol.* **2020**, *11*, 285. [CrossRef] [PubMed]
12. Sahu, A.K.; Verma, V.K.; Mutneja, E.; Malik, S.; Nag, T.C.; Dinda, A.K.; Arya, D.S.; Bhatia, J. Mangiferin attenuates cisplatin-induced acute kidney injury in rats mediating modulation of MAPK pathway. *Mol. Cell. Biochem.* **2019**, *452*, 141–152. [CrossRef] [PubMed]
13. Rahman, M.S.; Kim, Y.-S. PINK1-PRKN mitophagy suppression by Mangiferin promotes a brown-fat-phenotype via PKA-p38 MAPK signalling in murine C3H10T1/2 mesenchymal stem cells. *Metabolism* **2020**, 154228. [CrossRef] [PubMed]
14. Suchal, K.; Malik, S.; Khan, S.I.; Malhotra, R.K.; Goyal, S.N.; Bhatia, J.; Kumari, S.; Ojha, S.; Arya, D.S. Protective effect of mangiferin on myocardial ischemia-reperfusion injury in streptozotocin-induced diabetic rats: Role of AGE-RAGE/MAPK pathways. *Sci. Rep.* **2017**, *7*, 42027. [CrossRef] [PubMed]
15. Kennedy, D.O. Polyphenols and the human brain: Plant "secondary metabolite" ecologic roles and endogenous signaling functions drive benefits. *Adv. Nutr.* **2014**, *5*, 515–533. [CrossRef] [PubMed]
16. Spencer, J.P. Flavonoids and brain health: Multiple effects underpinned by common mechanisms. *Genes Nutr.* **2009**, *4*, 243–250. [CrossRef]
17. Williams, R.J.; Spencer, J.P. Flavonoids, cognition, and dementia: Actions, mechanisms, and potential therapeutic utility for Alzheimer disease. *Free Radic. Biol. Med.* **2012**, *52*, 35–45. [CrossRef]
18. Vauzour, D. Effect of flavonoids on learning memory and neurocognitive performance: Relevance and potential implications for Alzheimer's disease pathophysiology. *J. Sci. Food Agric.* **2014**, *94*, 1042–1056. [CrossRef]
19. Baptista, F.I.; Henriques, A.G.; Silva, A.M.; Wiltfang, J.; da Cruz e Silva, O.A. Flavonoids as therapeutic compounds targeting key proteins involved in Alzheimer's disease. *ACS Chem. Neurosci.* **2014**. [CrossRef]
20. Kennedy, D.O. *Plants and the Human Brain*; Oxford University Press: New York, NY, USA, 2014.
21. Hooper, L.; Kay, C.; Abdelhamid, A.; Kroon, P.A.; Cohn, J.S.; Rimm, E.B.; Cassidy, A. Effects of chocolate, cocoa, and flavan-3-ols on cardiovascular health: A systematic review and meta-analysis of randomized trials. *Am. J. Clin. Nutr.* **2012**, *95*, 740–751. [CrossRef]
22. Shrime, M.G.; Bauer, S.R.; McDonald, A.C.; Chowdhury, N.H.; Coltart, C.E.; Ding, E.L. Flavonoid-rich cocoa consumption affects multiple cardiovascular risk factors in a meta-analysis of short-term studies. *J. Nutr.* **2011**, *141*, 1982–1988. [CrossRef] [PubMed]
23. Lin, X.; Zhang, I.; Li, A.; Manson, J.E.; Sesso, H.D.; Wang, L.; Liu, S. Cocoa flavanol intake and biomarkers for cardiometabolic health: A systematic review and meta-analysis of randomized controlled trials. *J. Nutr.* **2016**, *146*, 2325. [CrossRef] [PubMed]
24. Scholey, A.B.; French, S.J.; Morris, P.J.; Kennedy, D.O.; Milne, A.L.; Haskell, C.F. Consumption of cocoa flavanols results in acute improvements in mood and cognitive performance during sustained mental effort. *J. Psychopharmacol.* **2010**, *24*, 1505–1514. [CrossRef] [PubMed]

25. Haskell-Ramsay, C.; Stuart, R.; Okello, E.; Watson, A. Cognitive and mood improvements following acute supplementation with purple grape juice in healthy young adults. *Eur. J. Nutr.* **2017**, *56*, 2621–2631. [CrossRef]
26. Ammar, A.; Trabelsi, K.; Boukhris, O.; Bouaziz, B.; Müller, P.; M Glenn, J.; Bott, N.T.; Müller, N.; Chtourou, H.; Driss, T. Effects of Polyphenol-Rich Interventions on Cognition and Brain Health in Healthy Young and Middle-Aged Adults: Systematic Review and Meta-Analysis. *J. Clin. Med.* **2020**, *9*, 1598. [CrossRef]
27. Desideri, G.; Kwik-Uribe, C.; Grassi, D.; Necozione, S.; Ghiadoni, L.; Mastroiacovo, D.; Raffaele, A.; Ferri, L.; Bocale, R.; Lechiara, M.C. Benefits in Cognitive Function, Blood Pressure, and Insulin Resistance Through Cocoa Flavanol Consumption in Elderly Subjects With Mild Cognitive ImpairmentNovelty and Significance The Cocoa, Cognition, and Aging (CoCoA) Study. *Hypertension* **2012**, *60*, 794–801. [CrossRef]
28. Mastroiacovo, D.; Kwik-Uribe, C.; Grassi, D.; Necozione, S.; Raffaele, A.; Pistacchio, L.; Righetti, R.; Bocale, R.; Lechiara, M.C.; Marini, C. Cocoa flavanol consumption improves cognitive function, blood pressure control, and metabolic profile in elderly subjects: The Cocoa, Cognition, and Aging (CoCoA) Study—A randomized controlled trial. *Am. J. Clin. Nutr.* **2014**, *101*, 538–548. [CrossRef]
29. Andreu, G.L.P.; Maurmann, N.; Reolon, G.K.; de Farias, C.B.; Schwartsmann, G.; Delgado, R.; Roesler, R. Mangiferin, a naturally occurring glucoxilxanthone improves long-term object recognition memory in rats. *Eur. J. Pharmacol.* **2010**, *635*, 124–128. [CrossRef]
30. Jung, K.; Lee, B.; Han, S.J.; Ryu, J.H.; Kim, D.-H. Mangiferin ameliorates scopolamine-induced learning deficits in mice. *Biol. Pharm. Bull.* **2009**, *32*, 242–246. [CrossRef]
31. Feng, X.; Xue, J.H.; Xie, K.X.; Liu, S.P.; Zhong, H.P.; Wang, C.C.; Feng, X.Q. Beneficial effect of Mangiferin against sleep deprivation-induced neurodegeneration and memory impairment in mice. *Biomed. Res.* **2017**, *28*, 769–777.
32. Jangra, A.; Lukhi, M.M.; Sulakhiya, K.; Baruah, C.C.; Lahkar, M. Protective effect of mangiferin against lipopolysaccharide-induced depressive and anxiety-like behaviour in mice. *Eur. J. Pharmacol.* **2014**, *740*, 337–345. [CrossRef] [PubMed]
33. Gelabert-Rebato, M.; Wiebe, J.C.; Martin-Rincon, M.; Gericke, N.; Perez-Valera, M.; Curtelin, D.; Galvan-Alvarez, V.; Lopez-Rios, L.; Morales-Alamo, D.; Calbet, J.A. Mangifera indica l. Leaf extract in combination with luteolin or quercetin enhances vo2peak and peak power output, and preserves skeletal muscle function during ischemia-reperfusion in humans. *Front. Physiol.* **2018**, *9*, 740. [CrossRef] [PubMed]
34. Gelabert-Rebato, M.; Wiebe, J.C.; Martin-Rincon, M.; Galvan-Alvarez, V.; Curtelin, D.; Perez-Valera, M.; Habib, J.J.; Pérez-López, A.; Vega, T.; Morales-Alamo, D. Enhancement of Exercise Performance by 48 Hours, and 15-Day Supplementation with Mangiferin and Luteolin in Men. *Nutrients* **2019**, *11*, 344. [CrossRef] [PubMed]
35. Gelabert-Rebato, M.; Martin-Rincon, M.; Galvan-Alvarez, V.; Gallego-Selles, A.; Martinez-Canton, M.; Vega-Morales, T.; Wiebe, J.C.; Fernandez-del Castillo, C.; Castilla-Hernandez, E.; Diaz-Tiberio, O. A Single Dose of The Mango Leaf Extract Zynamite® in Combination with Quercetin Enhances Peak Power Output During Repeated Sprint Exercise in Men and Women. *Nutrients* **2019**, *11*, 2592. [CrossRef]
36. Martin-Rincon, M.; Gelabert-Rebato, M.; Galvan-Alvarez, V.; Gallego-Selles, A.; Martinez-Canton, M.; Lopez-Rios, L.; Wiebe, J.C.; Martin-Rodriguez, S.; Arteaga-Ortiz, R.; Dorado, C. Supplementation with a Mango Leaf Extract (Zynamite®) in Combination with Quercetin Attenuates Muscle Damage and Pain and Accelerates Recovery after Strenuous Damaging Exercise. *Nutrients* **2020**, *12*, 614. [CrossRef]
37. Martín Rincón, M.; Galvan Alvarez, V.; Gelabert Rebato, M.; Gallego Selles, Á.; Martínez Cantón, M.; Martín Rodríguez, S.; Pérez Valera, M.; Morales Álamo, D.; López Calbet, J.A. Exercise-induced muscle pain is reduced and recovery accelerated by supplementation with mango leaf extract Zynamite® in combination with quercetin in men and women. In Proceedings of the International Sport Forum on Strength, Conditioning and Nutrition, Madrid, España, 15–16 November 2019.
38. Dimpfel, W.; Wiebe, J.; Gericke, N.; Schombert, L. Zynamite®(Mangifera indica Leaf Extract) and Caffeine Act in a Synergistic Manner on Electrophysiological Parameters of Rat Central Nervous System. *Food Nutr. Sci.* **2018**, *9*, 502.
39. López-Ríos, L.; Wiebe, J.; Vega-Morales, T.; Gericke, N. Central nervous system activities of extract *Mangifera indica* L. *J. Ethnopharmacol.* **2020**, 112996. [CrossRef]

40. Stonehouse, W.; Conlon, C.A.; Podd, J.; Hill, S.R.; Minihane, A.M.; Haskell, C.; Kennedy, D. DHA supplementation improved both memory and reaction time in healthy young adults: A randomized controlled trial. *Am. J. Clin. Nutr.* **2013**, *97*, 1134–1143. [CrossRef]
41. Kennedy, D.O.; Jackson, P.A.; Forster, J.; Khan, J.; Grothe, T.; Perrinjaquet-Moccetti, T.; Haskell-Ramsay, C.F. Acute effects of a wild green-oat (Avena sativa) extract on cognitive function in middle-aged adults: A double-blind, placebo-controlled, within-subjects trial. *Nutr. Neurosci.* **2017**, *20*, 135–151. [CrossRef]
42. Kennedy, D.; Wightman, E.; Khan, J.; Grothe, T.; Jackson, P. The Acute and Chronic Cognitive and Cerebral Blood-Flow Effects of Nepalese Pepper (Zanthoxylum armatum DC.) Extract—A Randomized, Double-Blind, Placebo-Controlled Study in Healthy Humans. *Nutrients* **2019**, *11*, 3022. [CrossRef]
43. Kennedy, D.O.; Wightman, E.L.; Forster, J.; Khan, J.; Haskell-Ramsay, C.F.; Jackson, P.A. Cognitive and mood effects of a nutrient enriched breakfast bar in healthy adults: A randomised, double-blind, placebo-controlled, parallel groups study. *Nutrients* **2017**, *9*, 1332. [CrossRef] [PubMed]
44. Kennedy, D.; Okello, E.; Chazot, P.; Howes, M.-J.; Ohiomokhare, S.; Jackson, P.; Haskell-Ramsay, C.; Khan, J.; Forster, J.; Wightman, E. Volatile terpenes and brain function: Investigation of the cognitive and mood effects of Mentha× piperita l. essential oil with in vitro properties relevant to central nervous system function. *Nutrients* **2018**, *10*, 1029. [CrossRef] [PubMed]
45. Kennedy, D.O.; Scholey, A.B. A glucose-caffeine 'energy drink' ameliorates subjective and performance deficits during prolonged cognitive demand. *Appetite* **2004**, *42*, 331–333. [CrossRef] [PubMed]
46. Reay, J.L.; Kennedy, D.O.; Scholey, A.B. Single doses of Panax ginseng (G115) reduce blood glucose levels and improve cognitive performance during sustained mental activity. *J. Psychopharmacol.* **2005**, *19*, 357–365. [CrossRef] [PubMed]
47. Heuchert, J.P.; McNair, D.M. *POMS 2 Manual. Profile of Mood States*; Multi-Health Systems Inc.: Toronto, ON, Canada, 2012.
48. Kennedy, D.O.; Bonnländer, B.; Lang, S.C.; Fischel, I.; Forster, J.; Khan, J.; Jackson, P.A.; Wightman, E.L. Acute and Chronic Effects of Green Oat (Avena sativa) Extract on Cognitive Function and Mood during a Laboratory Stressor in Healthy Adults: A Randomised, Double-Blind, Placebo-Controlled Study in Healthy Humans. *Nutrients* **2020**, *12*, 1598. [CrossRef]
49. Long, N.M.; Kuhl, B.A.; Chun, M.M. Memory and attention. *Stevens' Handbook of Experimental Psychology and Cognitive Neuroscience* **2018**, *1*, 1–37.
50. Philip, P.; Sagaspe, P.; Taillard, J.; Mandon, C.; Constans, J.; Pourtau, L.; Pouchieu, C.; Angelino, D.; Mena, P.; Martini, D. Acute Intake of a Grape and Blueberry Polyphenol-Rich Extract Ameliorates Cognitive Performance in Healthy Young Adults During a Sustained Cognitive Effort. *Antioxidants* **2019**, *8*, 650. [CrossRef]
51. Kennedy, D.O.; Wightman, E.L.; Reay, J.L.; Lietz, G.; Okello, E.J.; Wilde, A.; Haskell, C.F. Effects of resveratrol on cerebral blood flow variables and cognitive performance in humans: A double-blind, placebo-controlled, crossover investigation. *Am. J. Clin. Nutr.* **2010**, *91*, 1590–1597. [CrossRef]
52. Nehlig, A. Is caffeine a cognitive enhancer? *J. Alzheimers Dis.* **2010**, *20*, 85–94. [CrossRef]
53. Childs, E.; de Wit, H. Subjective, behavioral, and physiological effects of acute caffeine in light, nondependent caffeine users. *Psychopharmacology* **2006**, *185*, 514–523. [CrossRef]
54. McLellan, T.M.; Caldwell, J.A.; Lieberman, H.R. A review of caffeine's effects on cognitive, physical and occupational performance. *Neurosci. Biobehav. Rev.* **2016**, *71*, 294–312. [CrossRef] [PubMed]
55. Lieberman, H.R. Nutrition, brain function and cognitive performance. *Appetite* **2003**, *40*, 245–254. [CrossRef]
56. Chen, D.; Wang, C.Y.; Lambert, J.D.; Ai, N.; Welsh, W.J.; Yang, C.S. Inhibition of human liver catechol-O-methyltransferase by tea catechins and their metabolites: Structure–activity relationship and molecular-modeling studies. *Biochem. Pharmacol.* **2005**, *69*, 1523–1531. [CrossRef] [PubMed]
57. Cuyàs, E.; Verdura, S.; Lozano-Sánchez, J.; Viciano, I.; Llorach-Parés, L.; Nonell-Canals, A.; Bosch-Barrera, J.; Brunet, J.; Segura-Carretero, A.; Sanchez-Martinez, M. The extra virgin olive oil phenolic oleacein is a dual substrate-inhibitor of catechol-O-methyltransferase. *Food Chem. Toxicol.* **2019**, *128*, 35–45. [CrossRef]
58. Apud, J.A.; Mattay, V.; Chen, J.; Kolachana, B.S.; Callicott, J.H.; Rasetti, R.; Alce, G.; Iudicello, J.E.; Akbar, N.; Egan, M.F. Tolcapone improves cognition and cortical information processing in normal human subjects. *Neuropsychopharmacology* **2007**, *32*, 1011–1020. [CrossRef] [PubMed]
59. Schacht, J.P. COMT val158met moderation of dopaminergic drug effects on cognitive function: A critical review. *Pharm. J.* **2016**, *16*, 430–438. [CrossRef]

60. Valomon, A.; Holst, S.C.; Borrello, A.; Weigend, S.; Müller, T.; Berger, W.; Sommerauer, M.; Baumann, C.R.; Landolt, H.-P. Effects of COMT genotype and tolcapone on lapses of sustained attention after sleep deprivation in healthy young men. *Neuropsychopharmacology* **2018**, *43*, 1599–1607. [CrossRef]
61. Cameron, I.G.; Wallace, D.L.; Al-Zughoul, A.; Kayser, A.S.; D'Esposito, M. Effects of tolcapone and bromocriptine on cognitive stability and flexibility. *Psychopharmacology* **2018**, *235*, 1295–1305. [CrossRef]
62. Sethiya, N.K.; Mishra, S. Investigation of mangiferin, as a promising natural polyphenol xanthone on multiple targets of Alzheimer's disease. *J. Biol. Act. Prod. Nat.* **2014**, *4*, 111–119. [CrossRef]
63. Morais, T.C.; Lopes, S.C.; Carvalho, K.M.; Arruda, B.R.; de Souza, F.T.C.; Trevisan, M.T.S.; Rao, V.S.; Santos, F.A. Mangiferin, a natural xanthone, accelerates gastrointestinal transit in mice involving cholinergic mechanism. *World J. Gastroenterol. WJG* **2012**, *18*, 3207.
64. Decker, A.L.; Duncan, K. Acetylcholine and the complex interdependence of memory and attention. *Curr. Opin. Behav. Sci.* **2020**, *32*, 21–28. [CrossRef]
65. Lamport, D.J.; Pal, D.; Moutsiana, C.; Field, D.T.; Williams, C.M.; Spencer, J.P.; Butler, L.T. The effect of flavanol-rich cocoa on cerebral perfusion in healthy older adults during conscious resting state: A placebo controlled, crossover, acute trial. *Psychopharmacology* **2015**, *232*, 3227–3234. [CrossRef] [PubMed]
66. Decroix, L.; Tonoli, C.; Soares, D.D.; Tagougui, S.; Heyman, E.; Meeusen, R. Acute cocoa flavanol improves cerebral oxygenation without enhancing executive function at rest or after exercise. *Appl. Physiol. Nutr. Metab.* **2016**, *41*, 1225–1232. [CrossRef] [PubMed]
67. Francis, S.T.; Head, K.; Morris, P.G.; Macdonald, I.A. The effect of flavanol-rich cocoa on the fMRI response to a cognitive task in healthy young people. *J. Cardiovasc. Pharmacol.* **2006**, *47* (Suppl. 2), S215–S220. [CrossRef] [PubMed]
68. Sorond, F.A.; Lipsitz, L.A.; Hollenberg, N.K.; Fisher, N.D. Cerebral blood flow response to flavanol-rich cocoa in healthy elderly humans. *Neuropsychiatr. Dis. Treat.* **2008**, *4*, 433–440.
69. Wightman, E.L.; Reay, J.L.; Haskell, C.F.; Williamson, G.; Dew, T.P.; Kennedy, D.O. Effects of resveratrol alone or in combination with piperine on cerebral blood flow parameters and cognitive performance in human subjects: A randomised, double-blind, placebo-controlled, cross-over investigation. *Br. J. Nutr.* **2014**, *112*, 203–213. [CrossRef]

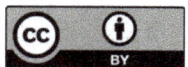

© 2020 by the authors. Licensee MDPI, Basel, Switzerland. This article is an open access article distributed under the terms and conditions of the Creative Commons Attribution (CC BY) license (http://creativecommons.org/licenses/by/4.0/).

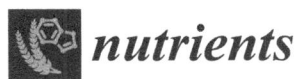

Article

Associations of Urinary Phytoestrogen Concentrations with Sleep Disorders and Sleep Duration among Adults

Jing Sun [1], Hong Jiang [2,*], Weijing Wang [1], Xue Dong [1] and Dongfeng Zhang [1]

1. Department of Epidemiology and Health Statistics, The School of Public Health of Qingdao University, 308 Ningxia Road, Qingdao 266071, China; sunjing1011@163.com (J.S.); wangwj793@126.com (W.W.); dongxue199411@126.com (X.D.); zhangdf1961@126.com (D.Z.)
2. Department of Physiology, Shandong Provincial Key Laboratory of Pathogenesis and Prevention of Neurological Disorders and State Key Disciplines: Physiology, School of Basic Medicine, Qingdao University, Qingdao 266071, China
* Correspondence: hongjiang@qdu.edu.cn

Received: 29 June 2020; Accepted: 13 July 2020; Published: 16 July 2020

Abstract: Current evidence on the relationship of phytoestrogens with sleep is limited and contradictory. In particular, studies on individual phytoestrogens and sleep have not been reported. Thus, this study aimed to appraise the associations of individual phytoestrogens with sleep disorders and sleep duration. This cross-sectional study comprising 4830 adults utilized data from the National Health and Nutrition Examination Survey 2005–2010. Phytoestrogens were tested in urine specimens. Sleep disorders and sleep duration were based on a self-reported doctor's diagnosis and usual sleep duration. The main analyses utilized logistic and multinomial logistic regression models and a restricted cubic spline. In the fully adjusted model, compared with tertile 1 (lowest), the odds ratios (95% confidence intervals (CIs)) of sleep disorders for the highest tertile of urinary concentrations of enterolactone, enterodiol, and O-desmethylangolensin were 0.64 (0.41–1.00), 1.54 (1.07–2.21), and 1.89 (1.26–2.85), respectively. Linear inverse, approximatively linear positive, and inverted L-shaped concentration–response relationships were found between enterolactone, enterodiol, and O-desmethylangolensin and sleep disorders, respectively. Compared with normal sleep (7–8 h/night), the relative risk ratio (RRR) (95% CI) of very short sleep for enterolactone was 0.56 (0.36–0.86), and the RRR (95% CI) of long sleep risk for genistein was 0.62 (0.39–0.99). Furthermore, negative associations of genistein with sleep disorders and enterolactone with long sleep risk, as well as positive associations of enterodiol with both long and very short sleep, were observed in the stratified analysis by age or gender. Finally, a notable finding was that urinary O-desmethylangolensin concentration was positively related to sleep disorders in both females aged 40–59 years and non-Hispanic Whites but inversely associated with sleep disorders in both females aged 60 years or over and other Hispanics. Our findings suggested that enterolactone and genistein might be beneficial for preventing sleep disorders or non-normal sleep duration among adults, and enterodiol might be adverse toward this goal. However, the association of O-desmethylangolensin with sleep disorders might be discrepant in different races and females of different ages.

Keywords: sleep disorders; sleep duration; urinary phytoestrogens; concentration–response; NHANES

---

1. Introduction

Sleep disorders, classified into insomnia, central disorders of hypersomnolence, sleep-related breathing disorders, parasomnias, sleep-related movement disorders, circadian rhythm sleep–wake disorders, and other sleep disorders [1], are common conditions and can seriously harm human health and quality of life [2]. Studies have found that poor sleep (short or long sleep duration, or other sleep problems) was associated with obesity, cardiovascular disease, diabetes, hypertension, cancer, and higher mortality [3–8]. Exploration of modifiable factors for reducing the risk of sleep disorders is urgently required. Estrogen has been a focus of attention due to its influences on the central nervous system that is involved in regulating sleep [9]. Randomized trials have revealed that estrogen therapy could reduce sleep disturbances and improve sleep quality [10–12]. Despite the significant beneficial effect on sleep, the use of estrogen therapy is still very cautious in virtue of its potentially serious health risks [13–17]. Therefore, as the naturally occurring mimetic agents of estrogen, phytoestrogens have aroused great interest in their possibility of being estrogen substitutes.

Phytoestrogens are a group of plant-derived bioactive compounds that have estrogenic and anti-estrogenic effects due to their structures resembling estradiol [18,19] and they are also considered to be endocrine disruptors [20]. The two principal groups of phytoestrogens comprise lignans and isoflavones. Lignans mainly originate from oilseeds, dried seaweeds, and whole-grain cereals, and are metabolized into enterolactone and enterodiol by bacteria in the colon [21,22]. Isoflavones, which are primarily derived from soya beans, soy products, and legumes, consist of genistin and daidzin, which can be hydrolyzed into genistein and daidzein, respectively, where daidzein is further metabolized into O-desmethylangolensin (O-DMA) or equol by gut microbiota [22]. Different individuals have different capabilities to produce phytoestrogens via microbial synthesis due to the complex interaction of the colonic environment with internal and external factors [23,24]; for example, only approximately 30–50% of individuals can produce equol via gut bacterial metabolism [25]. Additionally, these metabolites can also be directly obtained from some animal products, such as dairy [26,27].

Thus far, several trial studies have explored the relationship between total isoflavone supplementation and sleep in climacteric women or androgen-deprived prostate cancer patients, with mixed findings, including improvement of sleep problems [28–31], no significant association [32–34], and even insomnia aggravation [35]. Only two observational studies have evaluated the association of total isoflavone consumption with sleep status among general adults and results showed that total isoflavone consumption was positively related to sleep quality and optimal sleep duration in Japanese adults and inversely associated with long sleep duration in Chinese adults [36,37]. However, no epidemiological study to date has appraised the relationship between lignans and sleep. Only several animal experiments have found the sedative and hypnotic effects of the lignan component [38,39]. Moreover, individual phytoestrogens have unequal biological activities and estrogen receptor (ER) affinities [40,41]. Studies have reported divergent associations between individual phytoestrogens and disease [42–46]. Thus, individual phytoestrogens may also have diverse impacts on sleep, and investigating the relationships with sleep among individual phytoestrogens may be more meaningful. Meanwhile, investigating phytoestrogens via dietary evaluation made it difficult to include all food origins and did not take into account the metabolic transformation of intestinal flora, causing inexact individual exposure; therefore, it is necessary to assess phytoestrogens based on biomarkers to reflect the true exposure. Additionally, the concentration–response relationships of phytoestrogens with sleep were also unknown. Therefore, the present study aimed to: first, appraise the associations between the urinary concentrations of individual phytoestrogens and sleep disorder risk among U.S. adults by utilizing data from the National Health and Nutrition Examination Survey (NHANES) 2005–2010; second, to explore the concentration–response relationships of them; third, to explore the gender, age, and race differences in the associations; and finally, to evaluate the associations of individual phytoestrogens with sleep duration.

2. Materials and Methods

2.1. Study Population

The NHANES is a cross-sectional, complex, multistage, and stratified probability sampling design representing the non-institutionalized U.S. civilian population, which aims to investigate the health status and nutrition condition of Americans [47,48]. The NHANES collects data via examinations implemented in the mobile examination center (MEC) and via household interviews. All of the participants provided informed consent and the protocol of investigation was authorized by the Research Ethics Review Board of the National Center for Health Statistics.

This study chose three-cycle data (NHANES 2005–2006, 2007–2008, and 2009–2010) to create the current sample because the data of sleep and urinary phytoestrogens were measured simultaneously only in the three cycles. A total of 31,034 individuals were enrolled in the NHANES 2005–2010, where the number of participants aged 18 years and over was 18,318. A subsample of approximately one-third of all NHANES participants aged six years or over was chosen to measure urinary phytoestrogens, leaving 5496 participants. Among them, 666 individuals were further ruled out, including participants with missing sleep data ($n = 24$), lactating or pregnant females ($n = 199$), females with both ovaries removed ($n = 269$), and individuals using sedative-hypnotic drugs ($n = 174$). Ultimately, 4830 participants (age ≥ 18 years) with phytoestrogen data were analyzed in the current study (Figure 1).

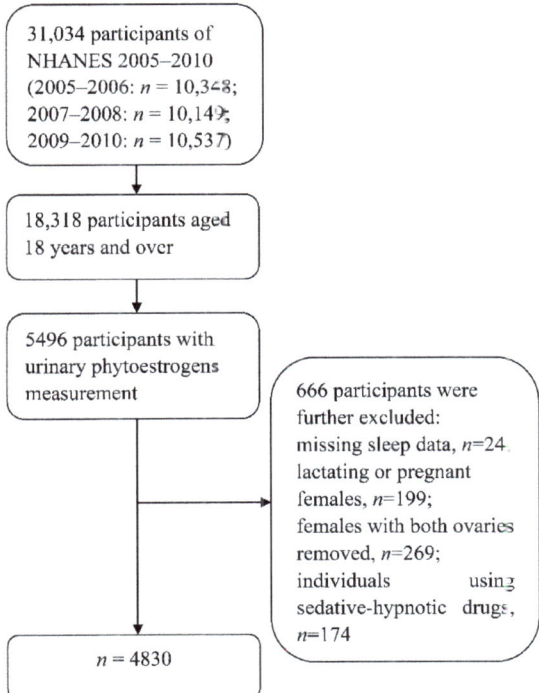

Figure 1. Flowchart of the screening process of eligible participants from the National Health and Nutrition Examination Survey 2005–2010.

2.2. Urinary Phytoestrogens Measurement

Spot urine specimens were collected in the MEC and urinary concentrations of individual phytoestrogens (enterolactone, enterodiol, daidzein, O-DMA, equol, and genistein) were tested in the one-third subsample of all NHANES participants aged six years or over by utilizing high-performance liquid chromatography–atmospheric pressure photoionization–tandem mass spectrometry during the NHANES 2005–2010. More details are available in the laboratory procedure manual [49]. Studies have revealed that phytoestrogen concentrations in spot urine are reliable biomarkers for phytoestrogen intake [23,50,51].

To correct for urine dilution, phytoestrogen concentrations were creatinine-standardized and expressed as µg/g creatinine [52]. Urine creatinine was measured by utilizing the Beckman CX3 during 2005–2006 but the Roche ModP was used since 2007; therefore, we adjusted creatinine 2005–2006 for the comparability of creatinine between 2005–2006 and 2007–2010 using the equations recommended by the NHANES [53].

2.3. Sleep Disorders and Sleep Duration Assessments

The sleep disorder investigations were administered by utilizing a computer-assisted personal interviewing system by trained interviewers in the home. Participants were classified into the sleep disorder groups based on a self-reported doctor diagnosis, and this classification method was used by prior published studies [54,55]. Sleep duration was categorized as 7–8 h/night (normal sleep), <5 h/night (very short sleep), 5–6 h/night (short sleep), and ≥9 h/night (long sleep) based on the self-reported usual sleep duration at night [54,56].

2.4. Covariates

The covariates gender, age, marital status, race, occupation, family income, educational level, body mass index (BMI), smoking status, alcohol consumption, use of female hormones, physical activity, caffeine intake, C-reactive protein, hypertension, depressive symptoms, and diabetes were chosen based on previous literature to control for potential confounding effects [12,36,57]. The details of the classification and criteria for covariates are displayed in Table S1.

2.5. Statistical Analysis

To explicate the complexity of the sampling design and create the estimated values of national representativeness, a primary sampling unit, strata information, and specific sampling weights for the one-third subsample were utilized in the present analyses. According to the analytical guideline [58], the new six-year weights were generated by dividing the two-year environmental weights by three and were applied in this study due to the combination of three two-year NHANES cycles.

The distribution types of continuous variables were identified using Kolmogorov–Smirnov normality tests. Numbers (percentages) and medians (interquartile ranges) were used to describe the qualitative data and non-normal quantitative data, respectively. Chi-square tests and Mann–Whitney *U* tests were performed to compare percentages for qualitative data and averages for non-normal quantitative data between the non-sleep disorders group and the sleep disorders group, respectively. Urinary concentrations of individual phytoestrogens were segmented into tertiles based on their distributions in the present population, with tertile 1 (lowest) being the referent. First, logistic regression analyses were conducted to appraise the relationships between urinary phytoestrogens and sleep disorders, along with calculating the odds ratios (ORs) and 95% confidence intervals (CIs). Six phytoestrogens were entered into model 1 simultaneously for controlling for potentially confounding effects. Model 2 additionally adjusted for gender and age, and model 3 was further adjusted for marital status, race, occupation, family income, educational level, BMI, smoking status, alcohol consumption, use of female hormones, physical activity, caffeine intake, C-reactive protein, hypertension, depressive symptoms, and diabetes. The concentration–response relationships of urinary phytoestrogens with sleep disorders were evaluated using restricted cubic spline functions of three knots (the 25th, 50th, and 75th percentiles of the exposure distributions) in model 3. Second, multinomial logistic regressions were utilized to evaluate the associations between urinary phytoestrogens and sleep duration in model 3, with normal sleep (7–8 h/night) being the referent. Third, considering the significant differences in sleep between different age groups and genders [59,60], we conducted stratified analyses by age (18–39, 40–59, and ≥60 years) and gender, as well as by age group separately for females and males, respectively. Finally, given that the intestinal metabolism of phytoestrogens may differ depending on the race [61], a stratified analysis by race (Mexican American, non-Hispanic Whites, non-Hispanic Blacks, and other Hispanics) was also performed. Statistical analyses were performed utilizing Stata 15.0 (Stata Corporation, College Station, TX, USA), and $p < 0.05$ (two-sided) suggested statistical significance.

3. Results

The characteristics of the participants in this study across sleep disorders are displayed in Table 1. In total, 4830 eligible individuals were analyzed, and the prevalence of sleep disorders was 6.25%. Except for family income and alcohol consumption, other characteristics were significantly different between the sleep disorders group and the non-sleep-disorders group. Individuals with the following characteristics were more likely to experience sleep disorders: older, male, non-Hispanic White, married or living with a partner, smoker, obese, hypertension, depressive symptoms, diabetes, higher education level, less physical activity, higher C-reactive protein concentration, higher caffeine intake, without work, and women using female hormones. Except for family income, alcohol consumption, and smoking status, other characteristics were significantly different between the male sleep disorders group and the male non-sleep-disorders group. However, there were significant differences between the female sleep disorders group and the female non-sleep-disorders group only in terms of age, BMI, use of female hormones, hypertension, depressive symptoms, and diabetes.

Table 2 presents the weighted ORs with 95% CIs for sleep disorders according to the tertiles of urinary phytoestrogen concentrations. In model 1, the urinary concentrations of enterolactone and genistein were inversely associated with sleep disorders, while the urinary O-DMA concentration was positively related to sleep disorders. After an additional adjustment for gender and age in model 2, the results were concordant with model 1. In the fully adjusted model (model 3), the negative association between the genistein concentration and sleep disorders was no longer significant, and the enterolactone concentration was still inversely associated with sleep disorders, while the urinary concentrations of enterodiol and O-DMA were positively related to sleep disorders. Compared with tertile 1 (lowest), the fully adjusted ORs (95% CIs) for sleep disorders for the highest tertile of urinary concentrations of enterolactone, enterodiol, and O-DMA were 0.64 (0.41–1.00), 1.54 (1.07–2.21), and 1.89 (1.26–2.85), respectively.

The concentration–response relationships of the urinary concentrations of enterolactone, enterodiol, and O-DMA with sleep disorders are depicted in Figures 2–4, respectively. The urinary enterolactone concentration was linearly negatively associated with sleep disorders (p-nonlinearity = 0.849). The association began to show statistical significance when the enterolactone concentration reached around 904 µg/g creatinine (OR: 0.66, 95% CI: 0.43–0.99) (Figure 2). However, an approximately linear positive relationship was observed between the urinary enterodiol concentration and sleep disorders (p-nonlinearity = 0.274), and when the enterodiol concentration reached around 86 µg/g creatinine (OR: 1.68, 95% CI: 1.00–2.83), the relationship began to present statistical significance (Figure 3). There was a nonlinear positive (inverted L-shaped) association between urinary O-DMA concentration and sleep disorders (p-nonlinearity = 0.033). The OR of sleep disorders increased with increasing urinary O-DMA concentrations, and it arrived at a plateau when the O-DMA concentration was above approximately 13 µg/g creatinine (OR: 1.90, 95% CI: 1.09–3.31) (Figure 4).

Table 1. Characteristics of the subjects (age ≥ 18 years) by sleep disorders (National Health and Nutrition Examination Survey 2005–2010).

Characteristics	Total			Males			Females		
	No Sleep Disorders	Sleep Disorders	p-Value	No Sleep Disorders	Sleep Disorders	p-Value	No Sleep Disorders	Sleep Disorders	p-Value
Number of individuals (%)	4528 (93.75)	302 (6.25)		2396 (92.80)	186 (7.20)		2132 (94.84)	116 (5.16)	
Gender (%)			0.003						
Female	2132 (47.08)	116 (38.41)		-	-		-	-	
Male	2396 (52.92)	186 (61.59)		-	-		-	-	
Age (%)			<0.001			<0.001			0.005
18–39 years	1846 (40.77)	71 (23.51)		957 (39.94)	40 (21.51)		889 (41.70)	31 (26.72)	
40–59 years	1378 (30.43)	109 (36.09)		707 (29.51)	66 (35.48)		671 (31.47)	43 (37.07)	
≥60 years	1304 (28.80)	122 (40.40)		732 (30.55)	80 (43.01)		572 (26.83)	42 (36.21)	
Race (%)			<0.001			<0.001			0.287
Mexican American	914 (20.19)	39 (12.91)		466 (19.45)	16 (8.60)		448 (21.01)	23 (19.83)	
Non-Hispanic White	2040 (45.05)	173 (57.28)		1118 (46.66)	116 (62.37)		922 (43.25)	57 (49.14)	
Non-Hispanic Black	975 (21.53)	54 (17.88)		529 (22.08)	34 (18.28)		446 (20.92)	20 (17.24)	
Other Hispanic	385 (8.50)	28 (9.27)		180 (7.51)	14 (7.53)		205 (9.62)	14 (12.07)	
Other race	214 (4.73)	8 (2.65)		103 (4.30)	6 (3.23)		111 (5.21)	2 (1.72)	
Education (%)			0.006			0.004			0.444
High school	1117 (24.69)	63 (20.86)		619 (25.86)	41 (22.04)		498 (23.37)	22 (18.97)	
Below high school	1317 (29.10)	71 (23.51)		708 (29.57)	39 (20.97)		609 (28.58)	32 (27.59)	
Above high school	2091 (46.21)	168 (55.63)		1067 (44.57)	106 (56.99)		1024 (48.05)	62 (53.45)	
Occupation (%)			0.002			<0.001			0.626
No work	1878 (41.48)	156 (51.66)		898 (37.49)	100 (53.76)		980 (45.97)	56 (48.28)	
Regular night or evening shift/rotating shift/other	735 (16.24)	41 (13.58)		428 (17.87)	22 (11.83)		307 (14.40)	19 (16.38)	
Regular daytime schedule	1914 (42.28)	105 (34.77)		1069 (44.63)	64 (34.41)		845 (39.63)	41 (35.34)	
Family income/year (%)			0.721			0.932			0.536
$20,000 and over	3019 (74.07)	201 (73.09)		1630 (75.74)	126 (75.45)		1389 (72.19)	75 (69.44)	
Below $20,000	1057 (25.93)	74 (26.91)		522 (24.26)	41 (24.55)		535 (27.81)	33 (30.56)	
Marital status (%)			0.032			0.006			0.712
Living with partner/married	2578 (59.40)	197 (65.67)		1454 (63.52)	136 (73.51)		1124 (54.80)	61 (53.04)	
Never married/widowed/separated/divorced	1762 (40.60)	103 (34.33)		835 (36.48)	49 (26.49)		927 (45.20)	54 (46.96)	
Body mass index (%)			<0.001			<0.001			0.009
18.5 to <25 kg/m²	1371 (30.56)	43 (14.63)		688 (28.97)	21 (11.67)		683 (32.35)	22 (19.30)	
<18.5 kg/m²	83 (1.85)	2 (0.68)		37 (1.56)	0 (0.00)		46 (2.18)	2 (1.75)	
25 to <30 kg/m²	1499 (33.42)	82 (27.89)		896 (37.73)	50 (27.78)		603 (28.56)	32 (28.07)	
≥30 kg/m²	1533 (34.17)	167 (56.80)		754 (31.75)	109 (60.56)		779 (36.90)	58 (50.88)	
Physical activity			0.047			0.017			0.234
Moderate	1267 (28.26)	88 (29.53)		573 (24.17)	54 (29.67)		694 (32.84)	34 (29.31)	
Vigorous	1720 (38.36)	94 (31.54)		1118 (47.15)	66 (36.26)		602 (28.49)	28 (24.14)	
Other	1497 (33.39)	116 (38.93)		680 (28.68)	62 (34.07)		817 (38.67)	54 (46.55)	
Smoked at least 100 cigarettes in life (%)	1948 (46.47)	163 (54.70)	0.006	1222 (55.37)	115 (62.84)	0.050	726 (36.57)	48 (41.74)	0.264
Had at least 12 alcohol drinks/year (%)	2810 (73.52)	196 (71.01)	0.363	1735 (84.63)	140 (82.35)	0.430	1075 (60.67)	56 (52.83)	0.109
Use of female hormones (%)	247 (5.94)	27 (9.28)	0.022	-	-	-	247 (14.00)	27 (25.71)	0.001
Hypertension (%)	1973 (44.91)	188 (63.09)	<0.001	1154 (49.34)	128 (70.33)	<0.001	819 (39.87)	60 (51.72)	0.011
Depressive symptoms (%)	240 (5.86)	57 (20.58)	<0.001	78 (3.54)	23 (13.29)	<0.001	162 (8.56)	34 (32.69)	<0.001
Diabetes (%)	432 (9.70)	60 (20.98)	<0.001	209 (8.89)	39 (22.29)	<0.001	223 (10.60)	21 (18.92)	0.006
C-reactive protein (mg/dL), median (interquartile range)	0.17 (0.36)	0.24 (0.44)	0.001	0.14 (0.27)	0.25 (0.41)	<0.001	0.21 (0.44)	0.22 (0.51)	0.225
Caffeine intake (mg/day), median (interquartile range)	92.00 (173.00)	128.00 (212.13)	0.001	103.50 (186.50)	132.75 (219.88)	0.012	82.00 (150.75)	103.25 (208.38)	0.057

The p-values were derived from Mann–Whitney U tests for non-normal continuous variables and chi-square tests for categorical variables.

Table 2. Weighted odds ratios (95% confidence intervals) for sleep disorders across tertiles of urinary phytoestrogens concentrations (National Health and Nutrition Examination Survey 2005–2010).

Phytoestrogen Concentrations (μg/g Creatinine)	Cases/Participants	Model 1 [a]	Model 2 [b]	Model 3 [c]
Enterolactone				
Tertile 1 (<160.53)	107/1612	1.00 (reference)	1.00 (reference)	1.00 (reference)
Tertile 2 (160.53 to <621.68)	96/1609	0.83 (0.54–1.25)	0.78 (0.52–1.18)	0.99 (0.63–1.56)
Tertile 3 (≥621.68)	99/1609	0.64 (0.42–0.96) *	0.57 (0.38–0.85) **	0.64 (0.41–1.00) *
Enterodiol				
Tertile 1 (<21.52)	91/1611	1.00 (reference)	1.00 (reference)	1.00 (reference)
Tertile 2 (21.52 to <70.27)	103/1609	1.21 (0.88–1.65)	1.18 (0.86–1.62)	1.28 (0.86–1.91)
Tertile 3 (≥70.27)	108/1610	1.34 (0.88–2.05)	1.35 (0.89–2.07)	1.54 (1.07–2.21) *
Daidzein				
Tertile 1 (<24.22)	83/1611	1.00 (reference)	1.00 (reference)	1.00 (reference)
Tertile 2 (24.22 to <108.62)	106/1609	1.46 (0.82–2.61)	1.48 (0.83–2.63)	1.18 (0.65–2.15)
Tertile 3 (≥108.62)	113/1610	1.30 (0.61–2.79)	1.32 (0.62–2.81)	1.12 (0.54–2.30)
O-Desmethylangolensin				
Tertile 1 (<1.04)	84/1624	1.00 (reference)	1.00 (reference)	1.00 (reference)
Tertile 2 (1.04 to <9.06)	102/1613	1.33 (0.88–2.02)	1.32 (0.86–2.03)	1.38 (0.84–2.27)
Tertile 3 (≥9.06)	116/1593	1.65 (1.05–2.61) *	1.68 (1.06–2.65) *	1.89 (1.26–2.85) **
Equol				
Tertile 1 (<3.75)	84/1613	1.00 (reference)	1.00 (reference)	1.00 (reference)
Tertile 2 (3.75 to <9.73)	119/1612	1.21 (0.83–1.74)	1.16 (0.79–1.71)	1.01 (0.66–1.56)
Tertile 3 (≥9.73)	99/1605	0.86 (0.57–1.30)	0.84 (0.55–1.28)	0.76 (0.52–1.12)
Genistein				
Tertile 1 (<12.35)	104/1626	1.00 (reference)	1.00 (reference)	1.00 (reference)
Tertile 2 (12.35 to <50.00)	85/1601	0.60 (0.40–0.91) *	0.58 (0.38–0.88) *	0.68 (0.41–1.12)
Tertile 3 (≥50.00)	113/1603	0.80 (0.46–1.38)	0.74 (0.42–1.29)	0.78 (0.41–1.46)

[a] Six phytoestrogens (tertiles) were entered into model 1 simultaneously. [b] Model 2 additionally adjusted for age and gender. [c] Model 3 further adjusted for race, education, marital status, occupation, family income, body mass index, physical activity, alcohol use, smoking status, depressive symptoms, diabetes, hypertension, use of female hormones, C-reactive protein (mg/dL), and caffeine intake (mg/day). * $p < 0.05$, ** $p < 0.01$.

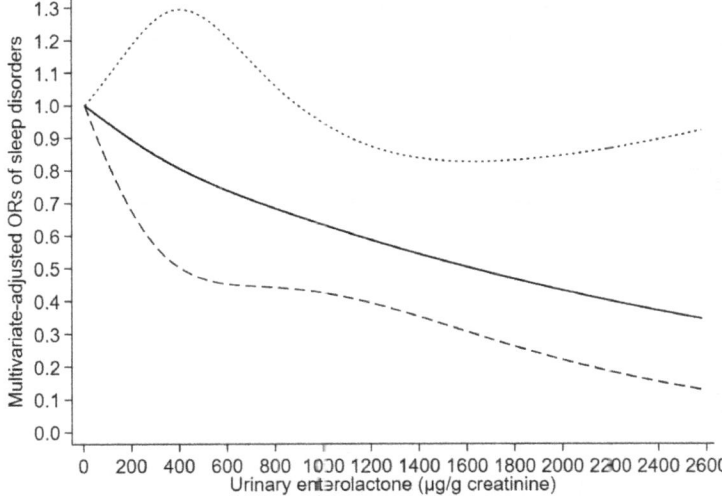

Figure 2. Concentration–response relationship of the urinary enterolactone concentration with sleep disorders. The solid line represents the estimated odds ratios (ORs) and the dashed lines represent their 95% confidence intervals. The relationship was adjusted for gender, age, marital status, race, occupation, family income, educational level, body mass index, smoking status, alcohol consumption, use of female hormones, physical activity, caffeine intake, C-reactive protein, hypertension, depressive symptoms, diabetes, and the other five phytoestrogens (tertiles).

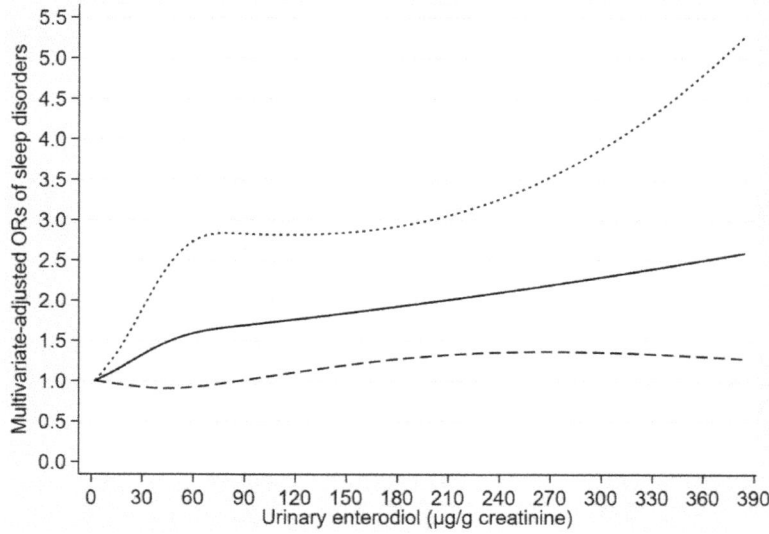

Figure 3. Concentration–response relationship of the urinary enterodiol concentration with sleep disorders. The solid line represents the estimated odds ratios (ORs) and the dashed lines represent their 95% confidence intervals. The relationship was adjusted for gender, age, marital status, race, occupation, family income, educational level, body mass index, smoking status, alcohol consumption, use of female hormones, physical activity, caffeine intake, C-reactive protein, hypertension, depressive symptoms, diabetes, and the other five phytoestrogens (tertiles).

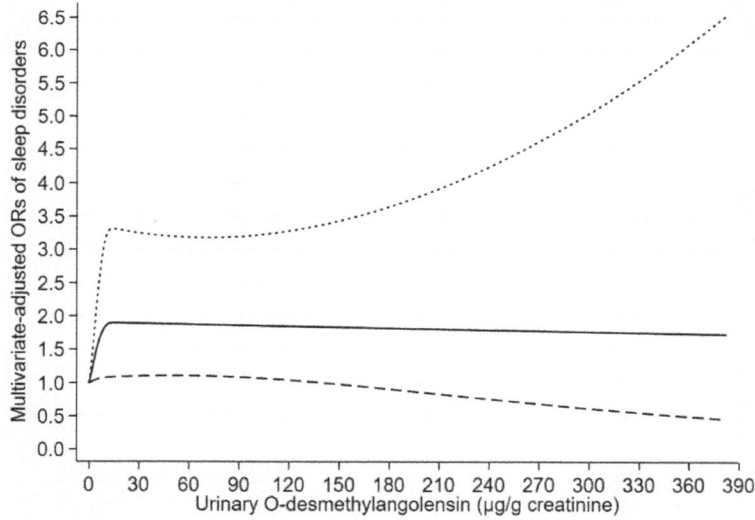

Figure 4. Concentration–response relationship of the urinary O-desmethylangolensin concentration with sleep disorders. The solid line represents the estimated odds ratios (ORs) and the dashed lines represent their 95% confidence intervals. The relationship was adjusted for gender, age, marital status, race, occupation, family income, educational level, body mass index, smoking status, alcohol consumption, use of female hormones, physical activity, caffeine intake, C-reactive protein, hypertension, depressive symptoms, diabetes, and the other five phytoestrogens (tertiles).

The associations of urinary phytoestrogen concentrations with sleep disorders stratified by age and gender are shown in Tables 3 and 4, respectively. In the fully adjusted model, the urinary enterolactone concentration was still inversely associated with sleep disorders in females (OR: 0.45, 95% CI: 0.21–0.94). Meanwhile, the urinary enterodiol concentration was still positively related to sleep disorders among middle-aged adults (40–59 years) (OR: 2.56, 95% CI: 1.12–5.84) and females (OR: 3.79, 95% CI: 1.83–7.87), and the O-DMA concentration was still positively associated with sleep disorders in young adults (18–39 years) (OR: 4.16, 95% CI: 1.58–10.97). Additionally, there was a negative association between the genistein concentration and sleep disorders in middle-aged adults (40–59 years) (OR: 0.34, 95% CI: 0.13–0.88). There were no significant associations between the urinary phytoestrogen concentrations and sleep disorders in males and older adults (≥60 years). To further describe the gender difference in the associations of the urinary concentrations of enterolactone and enterodiol with sleep disorders, the concentration–response relationships of them for males and females are presented in Figure 5a,b and Figure 6a,b, respectively. The urinary enterolactone concentration was linearly negatively associated with sleep disorders in females (p-nonlinearity = 0.283) (Figure 5a) and the enterodiol concentration was positively related to sleep disorders for females in a nonlinear manner (p-nonlinearity < 0.001) (Figure 6a), whereas the associations were not significant in males (Figures 5b and 6b).

Table 3. Weighted odds ratios (95% confidence intervals) for sleep disorders across tertiles of urinary phytoestrogens concentrations stratified by age (National Health and Nutrition Examination Survey 2005–2010).

Phytoestrogens Concentrations (µg/g Creatinine)	Cases/Participants	Model 1 [a]	Model 2 [b]	Model 3 [c]
Age (18–39 years)				
Enterolactone				
Tertile 1 (<160.53)	33/767	1.00 (reference)	1.00 (reference)	1.00 (reference)
Tertile 2 (160.53 to <621.68)	23/683	0.60 (0.26–1.38)	0.60 (0.26–1.38)	0.86 (0.36–2.02)
Tertile 3 (≥621.68)	15/467	0.40 (0.16–0.97) *	0.40 (0.16–1.01)	0.65 (0.27–1.56)
Enterodiol				
Tertile 1 (<21.52)	28/732	1.00 (reference)	1.00 (reference)	1.00 (reference)
Tertile 2 (21.52 to <70.27)	24/620	1.55 (0.79–3.03)	1.57 (0.81–3.05)	1.62 (0.73–3.57)
Tertile 3 (≥70.27)	19/565	1.35 (0.63–2.92)	1.39 (0.64–3.00)	1.21 (0.46–3.15)
Daidzein				
Tertile 1 (<24.22)	16/679	1.00 (reference)	1.00 (reference)	1.00 (reference)
Tertile 2 (24.22 to <108.62)	32/661	1.88 (0.77–4.57)	1.89 (0.78–4.58)	1.17 (0.58–2.36)
Tertile 3 (≥108.62)	23/577	0.86 (0.30–2.49)	0.87 (0.31–2.47)	0.88 (0.18–4.30)
O-Desmethylangolensin				
Tertile 1 (<1.04)	19/707	1.00 (reference)	1.00 (reference)	1.00 (reference)
Tertile 2 (1.04 to <9.06)	21/621	1.23 (0.59–2.58)	1.24 (0.59–2.60)	1.34 (0.68–2.66)
Tertile 3 (≥9.06)	31/589	3.27 (1.39–7.70) **	3.28 (1.40–7.68) **	4.16 (1.58–10.97) **
Equol				
Tertile 1 (<3.75)	27/694	1.00 (reference)	1.00 (reference)	1.00 (reference)
Tertile 2 (3.75 to <9.73)	22/631	0.89 (0.41–1.94)	0.89 (0.42–1.93)	0.78 (0.36–1.70)
Tertile 3 (≥9.73)	22/592	0.72 (0.32–1.64)	0.73 (0.32–1.65)	0.44 (0.16–1.15)
Genistein				
Tertile 1 (<12.35)	19/701	1.00 (reference)	1.00 (reference)	1.00 (reference)
Tertile 2 (12.35 to <50.00)	30/650	1.08 (0.52–2.24)	1.08 (0.52–2.24)	1.18 (0.45–3.09)
Tertile 3 (≥50.00)	22/566	1.20 (0.49–2.93)	1.20 (0.49–2.94)	1.29 (0.31–5.39)
Age (40–59 years)				
Enterolactone				
Tertile 1 (<160.53)	39/533	1.00 (reference)	1.00 (reference)	1.00 (reference)
Tertile 2 (160.53 to <621.68)	37/468	0.89 (0.48–1.66)	0.89 (0.48–1.64)	1.00 (0.54–1.83)
Tertile 3 (≥621.68)	33/486	0.63 (0.31–1.29)	0.67 (0.33–1.33)	0.58 (0.28–1.22)

Table 3. Cont.

Phytoestrogens Concentrations (μg/g Creatinine)	Cases/Participants	Model 1 [a]	Model 2 [b]	Model 3 [c]
Enterodiol				
Tertile 1 (<21.52)	30/470	1.00 (reference)	1.00 (reference)	1.00 (reference)
Tertile 2 (21.52 to <70.27)	37/515	0.97 (0.53–1.75)	1.00 (0.56–1.78)	1.33 (0.62–2.87)
Tertile 3 (≥70.27)	42/502	1.29 (0.69–2.40)	1.36 (0.73–2.53)	2.56 (1.12–5.84) *
Daidzein				
Tertile 1 (<24.22)	36/521	1.00 (reference)	1.00 (reference)	1.00 (reference)
Tertile 2 (24.22 to <108.62)	30/469	1.20 (0.49–2.94)	1.14 (0.47–2.79)	1.37 (0.46–4.05)
Tertile 3 (≥108.62)	43/497	1.37 (0.43–4.34)	1.32 (0.42–4.19)	1.22 (0.31–4.74)
O-Desmethylangolensin				
Tertile 1 (<1.04)	31/522	1.00 (reference)	1.00 (reference)	1.00 (reference)
Tertile 2 (1.04 to <9.06)	35/481	1.84 (0.89–3.80)	1.86 (0.90–3.83)	1.65 (0.64–4.27)
Tertile 3 (≥9.06)	43/484	1.90 (0.92–3.93)	2.00 (0.98–4.05)	1.92 (0.78–4.76)
Equol				
Tertile 1 (<3.75)	32/534	1.00 (reference)	1.00 (reference)	1.00 (reference)
Tertile 2 (3.75 to <9.73)	40/487	1.17 (0.62–2.19)	1.20 (0.64–2.26)	1.07 (0.46–2.51)
Tertile 3 (≥9.73)	37/466	0.90 (0.48–1.70)	0.95 (0.50–1.80)	1.07 (0.51–2.24)
Genistein				
Tertile 1 (<12.35)	47/526	1.00 (reference)	1.00 (reference)	1.00 (reference)
Tertile 2 (12.35 to <50.00)	19/474	0.35 (0.16–0.77) *	0.34 (0.15–0.78) *	0.34 (0.13–0.88) *
Tertile 3 (≥50.00)	43/487	0.65 (0.21–1.97)	0.65 (0.21–2.00)	0.50 (0.17–1.48)
Age (≥60 years)				
Enterolactone				
Tertile 1 (<160.53)	35/312	1.00 (reference)	1.00 (reference)	1.00 (reference)
Tertile 2 (160.53 to <621.68)	36/458	0.87 (0.46–1.63)	0.80 (0.42–1.53)	1.21 (0.53–2.77)
Tertile 3 (≥621.68)	51/656	0.60 (0.34–1.06)	0.58 (0.32–1.03)	0.84 (0.38–1.90)
Enterodiol				
Tertile 1 (<21.52)	33/409	1.00 (reference)	1.00 (reference)	1.00 (reference)
Tertile 2 (21.52 to <70.27)	42/474	1.21 (0.67–2.16)	1.22 (0.68–2.20)	1.01 (0.52–1.96)
Tertile 3 (≥70.27)	47/543	1.26 (0.67–2.37)	1.34 (0.71–2.50)	0.88 (0.43–1.78)
Daidzein				
Tertile 1 (<24.22)	31/411	1.00 (reference)	1.00 (reference)	1.00 (reference)
Tertile 2 (24.22 to <108.62)	44/479	1.93 (0.85–4.36)	1.88 (0.82–4.29)	1.27 (0.48–3.35)
Tertile 3 (≥108.62)	47/536	2.36 (0.65–8.53)	2.26 (0.63–8.16)	1.59 (0.43–5.93)
O-Desmethylangolensin				
Tertile 1 (<1.04)	34/395	1.00 (reference)	1.00 (reference)	1.00 (reference)
Tertile 2 (1.04 to <9.06)	46/511	0.73 (0.38–1.38)	0.75 (0.39–1.44)	0.78 (0.33–1.80)
Tertile 3 (≥9.06)	42/520	0.66 (0.34–1.29)	0.70 (0.35–1.39)	0.87 (0.34–2.28)
Equol				
Tertile 1 (<3.75)	25/385	1.00 (reference)	1.00 (reference)	1.00 (reference)
Tertile 2 (3.75 to <9.73)	57/494	1.41 (0.79–2.54)	1.41 (0.78–2.55)	1.01 (0.42–2.45)
Tertile 3 (≥9.73)	40/547	0.75 (0.36–1.56)	0.76 (0.37–1.59)	0.56 (0.25–1.24)
Genistein				
Tertile 1 (<12.35)	38/399	1.00 (reference)	1.00 (reference)	1.00 (reference)
Tertile 2 (12.35 to <50.00)	36/477	0.60 (0.29–1.26)	0.60 (0.29–1.25)	0.77 (0.29–2.06)
Tertile 3 (≥50.00)	48/550	0.51 (0.16–1.61)	0.53 (0.17–1.64)	0.86 (0.19–3.85)

[a] Six phytoestrogens (tertiles) were entered into model 1 simultaneously. [b] Model 2 additionally adjusted for gender. [c] Model 3 further adjusted for race, education, marital status, occupation, family income, body mass index, physical activity, alcohol use, smoking status, depressive symptoms, diabetes, hypertension, use of female hormones, C-reactive protein (mg/dL), and caffeine intake (mg/day). * $p < 0.05$, ** $p < 0.01$.

Table 4. Weighted odds ratios (95% confidence intervals) for sleep disorders across tertiles of urinary phytoestrogen concentrations stratified by gender (National Health and Nutrition Examination Survey 2005–2010).

Phytoestrogen Concentrations (μg/g Creatinine)	Cases/Participants	Model 1 [a]	Model 2 [b]	Model 3 [c]
Females				
Enterolactone				
Tertile 1 (<160.53)	40/698	1.00 (reference)	1.00 (reference)	1.00 (reference)
Tertile 2 (160.53 to <621.68)	36/706	0.52 (0.24–1.14)	0.53 (0.24–1.16)	0.56 (0.25–1.26)
Tertile 3 (≥621.68)	40/844	0.36 (0.19–0.68) **	0.32 (0.17–0.61) **	0.45 (0.21–0.94) *
Enterodiol				
Tertile 1 (<21.52)	28/649	1.00 (reference)	1.00 (reference)	1.00 (reference)
Tertile 2 (21.52 to <70.27)	33/728	1.90 (1.04–3.48) *	1.81 (0.98–3.32)	2.70 (1.60–4.55) ***
Tertile 3 (≥70.27)	55/871	2.89 (1.54–5.42) **	2.79 (1.46–5.31) **	3.79 (1.83–7.87) **
Daidzein				
Tertile 1 (<24.22)	21/708	1.00 (reference)	1.00 (reference)	1.00 (reference)
Tertile 2 (24.22 to <108.62)	51/745	2.16 (0.93–5.00)	2.33 (1.01–5.35) *	1.82 (0.77–4.30)
Tertile 3 (≥108.62)	44/795	1.71 (0.56–5.20)	1.82 (0.59–5.55)	1.44 (0.48–4.28)
O-Desmethylangolensin				
Tertile 1 (<1.04)	27/697	1.00 (reference)	1.00 (reference)	1.00 (reference)
Tertile 2 (1.04 to <9.06)	41/753	1.70 (0.82–3.52)	1.68 (0.79–3.57)	2.04 (0.95–4.37)
Tertile 3 (≥9.06)	48/798	2.00 (1.00–3.99)	1.94 (1.00–3.76)	2.09 (0.96–4.56)
Equol				
Tertile 1 (<3.75)	31/669	1.00 (reference)	1.00 (reference)	1.00 (reference)
Tertile 2 (3.75 to <9.73)	47/752	1.36 (0.74–2.48)	1.30 (0.71–2.37)	1.25 (0.57–2.73)
Tertile 3 (≥9.73)	38/827	0.85 (0.41–1.78)	0.80 (0.38–1.68)	0.62 (0.28–1.35)
Genistein				
Tertile 1 (<12.35)	33/720	1.00 (reference)	1.00 (reference)	1.00 (reference)
Tertile 2 (12.35 to <50.00)	39/723	0.60 (0.31–1.17)	0.57 (0.29–1.12)	0.59 (0.25–1.38)
Tertile 3 (≥50.00)	44/805	0.62 (0.27–1.42)	0.57 (0.25–1.30)	0.61 (0.23–1.57)
Males				
Enterolactone				
Tertile 1 (<160.53)	67/914	1.00 (reference)	1.00 (reference)	1.00 (reference)
Tertile 2 (160.53 to <621.68)	60/903	1.16 (0.67–1.99)	1.08 (0.63–1.85)	1.58 (0.86–2.91)
Tertile 3 (≥621.68)	59/765	1.11 (0.65–1.88)	0.93 (0.54–1.61)	0.92 (0.46–1.83)
Enterodiol				
Tertile 1 (<21.52)	63/962	1.00 (reference)	1.00 (reference)	1.00 (reference)
Tertile 2 (21.52 to <70.27)	70/881	0.99 (0.64–1.52)	0.94 (0.61–1.46)	0.92 (0.51–1.65)
Tertile 3 (≥70.27)	53/739	0.88 (0.52–1.50)	0.85 (0.51–1.42)	0.92 (0.56–1.53)
Daidzein				
Tertile 1 (<24.22)	62/903	1.00 (reference)	1.00 (reference)	1.00 (reference)
Tertile 2 (24.22 to <108.62)	55/864	1.10 (0.58–2.06)	1.07 (0.58–1.98)	0.88 (0.48–1.64)
Tertile 3 (≥108.62)	69/815	1.02 (0.41–2.52)	1.01 (0.42–2.45)	1.05 (0.44–2.50)
O-Desmethylangolensin				
Tertile 1 (<1.04)	57/927	1.00 (reference)	1.00 (reference)	1.00 (reference)
Tertile 2 (1.04 to <9.06)	61/860	1.17 (0.65–2.11)	1.15 (0.65–2.04)	1.05 (0.53–2.05)
Tertile 3 (≥9.06)	68/795	1.57 (0.88–2.80)	1.58 (0.89–2.80)	1.58 (0.89–2.79)
Equol				
Tertile 1 (<3.75)	53/944	1.00 (reference)	1.00 (reference)	1.00 (reference)
Tertile 2 (3.75 to <9.73)	72/860	1.12 (0.70–1.81)	1.06 (0.65–1.73)	0.79 (0.47–1.35)
Tertile 3 (≥9.73)	61/778	0.91 (0.54–1.54)	0.88 (0.52–1.48)	0.86 (0.47–1.58)
Genistein				
Tertile 1 (<12.35)	71/906	1.00 (reference)	1.00 (reference)	1.00 (reference)
Tertile 2 (12.35 to <50.00)	46/878	0.59 (0.36–0.97) *	0.57 (0.35–0.93) *	0.74 (0.41–1.33)
Tertile 3 (≥50.00)	69/798	1.04 (0.52–2.10)	0.96 (0.48–1.91)	0.96 (0.42–2.20)

[a] Six phytoestrogens (tertiles) were entered into model 1 simultaneously. [b] Model 2 additionally adjusted for age. [c] Model 3 further adjusted for race, education, marital status, occupation, family income, body mass index, physical activity, alcohol use, smoking status, depressive symptoms, diabetes, hypertension, use of female hormones (only in females), C-reactive protein (mg/dL), and caffeine intake (mg/day). * $p < 0.05$, ** $p < 0.01$, *** $p < 0.001$.

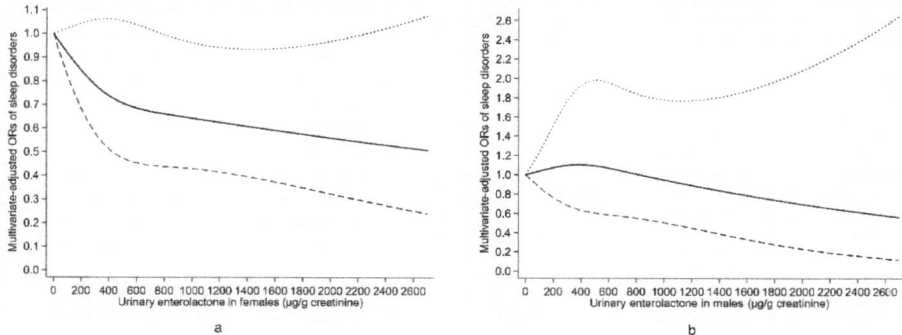

Figure 5. Concentration–response relationship of the urinary enterolactone concentration with sleep disorders for females (**a**) and males (**b**). The solid line represents the estimated odds ratios (ORs) and the dashed lines represent their 95% confidence intervals. The relationship adjusted for age, marital status, race, occupation, family income, educational level, body mass index, smoking status, alcohol consumption, use of female hormones (only in females), physical activity, caffeine intake, C-reactive protein, hypertension, depressive symptoms, diabetes, and the other five phytoestrogens (tertiles).

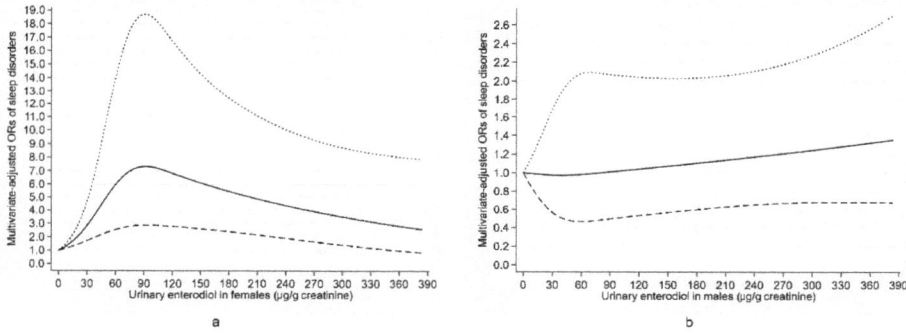

Figure 6. Concentration–response relationship of the urinary enterodiol concentration with sleep disorders for females (**a**) and males (**b**). The solid line represents the estimated odds ratios (ORs) and the dashed lines represent their 95% confidence intervals. The relationship adjusted for age, marital status, race, occupation, family income, educational level, body mass index, smoking status, alcohol consumption, use of female hormones (only in females), physical activity, caffeine intake, C-reactive protein, hypertension, depressive symptoms, diabetes, and the other five phytoestrogens (tertiles).

Furthermore, the associations between the urinary phytoestrogen concentrations and sleep disorders stratified by age group separately for males and females are shown in Table 5. The urinary O-DMA concentration was positively associated with sleep disorders in males aged 18–39 years (OR: 6.57, 95% CI: 2.06–20.99) and females aged 40–59 years (OR: 15.14, 95% CI: 2.99–76.65), whereas the O-DMA concentration was inversely related to sleep disorders in females aged 60 years or over (OR: 0.25, 95% CI: 0.10–0.58). The urinary enterodiol concentration was positively related to sleep disorders in females aged 18–39 (OR: 6.52, 95% CI: 1.69–25.23) and 40–59 years (OR: 13.66, 95% CI: 2.06–90.70). Furthermore, the urinary equol concentration was inversely associated with sleep disorders in females aged 18–39 years (OR: 0.08, 95% CI: 0.01–0.84), and daidzein concentration was positively related to sleep disorders in females aged 60 years or over (OR: 10.67, 95% CI: 1.88–60.44).

Table 5. Weighted odds ratios (95% confidence intervals) for sleep disorders across tertiles of urinary phytoestrogen concentrations stratified by age for males and females (National Health and Nutrition Examination Survey 2005–2010).

Phytoestrogen Concentrations (µg/g Creatinine)	Males		Females	
	Cases/Participants	Model 3 [a]	Cases/Participants	Model 3 [a]
Age (18–39 years)				
Enterolactone				
Tertile 1 (<160.53)	18/444	1.00 (reference)	15/323	1.00 (reference)
Tertile 2 (160.53 to <621.68)	13/353	1.65 (0.53–5.08)	10/330	0.54 (0.14–2.14)
Tertile 3 (≥621.68)	9/200	1.12 (0.27–4.69)	6/267	0.46 (0.10–2.14)
Enterodiol				
Tertile 1 (<21.52)	19/434	1.00 (reference)	9/298	1.00 (reference)
Tertile 2 (21.52 to <70.27)	12/328	0.90 (0.28–2.89)	12/292	6.52 (1.69–25.23) **
Tertile 3 (≥70.27)	9/235	1.28 (0.36–4.59)	10/330	1.84 (0.50–6.80)
Daidzein				
Tertile 1 (<24.22)	12/381	1.00 (reference)	4/298	1.00 (reference)
Tertile 2 (24.22 to <108.62)	16/327	0.86 (0.38–1.93)	16/334	2.35 (0.60–9.22)
Tertile 3 (≥108.62)	12/289	0.45 (0.09–2.25)	11/288	5.07 (0.52–49.84)
O-Desmethylangolensin				
Tertile 1 (<1.04)	10/395	1.00 (reference)	9/312	1.00 (reference)
Tertile 2 (1.04 to <9.06)	12/311	1.28 (0.39–4.18)	9/310	1.18 (0.37–3.72)
Tertile 3 (≥9.06)	18/291	6.57 (2.06–20.99) **	13/298	0.74 (0.12–4.45)
Equol				
Tertile 1 (<3.75)	15/396	1.00 (reference)	12/298	1.00 (reference)
Tertile 2 (3.75 to <9.73)	9/318	0.44 (0.15–1.33)	13/313	1.37 (0.38–4.88)
Tertile 3 (≥9.73)	16/283	0.74 (0.29–1.86)	6/309	0.08 (0.01–0.84) *
Genistein				
Tertile 1 (<12.35)	13/386	1.00 (reference)	6/315	1.00 (reference)
Tertile 2 (12.35 to <50.00)	15/337	1.60 (0.54–4.73)	15/313	1.10 (0.29–4.10)
Tertile 3 (≥50.00)	12/274	1.70 (0.37–7.85)	10/292	0.59 (0.12–2.81)
Age (40–59 years)				
Enterolactone				
Tertile 1 (<160.53)	25/304	1.00 (reference)	14/229	1.00 (reference)
Tertile 2 (160.53 to <621.68)	24/260	1.90 (0.74–4.88)	13/208	0.50 (0.16–1.53)
Tertile 3 (≥621.68)	17/209	1.15 (0.36–3.61)	16/277	0.32 (0.10–1.03)
Enterodiol				
Tertile 1 (<21.52)	23/272	1.00 (reference)	7/198	1.00 (reference)
Tertile 2 (21.52 to <70.27)	24/272	1.04 (0.32–3.42)	13/243	3.02 (1.10–8.30) *
Tertile 3 (≥70.27)	19/229	1.47 (0.43–5.00)	23/273	13.66 (2.06–90.70) **
Daidzein				
Tertile 1 (<24.22)	25/281	1.00 (reference)	11/240	1.00 (reference)
Tertile 2 (24.22 to <108.62)	15/262	2.04 (0.45–9.16)	15/207	1.65 (0.41–6.72)
Tertile 3 (≥108.62)	26/230	2.94 (0.38–22.73)	17/267	0.85 (0.13–5.75)
O-Desmethylangolensin				
Tertile 1 (<1.04)	25/297	1.00 (reference)	6/225	1.00 (reference)
Tertile 2 (1.04 to <9.06)	18/252	0.56 (0.18–1.79)	17/229	11.50 (2.14–61.72) **
Tertile 3 (≥9.06)	23/224	0.68 (0.21–2.20)	20/260	15.14 (2.99–76.65) **
Equol				
Tertile 1 (<3.75)	21/316	1.00 (reference)	11/218	1.00 (reference)
Tertile 2 (3.75 to <9.73)	27/251	0.88 (0.27–2.86)	13/236	0.95 (0.29–3.12)
Tertile 3 (≥9.73)	18/206	1.28 (0.43–3.80)	19/260	0.77 (0.26–2.31)
Genistein				
Tertile 1 (<12.35)	30/285	1.00 (reference)	17/241	1.00 (reference)
Tertile 2 (12.35 to <50.00)	10/256	0.29 (0.05–1.61)	9/218	0.20 (0.04–1.00)
Tertile 3 (≥50.00)	26/232	0.43 (0.06–3.03)	17/255	0.38 (0.07–2.05)
Age (≥60 years)				
Enterolactone				
Tertile 1 (<160.53)	24/166	1.00 (reference)	11/146	1.00 (reference)
Tertile 2 (160.53 to <621.68)	23/290	1.59 (0.63–4.04)	13/168	1.37 (0.43–4.40)
Tertile 3 (≥621.68)	33/356	0.77 (0.34–1.75)	18/300	1.47 (0.29–7.40)

Table 5. Cont.

Phytoestrogen Concentrations (µg/g Creatinine)	Males		Females	
	Cases/Participants	Model 3 [a]	Cases/Participants	Model 3 [a]
Enterodiol				
Tertile 1 (<21.52)	21/256	1.00 (reference)	12/153	1.00 (reference)
Tertile 2 (21.52 to <70.27)	34/281	0.98 (0.44–2.20)	8/193	1.18 (0.26–5.28)
Tertile 3 (≥70.27)	25/275	0.48 (0.20–1.16)	22/268	2.00 (0.71–5.57)
Daidzein				
Tertile 1 (<24.22)	25/241	1.00 (reference)	6/170	1.00 (reference)
Tertile 2 (24.22 to <108.62)	24/275	0.47 (0.16–1.39)	20/204	13.45 (2.89–62.50) **
Tertile 3 (≥108.62)	31/296	0.80 (0.13–4.79)	16/240	10.67 (1.88–60.44) **
O-Desmethylangolensin				
Tertile 1 (<1.04)	22/235	1.00 (reference)	12/160	1.00 (reference)
Tertile 2 (1.04 to <9.06)	31/297	1.16 (0.37–3.66)	15/214	0.27 (0.06–1.19)
Tertile 3 (≥9.06)	27/280	1.19 (0.33–4.37)	15/240	0.25 (0.10–0.58) **
Equol				
Tertile 1 (<3.75)	17/232	1.00 (reference)	8/153	1.00 (reference)
Tertile 2 (3.75 to <9.73)	36/291	0.69 (0.23–2.08)	21/203	2.05 (0.63–6.68)
Tertile 3 (≥9.73)	27/289	0.72 (0.28–1.83)	13/258	0.49 (0.12–1.97)
Genistein				
Tertile 1 (<12.35)	28/235	1.00 (reference)	10/164	1.00 (reference)
Tertile 2 (12.35 to <50.00)	21/285	0.75 (0.22–2.53)	15/192	0.71 (0.14–3.53)
Tertile 3 (≥50.00)	31/292	1.29 (0.16–10.26)	17/258	0.41 (0.06–2.82)

[a] Adjusted for education, marital status, occupation, family income, body mass index, physical activity, alcohol use, smoking status, depressive symptoms, diabetes, hypertension, use of female hormones (only in females), C-reactive protein (mg/dL), caffeine intake (mg/day), and the other five phytoestrogens (tertiles). * $p < 0.05$, ** $p < 0.01$.

The associations between the urinary phytoestrogen concentrations and sleep disorders stratified by race are displayed in Table 6. An interesting finding was that the urinary O-DMA concentration was positively related to sleep disorders in non-Hispanic Whites (OR: 2.16, 95% CI: 1.31–3.55) but inversely associated with sleep disorders in other Hispanics (OR: 0.13, 95% CI: 0.02–0.86). Furthermore, the urinary enterolactone concentration was negatively related to sleep disorders (OR: 0.56, 95% CI: 0.33–0.95), while the enterodiol concentration was positively associated with sleep disorders (OR: 1.89, 95% CI: 1.13–3.13) in non-Hispanic Whites and the equol concentration was positively related to sleep disorders in other Hispanics (OR: 3.22, 95% CI: 1.11–9.30).

Table 6. Weighted odds ratios (95% confidence intervals) for sleep disorders across tertiles of urinary phytoestrogen concentrations stratified by race (National Health and Nutrition Examination Survey 2005–2010).

Phytoestrogen Concentrations (µg/g Creatinine)	Cases/Participants	Model 3 [a]
Mexican American		
Enterolactone		
Tertile 1 (<160.53)	9/298	1.00 (reference)
Tertile 2 (160.53 to <621.68)	11/347	2.24 (0.28–17.56)
Tertile 3 (≥621.68)	19/308	2.47 (0.54–11.42)
Enterodiol		
Tertile 1 (<21.52)	9/366	1.00 (reference)
Tertile 2 (21.52 to <70.27)	15/315	1.64 (0.85–3.17)
Tertile 3 (≥70.27)	15/272	1.91 (0.56–6.50)
Daidzein		
Tertile 1 (<24.22)	10/359	1.00 (reference)
Tertile 2 (24.22 to <108.62)	12/292	0.72 (0.14–3.83)
Tertile 3 (≥108.62)	17/302	1.03 (0.11–9.46)
O-Desmethylangolensin		
Tertile 1 (<1.04)	7/401	1.00 (reference)
Tertile 2 (1.04 to <9.06)	18/312	2.00 (0.53–7.61)
Tertile 3 (≥9.06)	14/240	2.16 (0.73–6.39)

Table 6. Cont.

Phytoestrogen Concentrations (μg/g Creatinine)	Cases/Participants	Model 3 [a]
Equol		
Tertile 1 (<3.75)	13/421	1.00 (reference)
Tertile 2 (3.75 to <9.73)	17/331	0.64 (0.17–2.45)
Tertile 3 (≥9.73)	9/201	0.37 (0.09–1.48)
Genistein		
Tertile 1 (<12.35)	10/341	1.00 (reference)
Tertile 2 (12.35 to <50.00)	13/314	2.26 (0.35–14.60)
Tertile 3 (≥50.00)	16/298	2.00 (0.14–28.91)
Non-Hispanic White		
Enterolactone		
Tertile 1 (<160.53)	57/673	1.00 (reference)
Tertile 2 (160.53 to <621.68)	59/681	1.00 (0.60–1.67)
Tertile 3 (≥621.68)	57/859	0.56 (0.33–0.95) *
Enterodiol		
Tertile 1 (<21.52)	43/606	1.00 (reference)
Tertile 2 (21.52 to <70.27)	62/765	1.52 (0.88–2.63)
Tertile 3 (≥70.27)	68/842	1.89 (1.13–3.13) *
Daidzein		
Tertile 1 (<24.22)	45/684	1.00 (reference)
Tertile 2 (24.22 to <108.62)	62/771	1.12 (0.55–2.29)
Tertile 3 (≥108.62)	66/758	0.95 (0.41–2.21)
O-Desmethylangolensin		
Tertile 1 (<1.04)	44/638	1.00 (reference)
Tertile 2 (1.04 to <9.06)	60/798	1.48 (0.76–2.90)
Tertile 3 (≥9.06)	69/777	2.16 (1.31–3.55) **
Equol		
Tertile 1 (<3.75)	39/493	1.00 (reference)
Tertile 2 (3.75 to <9.73)	67/729	0.97 (0.57–1.64)
Tertile 3 (≥9.73)	67/991	0.76 (0.47–1.22)
Genistein		
Tertile 1 (<12.35)	60/696	1.00 (reference)
Tertile 2 (12.35 to <50.00)	48/766	0.63 (0.34–1.16)
Tertile 3 (≥50.00)	65/751	0.86 (0.42–1.76)
Non-Hispanic Black		
Enterolactone		
Tertile 1 (<160.53)	20/388	1.00 (reference)
Tertile 2 (160.53 to <621.68)	17/385	1.11 (0.48–2.55)
Tertile 3 (≥621.68)	17/256	0.86 (0.26–2.89)
Enterodiol		
Tertile 1 (<21.52)	23/423	1.00 (reference)
Tertile 2 (21.52 to <70.27)	16/338	0.81 (0.29–2.25)
Tertile 3 (≥70.27)	15/268	0.79 (0.40–1.57)
Daidzein		
Tertile 1 (<24.22)	16/371	1.00 (reference)
Tertile 2 (24.22 to <108.62)	24/331	2.05 (0.57–7.36)
Tertile 3 (≥108.62)	14/327	0.91 (0.16–5.32)
O-Desmethylangolensin		
Tertile 1 (<1.04)	15/338	1.00 (reference)
Tertile 2 (1.04 to <9.06)	17/331	2.53 (0.86–7.50)
Tertile 3 (≥9.06)	22/360	2.23 (0.49–10.14)
Equol		
Tertile 1 (<3.75)	20/486	1.00 (reference)
Tertile 2 (3.75 to <9.73)	23/327	0.99 (0.44–2.26)
Tertile 3 (≥9.73)	11/216	0.54 (0.17–1.75)
Genistein		
Tertile 1 (<12.35)	24/411	1.00 (reference)
Tertile 2 (12.35 to <50.00)	16/313	0.51 (0.20–1.28)
Tertile 3 (≥50.00)	14/305	0.73 (0.18–3.02)

Table 6. Cont.

Phytoestrogen Concentrations (µg/g Creatinine)	Cases/Participants	Model 3 [a]
Other Hispanic		
Enterolactone		
Tertile 1 (<160.53)	16/159	1.00 (reference)
Tertile 2 (160.53 to <621.68)	8/135	1.34 (0.38–4.75)
Tertile 3 (≥621.68)	4/119	0.45 (0.03–6.95)
Enterodiol		
Tertile 1 (<21.52)	13/159	1.00 (reference)
Tertile 2 (21.52 to <70.27)	6/123	0.25 (0.05–1.31)
Tertile 3 (≥70.27)	9/131	2.76 (0.49–15.59)
Daidzein		
Tertile 1 (<24.22)	9/147	1.00 (reference)
Tertile 2 (24.22 to <108.62)	7/141	1.43 (0.21–9.83)
Tertile 3 (≥108.62)	12/125	18.97 (0.50–719.28)
O-Desmethylangolensin		
Tertile 1 (<1.04)	15/171	1.00 (reference)
Tertile 2 (1.04 to <9.06)	6/120	0.13 (0.02–0.86) *
Tertile 3 (≥9.06)	7/122	0.10 (0.01–1.32)
Equol		
Tertile 1 (<3.75)	8/130	1.00 (reference)
Tertile 2 (3.75 to <9.73)	8/137	0.46 (0.13–1.70)
Tertile 3 (≥9.73)	12/146	3.22 (1.11–9.30) *
Genistein		
Tertile 1 (<12.35)	7/132	1.00 (reference)
Tertile 2 (12.35 to <50.00)	6/144	0.58 (0.12–2.72)
Tertile 3 (≥50.00)	15/137	0.30 (0.03–2.91)

[a] Adjusted for age, gender, education, marital status, occupation, family income, body mass index, physical activity, alcohol use, smoking status, depressive symptoms, diabetes, hypertension, use of female hormones, C-reactive protein (mg/dL), caffeine intake (mg/day), and the other five phytoestrogens (tertiles). * $p < 0.05$, ** $p < 0.01$.

Table 7 presents the weighted relative risk ratios (RRRs) with 95% CIs of sleep duration according to tertiles of the urinary phytoestrogen concentrations. In the fully adjusted model, compared with normal sleep (7–8 h/night), the urinary enterolactone concentration was negatively associated with very short sleep (<5 h/night) (RRR: 0.56, 95% CI: 0.36–0.86), and the genistein concentration was inversely related to a long sleep risk (≥9 h/night) (RRR: 0.62, 95% CI: 0.39–0.99).

The associations of urinary phytoestrogen concentrations with sleep duration stratified by age and gender are shown in Tables 8 and 9, respectively. In the fully adjusted model, compared with normal sleep, the urinary enterolactone concentration was still negatively associated with very short sleep among young adults (18–39 years) (RRR: 0.24, 95% CI: 0.09–0.61) and a long sleep risk among older adults (≥60 years) (RRR: 0.49, 95% CI: 0.29–0.84). The urinary genistein concentration was still inversely associated with a long sleep risk in middle-aged adults (40–59 years) (RRR: 0.10, 95% CI: 0.02–0.56) and males (RRR: 0.51, 95% CI: 0.30–0.87). The urinary enterodiol concentration was positively related to very short sleep among young adults (18–39 years) (RRR: 2.73, 95% CI: 1.20–6.21) and a long sleep risk in females (RRR: 2.14, 95% CI: 1.11–4.13).

Table 7. Weighted relative risk ratios (95% confidence intervals) for sleep duration (reference, 7–8 h/night) across tertiles of the urinary phytoestrogen concentrations (National Health and Nutrition Examination Survey 2005–2010).

Phytoestrogen Concentrations (μg/g Creatinine)	Model 3 [a]		
	Very Short Sleep (<5 h/Night)	Short Sleep (5–6 h/Night)	Long Sleep (≥9 h/Night)
Enterolactone			
Tertile 1 (<160.53)	1.00 (reference)	1.00 (reference)	1.00 (reference)
Tertile 2 (160.53 to <621.68)	0.98 (0.64–1.50)	1.15 (0.86–1.54)	1.46 (0.93–2.28)
Tertile 3 (≥621.68)	0.56 (0.36–0.86) **	0.94 (0.69–1.27)	0.78 (0.45–1.33)
Enterodiol			
Tertile 1 (<21.52)	1.00 (reference)	1.00 (reference)	1.00 (reference)
Tertile 2 (21.52 to <70.27)	1.35 (0.76–2.42)	1.09 (0.84–1.40)	1.04 (0.65–1.67)
Tertile 3 (≥70.27)	0.97 (0.54–1.76)	1.04 (0.77–1.39)	1.46 (0.88–2.40)
Daidzein			
Tertile 1 (<24.22)	1.00 (reference)	1.00 (reference)	1.00 (reference)
Tertile 2 (24.22 to <108.62)	1.02 (0.49–2.13)	1.08 (0.85–1.37)	1.10 (0.63–1.93)
Tertile 3 (≥108.62)	1.49 (0.48–4.63)	1.29 (0.83–2.03)	1.15 (0.54–2.43)
O-Desmethylangolensin			
Tertile 1 (<1.04)	1.00 (reference)	1.00 (reference)	1.00 (reference)
Tertile 2 (1.04 to <9.06)	1.43 (0.83–2.47)	1.01 (0.82–1.26)	1.05 (0.67–1.64)
Tertile 3 (≥9.06)	0.82 (0.36–1.88)	0.86 (0.61–1.21)	1.44 (0.80–2.56)
Equol			
Tertile 1 (<3.75)	1.00 (reference)	1.00 (reference)	1.00 (reference)
Tertile 2 (3.75 to <9.73)	1.01 (0.71–1.44)	1.04 (0.81–1.33)	1.06 (0.69–1.62)
Tertile 3 (≥9.73)	0.89 (0.50–1.58)	1.05 (0.84–1.31)	0.92 (0.60–1.41)
Genistein			
Tertile 1 (<12.35)	1.00 (reference)	1.00 (reference)	1.00 (reference)
Tertile 2 (12.35 to <50.00)	0.94 (0.47–1.89)	1.10 (0.85–1.43)	0.62 (0.39–0.99) *
Tertile 3 (≥50.00)	1.05 (0.44–2.53)	0.95 (0.65–1.40)	0.62 (0.33–1.15)

[a] Adjusted for age, gender, race, education, marital status, occupation, family income, body mass index, physical activity, alcohol use, smoking status, depressive symptoms, diabetes, hypertension, use of female hormones, C-reactive protein (mg/dL), caffeine intake (mg/day), and the other five phytoestrogens (tertiles). * $p < 0.05$, ** $p < 0.01$.

Table 8. Weighted relative risk ratios (95% confidence intervals) for sleep duration (reference, 7–8 h/night) across tertiles of the urinary phytoestrogen concentrations stratified by age (National Health and Nutrition Examination Survey 2005–2010).

Phytoestrogen Concentrations (μg/g Creatinine)	Model 3 [a]		
	Very Short Sleep (<5 h/Night)	Short Sleep (5–6 h/Night)	Long Sleep (≥9 h/Night)
Age (18–39 years)			
Enterolactone			
Tertile 1 (<160.53)	1.00 (reference)	1.00 (reference)	1.00 (reference)
Tertile 2 (160.53 to <621.68)	0.69 (0.30–1.59)	0.96 (0.62–1.48)	2.21 (0.99–4.90)
Tertile 3 (≥621.68)	0.24 (0.09–0.61) **	0.78 (0.45–1.36)	1.33 (0.53–3.33)
Enterodiol			
Tertile 1 (<21.52)	1.00 (reference)	1.00 (reference)	1.00 (reference)
Tertile 2 (21.52 to <70.27)	2.73 (1.20–6.21) *	1.20 (0.72–2.01)	0.72 (0.33–1.58)
Tertile 3 (≥70.27)	0.81 (0.25–2.63)	1.00 (0.59–1.69)	1.63 (0.71–3.77)
Daidzein			
Tertile 1 (<24.22)	1.00 (reference)	1.00 (reference)	1.00 (reference)
Tertile 2 (24.22 to <108.62)	1.24 (0.28–5.41)	1.05 (0.72–1.52)	0.58 (0.19–1.73)
Tertile 3 (≥108.62)	1.94 (0.19–19.60)	1.34 (0.65–2.74)	1.09 (0.35–3.36)

Table 8. Cont.

Phytoestrogen Concentrations (μg/g Creatinine)	Model 3 [a]		
	Very Short Sleep (<5 h/Night)	Short Sleep (5–6 h/Night)	Long Sleep (≥9 h/Night)
O-Desmethylangolensin			
Tertile 1 (<1.04)	1.00 (reference)	1.00 (reference)	1.00 (reference)
Tertile 2 (1.04 to <9.06)	1.75 (0.54–5.73)	1.03 (0.69–1.53)	0.64 (0.27–1.52)
Tertile 3 (≥9.06)	1.21 (0.24–6.20)	0.84 (0.52–1.34)	1.28 (0.54–3.08)
Equol			
Tertile 1 (<3.75)	1.00 (reference)	1.00 (reference)	1.00 (reference)
Tertile 2 (3.75 to <9.73)	1.67 (0.70–4.00)	1.09 (0.71–1.67)	0.88 (0.44–1.76)
Tertile 3 (≥9.73)	0.69 (0.23–2.03)	1.03 (0.67–1.59)	0.68 (0.32–1.45)
Genistein			
Tertile 1 (<12.35)	1.00 (reference)	1.00 (reference)	1.00 (reference)
Tertile 2 (12.35 to <50.00)	1.52 (0.46–5.00)	1.21 (0.79–1.83)	1.35 (0.59–3.08)
Tertile 3 (≥50.00)	1.61 (0.36–7.19)	0.91 (0.46–1.79)	0.92 (0.31–2.71)
Age (40-59 years)			
Enterolactone			
Tertile 1 (<160.53)	1.00 (reference)	1.00 (reference)	1.00 (reference)
Tertile 2 (160.53 to <621.68)	1.32 (0.70–2.49)	1.44 (0.87–2.38)	1.98 (0.98–4.03)
Tertile 3 (≥621.68)	0.87 (0.37–2.05)	1.25 (0.80–1.94)	0.55 (0.19–1.58)
Enterodiol			
Tertile 1 (<21.52)	1.00 (reference)	1.00 (reference)	1.00 (reference)
Tertile 2 (21.52 to <70.27)	0.95 (0.40–2.29)	0.97 (0.65–1.44)	0.69 (0.24–1.94)
Tertile 3 (≥70.27)	0.59 (0.23–1.55)	0.93 (0.65–1.33)	1.45 (0.69–3.07)
Daidzein			
Tertile 1 (<24.22)	1.00 (reference)	1.00 (reference)	1.00 (reference)
Tertile 2 (24.22 to <108.62)	0.77 (0.26–2.27)	1.12 (0.64–1.96)	2.42 (0.96–6.12)
Tertile 3 (≥108.62)	1.69 (0.39–7.36)	1.45 (0.62–3.42)	3.92 (0.55–27.81)
O-Desmethylangolensin			
Tertile 1 (<1.04)	1.00 (reference)	1.00 (reference)	1.00 (reference)
Tertile 2 (1.04 to <9.06)	1.37 (0.59–3.17)	0.87 (0.59–1.26)	1.54 (0.58–4.11)
Tertile 3 (≥9.06)	0.43 (0.12–1.60)	0.71 (0.35–1.44)	1.41 (0.56–3.58)
Equol			
Tertile 1 (<3.75)	1.00 (reference)	1.00 (reference)	1.00 (reference)
Tertile 2 (3.75 to <9.73)	0.41 (0.14–1.22)	0.98 (0.65–1.48)	1.42 (0.68–2.96)
Tertile 3 (≥9.73)	0.65 (0.25–1.73)	0.95 (0.67–1.36)	1.14 (0.37–3.55)
Genistein			
Tertile 1 (<12.35)	1.00 (reference)	1.00 (reference)	1.00 (reference)
Tertile 2 (12.35 to <50.00)	0.73 (0.27–2.01)	1.09 (0.68–1.76)	0.14 (0.05–0.40) ***
Tertile 3 (≥50.00)	0.85 (0.23–3.17)	1.00 (0.53–1.86)	0.10 (0.02–0.56) *
Age (≥60 years)			
Enterolactone			
Tertile 1 (<160.53)	1.00 (reference)	1.00 (reference)	1.00 (reference)
Tertile 2 (160.53 to <621.68)	1.75 (0.62–4.94)	1.07 (0.61–1.87)	0.61 (0.29–1.30)
Tertile 3 (≥621.68)	1.27 (0.52–3.10)	0.81 (0.52–1.27)	0.49 (0.29–0.84) *
Enterodiol			
Tertile 1 (<21.52)	1.00 (reference)	1.00 (reference)	1.00 (reference)
Tertile 2 (21.52 to <70.27)	0.45 (0.16–1.30)	1.09 (0.65–1.84)	1.56 (0.82–2.96)
Tertile 3 (≥70.27)	1.38 (0.63–3.02)	1.11 (0.66–1.88)	1.64 (0.92–2.93)
Daidzein			
Tertile 1 (<24.22)	1.00 (reference)	1.00 (reference)	1.00 (reference)
Tertile 2 (24.22 to <108.62)	0.94 (0.11–7.95)	1.07 (0.61–1.88)	1.35 (0.68–2.68)
Tertile 3 (≥108.62)	0.62 (0.04–10.32)	1.08 (0.46–2.55)	0.62 (0.26–1.48)

Table 8. Cont.

Phytoestrogen Concentrations (µg/g Creatinine)	Model 3 [a]		
	Very Short Sleep (<5 h/Night)	Short Sleep (5–6 h/Night)	Long Sleep (≥9 h/Night)
O-Desmethylangolensin			
Tertile 1 (<1.04)	1.00 (reference)	1.00 (reference)	1.00 (reference)
Tertile 2 (1.04 to <9.06)	1.21 (0.47–3.14)	1.53 (0.92–2.53)	1.33 (0.72–2.45)
Tertile 3 (≥9.06)	0.75 (0.17–3.22)	1.21 (0.64–2.27)	1.38 (0.66–2.89)
Equol			
Tertile 1 (<3.75)	1.00 (reference)	1.00 (reference)	1.00 (reference)
Tertile 2 (3.75 to <9.73)	1.26 (0.52–3.06)	0.95 (0.54–1.67)	1.07 (0.48–2.40)
Tertile 3 (≥9.73)	1.93 (0.81–4.62)	1.10 (0.66–1.86)	1.16 (0.59–2.26)
Genistein			
Tertile 1 (<12.35)	1.00 (reference)	1.00 (reference)	1.00 (reference)
Tertile 2 (12.35 to <50.00)	0.89 (0.14–5.68)	0.84 (0.47–1.51)	0.50 (0.23–1.09)
Tertile 3 (≥50.00)	1.77 (0.15–21.09)	0.73 (0.37–1.42)	1.32 (0.59–2.94)

[a] Adjusted for gender, race, education, marital status, occupation, family income, body mass index, physical activity, alcohol use, smoking status, depressive symptoms, diabetes, hypertension, use of female hormones, C-reactive protein (mg/dL), caffeine intake (mg/day), and the other five phytoestrogens (tertiles). * $p < 0.05$, ** $p < 0.01$, *** $p < 0.001$.

Table 9. Weighted relative risk ratios (95% confidence intervals) for sleep duration (reference, 7–8 h/night) across tertiles of the urinary phytoestrogen concentrations stratified by gender (National Health and Nutrition Examination Survey 2005–2010).

Phytoestrogen Concentrations (µg/g Creatinine)	Model 3 [a]		
	Very Short Sleep (<5 h/Night)	Short Sleep (5–6 h/Night)	Long Sleep (≥9 h/Night)
Females			
Enterolactone			
Tertile 1 (<160.53)	1.00 (reference)	1.00 (reference)	1.00 (reference)
Tertile 2 (160.53 to <621.68)	0.69 (0.38–1.27)	0.99 (0.63–1.55)	1.55 (0.83–2.87)
Tertile 3 (≥621.68)	0.61 (0.31–1.20)	0.91 (0.62–1.35)	0.74 (0.35–1.54)
Enterodiol			
Tertile 1 (<21.52)	1.00 (reference)	1.00 (reference)	1.00 (reference)
Tertile 2 (21.52 to <70.27)	1.39 (0.70–2.77)	0.77 (0.53–1.13)	1.03 (0.56–1.90)
Tertile 3 (≥70.27)	0.91 (0.42–1.99)	0.99 (0.61–1.59)	2.14 (1.11–4.13) *
Daidzein			
Tertile 1 (<24.22)	1.00 (reference)	1.00 (reference)	1.00 (reference)
Tertile 2 (24.22 to <108.62)	1.50 (0.58–3.89)	0.85 (0.57–1.28)	0.79 (0.34–1.86)
Tertile 3 (≥108.62)	1.69 (0.35–8.12)	0.72 (0.41–1.28)	0.75 (0.27–2.10)
O-Desmethylangolensin			
Tertile 1 (<1.04)	1.00 (reference)	1.00 (reference)	1.00 (reference)
Tertile 2 (1.04 to <9.06)	1.33 (0.63–2.80)	1.25 (0.83–1.87)	1.19 (0.64–2.20)
Tertile 3 (≥9.06)	0.87 (0.32–2.39)	1.23 (0.77–1.97)	2.23 (0.95–5.26)
Equol			
Tertile 1 (<3.75)	1.00 (reference)	1.00 (reference)	1.00 (reference)
Tertile 2 (3.75 to <9.73)	0.90 (0.44–1.85)	0.95 (0.71–1.27)	1.12 (0.64–1.97)
Tertile 3 (≥9.73)	0.54 (0.25–1.16)	0.76 (0.53–1.09)	0.74 (0.39–1.40)
Genistein			
Tertile 1 (<12.35)	1.00 (reference)	1.00 (reference)	1.00 (reference)
Tertile 2 (12.35 to <50.00)	0.58 (0.26–1.31)	1.50 (0.93–2.41)	0.70 (0.34–1.45)
Tertile 3 (≥50.00)	0.70 (0.17–2.85)	1.37 (0.76–2.46)	0.70 (0.29–1.69)

Table 9. Cont.

Phytoestrogen Concentrations (μg/g Creatinine)	Model 3 [a]		
	Very Short Sleep (<5 h/Night)	Short Sleep (5–6 h/Night)	Long Sleep (≥9 h/Night)
Males			
Enterolactone			
Tertile 1 (<160.53)	1.00 (reference)	1.00 (reference)	1.00 (reference)
Tertile 2 (160.53 to <621.68)	1.48 (0.70–3.13)	1.29 (0.89–1.88)	1.20 (0.65–2.23)
Tertile 3 (≥621.68)	0.50 (0.23–1.13)	0.94 (0.62–1.42)	0.89 (0.44–1.82)
Enterodiol			
Tertile 1 (<21.52)	1.00 (reference)	1.00 (reference)	1.00 (reference)
Tertile 2 (21.52 to <70.27)	1.31 (0.60–2.87)	1.40 (0.99–1.99)	1.05 (0.56–1.98)
Tertile 3 (≥70.27)	0.95 (0.39–2.28)	1.06 (0.73–1.54)	0.93 (0.47–1.84)
Daidzein			
Tertile 1 (<24.22)	1.00 (reference)	1.00 (reference)	1.00 (reference)
Tertile 2 (24.22 to <108.62)	0.63 (0.23–1.76)	1.28 (0.87–1.88)	1.72 (0.82–3.59)
Tertile 3 (≥108.62)	1.14 (0.24–5.40)	1.87 (0.95–3.65)	1.79 (0.68–4.72)
O-Desmethylangolensin			
Tertile 1 (<1.04)	1.00 (reference)	1.00 (reference)	1.00 (reference)
Tertile 2 (1.04 to <9.06)	1.59 (0.65–3.87)	0.90 (0.69–1.16)	0.94 (0.50–1.76)
Tertile 3 (≥9.06)	0.75 (0.21–2.68)	0.70 (0.46–1.04)	0.83 (0.38–1.82)
Equol			
Tertile 1 (<3.75)	1.00 (reference)	1.00 (reference)	1.00 (reference)
Tertile 2 (3.75 to <9.73)	1.07 (0.64–1.79)	1.06 (0.74–1.51)	0.95 (0.49–1.82)
Tertile 3 (≥9.73)	1.22 (0.66–2.26)	1.29 (0.92–1.81)	1.18 (0.62–2.27)
Genistein			
Tertile 1 (<12.35)	1.00 (reference)	1.00 (reference)	1.00 (reference)
Tertile 2 (12.35 to <50.00)	1.55 (0.61–3.93)	0.90 (0.63–1.29)	0.51 (0.30–0.87) *
Tertile 3 (≥50.00)	1.78 (0.68–4.62)	0.81 (0.51–1.27)	0.51 (0.25–1.02)

[a] Adjusted for age, race, education, marital status, occupation, family income, body mass index, physical activity, alcohol use, smoking status, depressive symptoms, diabetes, hypertension, use of female hormones (only in females), C-reactive protein (mg/dL), caffeine intake (mg/day), and the other five phytoestrogens (tertiles). * $p < 0.05$.

4. Discussion

To our knowledge, the current study was the first evaluation of the associations between the urinary concentrations of individual phytoestrogens (enterolactone, enterodiol, daidzein, O-DMA, equol, and genistein) and sleep disorders and sleep duration among general American adults. This study was based on data from the NHANES 2005–2010 and found that the urinary enterolactone concentration was linearly inversely associated with the risk of sleep disorders, while the enterodiol concentration was positively related to sleep disorders in an approximately linear manner and the O-DMA concentration was positively associated with sleep disorders in a nonlinear (inverted L-shaped) manner. The urinary enterolactone concentration was negatively associated with very short sleep, and the genistein concentration was inversely related to a long sleep risk. Furthermore, a negative association of the urinary genistein concentration with sleep disorders was observed in middle-aged adults (40–59 years). The urinary enterolactone concentration was inversely associated with a long sleep risk among older adults (≥60 years), while the enterodiol concentration was positively related to a long sleep risk in females and very short sleep in young adults (18–39 years). Finally, an interesting finding was that the urinary O-DMA concentration was positively related to sleep disorders in both females aged 40–59 years and non-Hispanic Whites, but was inversely associated with sleep disorders in both females aged 60 years or over and other Hispanics.

There has been no epidemiological study that has appraised the relationship of total lignans or individual lignans (enterolactone or enterodiol) with sleep disorders to date. However, animal experiments have indicated that a lignan component could increase sleep duration and decrease sleep latency via modulating the γ-aminobutyric acid (GABA)-ergic system [38,39], which supports our findings that enterolactone was negatively associated with sleep disorders and very short sleep, and enterodiol was positively related to a long sleep risk in females. We also found that enterolactone was inversely associated with a long sleep risk among older adults (≥60 years), while enterodiol was positively associated with sleep disorders in the whole population and very short sleep in young adults (18–39 years). This seems to suggest that enterolactone might be beneficial for preventing both long and very short sleep, whereas enterodiol might be adverse toward this goal. However, further comparisons were difficult due to limited prior studies.

Some studies have evaluated the association between total isoflavone consumption and sleep but the results were contradictory. A study with a cross-sectional design performed in Japanese adults found that the intake of isoflavone was positively related to sleep quality and optimal sleep duration [36]. Another longitudinal study of Chinese adults reported that isoflavone intake was inversely related to falling asleep in the daytime in females and long sleep duration in both genders [37], which was similar to our result regarding genistein and a long sleep risk. Several trial studies also showed that isoflavone supplementation alleviated insomnia or sleep disorders among climacteric women [28–31]. However, other trial studies of isoflavone supplementation in climacteric women or androgen-deprived males found no significant improvement in insomnia or sleep quality [32–34]. Meanwhile, another randomized, placebo-controlled, double-blinded trial over six months performed on climacteric women indicated that insomnia was more frequent in the isoflavone supplementation group [35], and the longitudinal study reported that soy milk (one of the main food sources for isoflavone intake in the study) was positively related to falling asleep in the daytime among males [37]. Similarly, we found a positive association between O-DMA and sleep disorders.

Thus far, little is known about individual isoflavones (daidzein, O-DMA, equol, and genistein) and sleep. The current study found discrepant associations of them with sleep disorders, where O-DMA was positively associated with sleep disorders, and genistein was negatively associated with sleep disorders in middle-aged adults (40–59 years). Likewise, there were also differential relationships between them and sleep duration, where only genistein was significantly inversely related to a long sleep risk, and no significant associations were found between daidzein, O-DMA, and equol and sleep duration in this study. Variable abilities in different individuals regarding the metabolic transformation of isoflavones [23], diverse biologic activities, and ER affinities of these metabolites (O-DMA and equol), as well as other individual isoflavones (daidzein and genistein) [40,41], and discrepant associations between them and sleep disorders or sleep duration may partially lead to the contradictory findings of prior studies focusing only on total isoflavones. Furthermore, potential gender, age, and race differences regarding these associations may also partially contribute to the prior contradictory findings.

The underlying mechanisms of the associations of phytoestrogens with sleep are unclear, where the following are several possible explanations. Estrogen can influence the synthesis and transport of serotonin [62] that is involved in the regulation of wakefulness and sleep [63], and studies have revealed that estrogen therapy alleviates sleep disturbances and improves sleep quality [10,11]. Therefore, phytoestrogens may affect the sleep–wake cycle through their estrogenic or anti-estrogenic effects [19], which may also explain the discrepant relationships of individual phytoestrogens with sleep disorders or sleep duration. A notable finding in our study was that the urinary O-DMA concentration was positively related to sleep disorders in females aged 40–59 years but was inversely associated with sleep disorders in females aged 60 years or over, which may be partly attributed to the anti-estrogenic and estrogenic effects of phytoestrogens, depending on the level of endogenous estrogen [64]. We also found that the urinary O-DMA concentration was positively related to sleep disorders in non-Hispanic Whites but was inversely associated with sleep disorders in other Hispanics, which may be partially due to the race difference in the compositions of gut microbiota and daidzein-metabolizing phenotypes [61,65]. Equol has estrogenic activities [66], which may partly contribute to the inverse association of equol with sleep disorders in females aged 18–39 years, while the mechanisms for the positive association between equol and sleep disorders in other Hispanics need to be investigated. Furthermore, the inter-individual variation of phytoestrogen metabolism by gut microbiota [67] may also contribute to the complexity of these results. The above-mentioned mechanisms may partly explain our findings, and further studies on the related mechanisms remain necessary.

This study has several advantages. First, the phytoestrogen assessments were based on urinary biomarkers, which reflected all food origins of phytoestrogens and took into account the metabolic transformation of intestinal flora, representing true and biologically effective exposures. Second, the relationships with sleep disorders or sleep duration were evaluated for individual phytoestrogens (enterolactone, enterodiol, daidzein, O-DMA, equol, and genistein), which made up for the fact that previous epidemiological studies did not investigate the relationship of lignans with sleep and focused only on total isoflavones while ignoring the potential differences of individual isoflavones. Third, our findings were based on data from the NHANES, which was carefully designed, of high quality, and nationally representative. Fourth, concentration–response relationships between individual phytoestrogens and sleep disorders were appraised in this study. Fifth, we further explored gender, age, and race differences in the associations of individual phytoestrogens with sleep disorders. Additionally, we adjusted for a wide range of confounders to control for potential confounding bias.

However, several potential limitations should also be considered. First of all, the cross-sectional design precludes the possibility of causal inference. Second, although phytoestrogen concentrations in spot urine are reliable biomarkers for phytoestrogen intake [23,50,51], it might be difficult to accurately reflect long-term intake information because spot urine was collected only once. Nonetheless, studies have demonstrated that phytoestrogen concentrations in spot urine are relatively stable and significantly related to dietary phytoestrogen intake over the long term [68,69]. Third, the sleep disorders assessment was via a self-reported doctor diagnosis, which might involve recall bias, and self-reported usual sleep duration might be not objective enough; however, objective sleep measurement, such as polysomnography, may be difficult to implement in large-scale surveys. Fourth, although three-cycle data with national representativeness were combined and the sample was relatively large, the case group might still be not enough due to the lower prevalence, which might lead to bias. Furthermore, although we adjusted multiple covariates, measurement errors and other factors affecting sleep quality might influence the present findings. However, the present results were approximate in the three models, suggesting that the results might be robust and exposure factors might be independently associated with sleep. Finally, we could not further explore the relationships between phytoestrogens and specific types of sleep disorders in virtue of the limited sleep disorders data.

5. Conclusions

The current findings suggested that the urinary enterolactone concentration was linearly inversely associated with the risk of sleep disorders among American adults, whereas the enterodiol and O-DMA concentrations were positively related to sleep disorders in approximately linear and inverted L-shaped manners, respectively. Meanwhile, the urinary enterolactone concentration was negatively associated with very short sleep and the genistein concentration was inversely related to a long sleep risk. Furthermore, a negative association of urinary genistein concentration with sleep disorders was observed in middle-aged adults. The urinary enterolactone concentration was inversely associated with a long sleep risk among older adults, while the enterodiol concentration was positively related to a long sleep risk in females and very short sleep in young adults. Finally, a notable finding was that the association of the urinary O-DMA concentration with sleep disorders was different between females aged 40–59 years and females aged 60 years or over, as well as between non-Hispanic Whites and other Hispanics. It may be meaningful and vital to choose more specific individual phytoestrogens, not choosing total lignans or isoflavones for preventing or improving sleep problems, and to match target groups given the potentially differential associations of individual phytoestrogens with sleep, as well as the gender, age, and race differences in the associations. Prospective cohort or trial studies evaluating the relationships of individual phytoestrogens with sleep are warranted to confirm the current findings.

Supplementary Materials: The following are available online at http://www.mdpi.com/2072-6643/12/7/2103/s1, Table S1. The classifications of the covariates.

Author Contributions: Conceptualization, J.S. and D.Z.; methodology, J.S., W.W., and D.Z.; data curation, J.S., X.D., and H.J.; writing—original draft preparation, J.S.; writing—review and editing, H.J. and D.Z. All authors have read and agreed to the published version of the manuscript.

Funding: This research received no external funding.

Acknowledgments: This study used data from the National Health and Nutrition Examination Survey (NHANES). The authors would like to thank all participants and contributors to the NHANES. This work was supported by the Taishan Scholars Construction Project.

Conflicts of Interest: The authors declare no conflict of interest.

References

1. Sateia, M.J. International classification of sleep disorders-third edition: Highlights and modifications. *Chest* **2014**, *146*, 1387–1394. [CrossRef] [PubMed]
2. Pavlova, M.K.; Latreille, V. Sleep Disorders. *Am. J. Med.* **2019**, *132*, 292–299. [CrossRef] [PubMed]
3. Taheri, S.; Lin, L.; Austin, D.; Young, T.; Mignot, E. Short sleep duration is associated with reduced leptin, elevated ghrelin, and increased body mass index. *PLoS Med.* **2004**, *1*, e62. [CrossRef] [PubMed]
4. Hoevenaar-Blom, M.P.; Spijkerman, A.M.; Kromhout, D.; Verschuren, W.M. Sufficient sleep duration contributes to lower cardiovascular disease risk in addition to four traditional lifestyle factors: The MORGEN study. *Eur. J. Prev. Cardiol.* **2014**, *21*, 1367–1375. [CrossRef]
5. Ayas, N.T.; White, D.P.; Al-Delaimy, W.K.; Manson, J.E.; Stampfer, M.J.; Speizer, F.E.; Patel, S.; Hu, F.B. A prospective study of self-reported sleep duration and incident diabetes in women. *Diabetes Care* **2003**, *26*, 380–384. [CrossRef] [PubMed]
6. Meng, L.; Zheng, Y.; Hui, R. The relationship of sleep duration and insomnia to risk of hypertension incidence: A meta-analysis of prospective cohort studies. *Hypertens. Res.* **2013**, *36*, 985–995. [CrossRef]
7. Gozal, D.; Farre, R.; Nieto, F.J. Obstructive sleep apnea and cancer: Epidemiologic links and theoretical biological constructs. *Sleep Med. Rev.* **2016**, *27*, 43–55. [CrossRef]
8. Yin, J.; Jin, X.; Shan, Z.; Li, S.; Huang, H.; Li, P.; Peng, X.; Peng, Z.; Yu, K.; Bao, W.; et al. Relationship of sleep duration with all-cause mortality and cardiovascular events: A systematic review and dose-response meta-analysis of prospective cohort studies. *J. Am. Heart Assoc.* **2017**, *6*. [CrossRef]
9. McEwen, B.S.; Alves, S.E. Estrogen actions in the central nervous system. *Endocr. Rev.* **1999**, *20*, 279–307. [CrossRef]
10. Wiklund, I.; Karlberg, J.; Mattsson, L.A. Quality of life of postmenopausal women on a regimen of transdermal estradiol therapy: A double-blind placebo-controlled study. *Am. J. Obstet. Gynecol.* **1993**, *168*, 824–830. [CrossRef]
11. Ensrud, K.E.; Guthrie, K.A.; Hohensee, C.; Caan, B.; Carpenter, J.S.; Freeman, E.W.; LaCroix, A.Z.; Landis, C.A.; Manson, J.; Newton, K.M.; et al. Effects of estradiol and venlafaxine on insomnia symptoms and sleep quality in women with hot flashes. *Sleep* **2015**, *38*, 97–108. [CrossRef]
12. Polo-Kantola, P.; Erkkola, R.; Helenius, H.; Irjala, K.; Polo, O. When does estrogen replacement therapy improve sleep quality? *Am. J. Obstet. Gynecol.* **1998**, *178*, 1002–1009. [CrossRef]
13. Canonico, M.; Plu-Bureau, G.; Lowe, G.D.; Scarabin, P.Y. Hormone replacement therapy and risk of venous thromboembolism in postmenopausal women: Systematic review and meta-analysis. *Brit. Med. J.* **2008**, *336*, 1227–1231. [CrossRef] [PubMed]
14. Furness, S.; Roberts, H.; Marjoribanks, J.; Lethaby, A. Hormone therapy in postmenopausal women and risk of endometrial hyperplasia. *Cochrane Database Syst. Rev.* **2012**. [CrossRef] [PubMed]
15. Benson, V.S.; Kirichek, O.; Beral, V.; Green, J. Menopausal hormone therapy and central nervous system tumor risk: Large UK prospective study and meta-analysis. *Int. J. Cancer* **2015**, *136*, 2369–2377. [CrossRef]
16. Greiser, C.M.; Greiser, E.M.; Doren, M. Menopausal hormone therapy and risk of breast cancer: A meta-analysis of epidemiological studies and randomized controlled trials. *Hum. Reprod. Update* **2005**, *11*, 561–573. [CrossRef]
17. Greiser, C.M.; Greiser, E.M.; Doren, M. Menopausal hormone therapy and risk of ovarian cancer: Systematic review and meta-analysis. *Hum. Reprod. Update* **2007**, *13*, 453–463. [CrossRef]

18. Nie, Q.; Xing, M.; Hu, J.; Hu, X.; Nie, S.; Xie, M. Metabolism and health effects of phyto-estrogens. *Crit. Rev. Food Sci. Nutr.* **2017**, *57*, 2432–2454. [CrossRef]
19. Mueller, S.O.; Simon, S.; Chae, K.; Metzler, M.; Korach, K.S. Phytoestrogens and their human metabolites show distinct agonistic and antagonistic properties on estrogen receptor alpha (ERalpha) and ERbeta in human cells. *Toxicol. Sci.* **2004**, *80*, 14–25. [CrossRef]
20. Patisaul, H.B.; Jefferson, W. The pros and cons of phytoestrogens. *Front. Neuroendocrinol.* **2010**, *31*, 400–419. [CrossRef]
21. Thompson, L.U.; Robb, P.; Serraino, M.; Cheung, F. Mammalian lignan production from various foods. *Nutr. Cancer* **1991**, *16*, 43–52. [CrossRef] [PubMed]
22. Knight, D.C.; Eden, J.A. Phytoestrogens—A short review. *Maturitas* **1995**, *22*, 167–175. [CrossRef]
23. Lampe, J.W. Isoflavonoid and lignan phytoestrogens as dietary biomarkers. *J. Nutr.* **2003**, *133* (Suppl. 3), 956s–964s. [CrossRef] [PubMed]
24. Lampe, J.W.; Atkinson, C.; Hullar, M.A. Assessing exposure to lignans and their metabolites in humans. *J. AOAC Int.* **2006**, *89*, 1174–1181. [CrossRef] [PubMed]
25. Atkinson, C.; Frankenfeld, C.L.; Lampe, J.W. Gut bacterial metabolism of the soy isoflavone daidzein: Exploring the relevance to human health. *Exp. Biol. Med.* **2005**, *230*, 155–170. [CrossRef]
26. Kuhnle, G.G.; Dell'Aquila, C.; Aspinall, S.M.; Runswick, S.A.; Mulligan, A.A.; Bingham, S.A. Phytoestrogen content of foods of animal origin: Dairy products, eggs, meat, fish, and seafood. *J. Agric. Food Chem.* **2008**, *56*, 10099–10104. [CrossRef] [PubMed]
27. Frankenfeld, C.L. Dairy consumption is a significant correlate of urinary equol concentration in a representative sample of US adults. *Am. J. Clin. Nutr.* **2011**, *93*, 1109–1116. [CrossRef] [PubMed]
28. Albert, A.; Altabre, C.; Baró, F.; Buendía, E.; Cabero, A.; Cancelo, M.J.; Castelo-Branco, C.; Chantre, P.; Duran, M.; Haya, J.; et al. Efficacy and safety of a phytoestrogen preparation derived from Glycine max (L.) Merr in climacteric symptomatology: A multicentric, open, prospective and non-randomized trial. *Phytomedicine* **2002**, *9*, 85–92. [CrossRef]
29. Hachul, H.; Brandao, L.C.; D'Almeida, V.; Bittencourt, L.R.; Baracat, E.C.; Tufik, S. Isoflavones decrease insomnia in postmenopause. *Menopause* **2011**, *18*, 178–184. [CrossRef] [PubMed]
30. Davinelli, S.; Scapagnini, G.; Marzatico, F.; Nobile, V.; Ferrara, N.; Corbi, G. Influence of equol and resveratrol supplementation on health-related quality of life in menopausal women: A randomized, placebo-controlled study. *Maturitas* **2017**, *96*, 77–83. [CrossRef] [PubMed]
31. Hirose, A.; Terauchi, M.; Akiyoshi, M.; Owa, Y.; Kato, K.; Kubota, T. Low-dose isoflavone aglycone alleviates psychological symptoms of menopause in Japanese women: A randomized, double-blind, placebo-controlled study. *Arch. Gynecol. Obstet.* **2016**, *293*, 609–615. [CrossRef] [PubMed]
32. Uesugi, S.; Watanabe, S.; Ishiwata, N.; Uehara, M.; Ouchi, K. Effects of isoflavone supplements on bone metabolic markers and climacteric symptoms in Japanese women. *Biofactors* **2004**, *22*, 221–228. [CrossRef] [PubMed]
33. Sharma, P.; Wisniewski, A.; Braga-Basaria, M.; Xu, X.; Yep, M.; Denmeade, S.; Dobs, A.S.; DeWeese, T.; Carducci, M.; Basaria, S. Lack of an effect of high dose isoflavones in men with prostate cancer undergoing androgen deprivation therapy. *J. Urol.* **2009**, *182*, 2265–2272. [CrossRef] [PubMed]
34. Costa, J.G.; Giolo, J.S.; Mariano, I.M.; Batista, J.P.; Ribeiro, A.; Souza, T.; de Oliveira, E.P.; Resende, A.; Puga, G.M. Combined exercise training reduces climacteric symptoms without the additive effects of isoflavone supplementation: A clinical, controlled, randomised, double-blind study. *Nutr. Health* **2017**, *23*, 271–279. [CrossRef]
35. Balk, J.L.; Whiteside, D.A.; Naus, G.; DeFerrari, E.; Roberts, J.M. A pilot study of the effects of phytoestrogen supplementation on postmenopausal endometrium. *J. Soc. Gynecol. Investig.* **2002**, *9*, 238–242. [CrossRef]
36. Cui, Y.; Niu, K.; Huang, C.; Momma, H.; Guan, L.; Kobayashi, Y.; Guo, H.; Chujo, M.; Otomo, A.; Nagatomi, R. Relationship between daily isoflavone intake and sleep in Japanese adults: A cross-sectional study. *Nutr. J.* **2015**, *14*, 127. [CrossRef]
37. Cao, Y.; Taylor, A.W.; Zhen, S.; Adams, R.; Appleton, S.; Shi, Z. Soy isoflavone intake and sleep parameters over 5 years among Chinese adults: Longitudinal analysis from the Jiangsu Nutrition Study. *J. Acad. Nutr. Diet.* **2017**, *117*, 536–544 e532. [CrossRef]

38. Zhu, H.; Zhang, L.; Wang, G.; He, Z.; Zhao, Y.; Xu, Y.; Gao, Y.; Zhang, L. Sedative and hypnotic effects of supercritical carbon dioxide fluid extraction from Schisandra chinensis in mice. *J. Food Drug Anal.* **2016**, *24*, 831–838. [CrossRef]
39. Li, N.; Liu, J.; Wang, M.; Yu, Z.; Zhu, K.; Gao, J.; Wang, C.; Sun, J.; Chen, J.; Li, H. Sedative and hypnotic effects of Schisandrin B through increasing GABA/Glu ratio and upregulating the expression of $GABA_A$ in mice and rats. *Biomed. Pharmacother.* **2018**, *103*, 509–516. [CrossRef]
40. Hu, C.; Yuan, Y.V.; Kitts, D.D. Antioxidant activities of the flaxseed lignan secoisolariciresinol diglucoside, its aglycone secoisolariciresinol and the mammalian lignans enterodiol and enterolactone in vitro. *Food Chem. Toxicol.* **2007**, *45*, 2219–2227. [CrossRef]
41. Muthyala, R.S.; Ju, Y.H.; Sheng, S.; Williams, L.D.; Doerge, D.R.; Katzenellenbogen, B.S.; Helferich, W.G.; Katzenellenbogen, J.A. Equol, a natural estrogenic metabolite from soy isoflavones: Convenient preparation and resolution of R- and S-equols and their differing binding and biological activity through estrogen receptors alpha and beta. *Bioorg. Med. Chem.* **2004**, *12*, 1559–1567. [CrossRef]
42. Montalesi, E.; Cipolletti, M.; Cracco, P.; Ficcchetti, M.; Marino, M. Divergent effects of daidzein and its metabolites on estrogen-induced survival of breast cancer cells. *Cancers* **2020**, *12*, 167. [CrossRef] [PubMed]
43. Carreau, C.; Flouriot, G.; Bennetau-Pelissero, C.; Potier, M. Enterodiol and enterolactone, two major diet-derived polyphenol metabolites have different impact on ERalpha transcriptional activation in human breast cancer cells. *J. Steroid Biochem. Mol. Biol.* **2008**, *110*, 176–185. [CrossRef]
44. Reger, M.K.; Zollinger, T.W.; Liu, Z.; Jones, J.; Zhang, J. Urinary phytoestrogens and cancer, cardiovascular, and all-cause mortality in the continuous National Health and Nutrition Examination Survey. *Eur. J. Nutr.* **2016**, *55*, 1029–1040. [CrossRef]
45. Richard, A.; Rohrmann, S.; Mohler-Kuo, M.; Rodgers, S.; Moffat, R.; Güth, U.; Eichholzer, M. Urinary phytoestrogens and depression in perimenopausal US women: NHANES 2005–2008. *J. Affect. Disord.* **2014**, *156*, 200–205. [CrossRef] [PubMed]
46. Xu, C.; Liu, Q.; Zhang, Q.; Gu, A.; Jiang, Z.Y. Urinary enterolactone is associated with obesity and metabolic alteration in men in the US National Health and Nutrition Examination Survey 2001-10. *Br. J. Nutr.* **2015**, *113*, 683–690. [CrossRef] [PubMed]
47. Centers for Disease Control and Prevention. National Health and Nutrition Examination Survey. Available online: https://www.cdc.gov/nchs/nhanes/index.htm (accessed on 28 April 2020).
48. Zipf, G.; Chiappa, M.; Porter, K.S.; Ostchega, Y.; Lewis, B.G.; Dostal, J. National health and nutrition examination survey: Plan and operations, 1999–2010. *Vital Health Stat 1* **2013**, *56*, 1–37.
49. Centers for Disease Control and Prevention, National Health and Nutrition Examination Survey. Laboratory Procedure Manual, Phytoestrogens. Available online: http://www.cdc.gov/nchs/data/nhanes/nhanes_09_10/Phyto_F_met_phytoestrogens.pdf (accessed on 28 April 2020).
50. Grace, P.B.; Taylor, J.I.; Low, Y.L.; Luben, R.N.; Mulligan, A.A.; Botting, N.P.; Dowsett, M.; Welch, A.A.; Khaw, K.T.; Wareham, N.J.; et al. Phytoestrogen concentrations in serum and spot urine as biomarkers for dietary phytoestrogen intake and their relation to breast cancer risk in European prospective investigation of cancer and nutrition-norfolk. *Cancer Epidemiol. Biomarkers Prev.* **2004**, *13*, 698–708.
51. Seow, A.; Shi, C.Y.; Franke, A.A.; Hankin, J.H.; Lee, H.P.; Yu, M.C. Isoflavonoid levels in spot urine are associated with frequency of dietary soy intake in a population-based sample of middle-aged and older Chinese in Singapore. *Cancer Epidemiol. Biomarkers Prev.* **1998**, *7*, 135–140.
52. Struja, T.; Richard, A.; Linseisen, J.; Eichholzer, M.; Rohrmann, S. The association between urinary phytoestrogen excretion and components of the metabolic syndrome in NHANES. *Eur. J. Nutr.* **2014**, *53*, 1371–1381. [CrossRef]
53. National Health and Nutrition Examination Survey 2007–2008 Data Documentation. Analytic Notes. Available online: https://wwwn.cdc.gov/Nchs/Nhanes/2007-2008/ALB_CR_E.htm (accessed on 28 April 2020).
54. Beydoun, H.A.; Beydoun, M.A.; Jeng, H.A.; Zonderman, A.B.; Eid, S.M. Bisphenol—A and sleep adequacy among adults in the national health and nutrition examination surveys. *Sleep* **2016**, *39*, 467–476. [CrossRef] [PubMed]
55. Patel, P.; Shiff, B.; Kohn, T.P.; Ramasamy, R. Impaired sleep is associated with low testosterone in US adult males: Results from the National Health and Nutrition Examination Survey. *World J. Urol.* **2019**, *37*, 1449–1453. [CrossRef] [PubMed]

56. Grandner, M.A.; Jackson, N.; Gerstner, J.R.; Knutson, K.L. Dietary nutrients associated with short and long sleep duration. Data from a nationally representative sample. *Appetite* **2013**, *64*, 71–80. [CrossRef] [PubMed]
57. Scinicariello, F.; Buser, M.C.; Feroe, A.G.; Attanasio, R. Antimony and sleep-related disorders: NHANES 2005-2008. *Environ. Res* **2017**, *156*, 247–252. [CrossRef] [PubMed]
58. Centers for Disease Control and Prevention. Continuous NHANES Web Tutorial. Available online: https://www.cdc.gov/nchs/tutorials/NHANES/index_continuous.htm (accessed on 28 April 2020).
59. Vaz Fragoso, C.A.; Van Ness, P.H.; Araujo, K.L.; Iannone, L.P.; Klar Yaggi, H. Age-related differences in sleep-wake symptoms of adults undergoing polysomnography. *J. Am. Geriatr. Soc.* **2015**, *63*, 1845–1851. [CrossRef] [PubMed]
60. Roehrs, T.; Kapke, A.; Roth, T.; Breslau, N. Sex differences in the polysomnographic sleep of young adults: A community-based study. *Sleep Med.* **2006**, *7*, 49–53. [CrossRef]
61. Atkinson, C.; Newton, K.M.; Bowles, E.J.; Yong, M.; Lampe, J.W. Demographic, anthropometric, and lifestyle factors and dietary intakes in relation to daidzein-metabolizing phenotypes among premenopausal women in the United States. *Am. J. Clin. Nutr.* **2008**, *87*, 679–687. [CrossRef]
62. Sherwin, B.B. Hormones, mood, and cognitive functioning in postmenopausal women. *Obstet. Gynecol.* **1996**, *87*, 20s–26s. [CrossRef]
63. Zeitzer, J.M.; Maidment, N.T.; Behnke, E.J.; Ackerson, L.C.; Fried, I.; Engel, J.; Jr Wilson, C.L. Ultradian sleep-cycle variation of serotonin in the human lateral ventricle. *Neurology* **2002**, *59*, 1272–1274. [CrossRef] [PubMed]
64. Brzezinski, A.; Debi, A. Phytoestrogens: The "natural" selective estrogen receptor modulators? *Eur. J. Obstet. Gynecol. Reprod. Biol.* **1999**, *85*, 47–51. [CrossRef]
65. Deschasaux, M.; Bouter, K.E.; Prodan, A.; Levin, E.; Groen, A.K.; Herrema, H.; Tremaroli, V.; Bakker, G.J.; Attaye, I.; Pinto-Sietsma, S.J.; et al. Depicting the composition of gut microbiota in a population with varied ethnic origins but shared geography. *Nat. Med.* **2018**, *24*, 1526–1531. [CrossRef] [PubMed]
66. Setchell, K.D.; Clerici, C. Equol: History, chemistry, and formation. *J. Nutr.* **2010**, *140*, 1355S–1362S. [CrossRef]
67. Gaya, P.; Medina, M.; Sánchez-Jiménez, A.; Landete, J.M. Phytoestrogen metabolism by adult human gut microbiota. *Molecules* **2016**, *21*, 1034. [CrossRef]
68. Lee, S.A.; Wen, W.; Xiang, Y.B.; Barnes, S.; Liu, D.; Cai, Q.; Zheng, W.; Shu, X.O. Assessment of dietary isoflavone intake among middle-aged Chinese men. *J. Nutr.* **2007**, *137*, 1011–1016. [CrossRef] [PubMed]
69. Shi, L.; Ryan, H.H.; Jones, E.; Simas, T.A.; Lichtenstein, A.H.; Sun, Q.; Hayman, L.L. Urinary isoflavone concentrations are inversely associated with cardiometabolic risk markers in pregnant U.S. women. *J. Nutr.* **2014**, *144*, 344–351. [CrossRef] [PubMed]

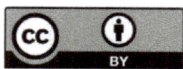

© 2020 by the authors. Licensee MDPI, Basel, Switzerland. This article is an open access article distributed under the terms and conditions of the Creative Commons Attribution (CC BY) license (http://creativecommons.org/licenses/by/4.0/).

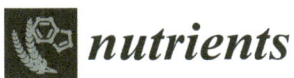

Article

Rice Bran Phenolic Extracts Modulate Insulin Secretion and Gene Expression Associated with β-Cell Function

Nancy Saji [1,2], Nidhish Francis [1,3], Lachlan J. Schwarz [1,4], Christopher L. Blanchard [1,2] and Abishek B. Santhakumar [1,2,*]

1. Australian Research Council (ARC) Industrial Transformation Training Centre (ITTC) for Functional Grains, Graham Centre for Agricultural Innovation Charles Sturt University, Wagga Wagga, NSW 2650, Australia; nsaji@csu.edu.au (N.S.); nfrancis@csu.edu.au (N.F.); lschwarz@csu.edu.au (L.J.S.); CBlanchard@csu.edu.au (C.L.B.)
2. School of Biomedical Sciences, Charles Sturt University, Locked Bag 588, Wagga Wagga, NSW 2678, Australia
3. School of Animal and Veterinary Sciences, Charles Sturt University, Locked Bag 588, Wagga Wagga, NSW 2678, Australia
4. School of Agricultural and Wine Sciences, Charles Sturt University, Locked Bag 588, Wagga Wagga, NSW 2678, Australia
* Correspondence: asanthakumar@csu.edu.au; Tel.: +61-2-6933-2678

Received: 10 May 2020; Accepted: 20 June 2020; Published: 24 June 2020

Abstract: Oxidative stress is known to modulate insulin secretion and initiate gene alterations resulting in impairment of β-cell function and type 2 diabetes mellitus (T2DM). Rice bran (RB) phenolic extracts contain bioactive properties that may target metabolic pathways associated with the pathogenesis of T2DM. This study aimed to examine the effect of stabilized RB phenolic extracts on the expression of genes associated with β-cell function such as glucose transporter 2 (*Glut2*), pancreatic and duodenal homeobox 1 (*Pdx1*), sirtuin 1 (*Sirt1*), mitochondrial transcription factor A (*Tfam*), and insulin 1 (*Ins1*) in addition to evaluating its impact on glucose-stimulated insulin secretion. It was observed that treatment with different concentrations of RB phenolic extracts (25–250 µg/mL) significantly increased the expression of *Glut2*, *Pdx1*, *Sirt1*, *Tfam*, and *Ins1* genes and glucose-stimulated insulin secretion under both normal and high glucose conditions. RB phenolic extracts favourably modulated the expression of genes involved in β-cell dysfunction and insulin secretion via several mechanisms such as synergistic action of polyphenols targeting signalling molecules, decreasing free radical damage by its antioxidant activity, and stimulation of effectors or survival factors of insulin secretion.

Keywords: rice bran; phenolic extracts; β-cell function; gene expression; insulin secretion

1. Introduction

Glucose homeostasis is regulated by a sequence of events within the pancreatic β-cells, which result in the secretion of insulin [1]. Typically, in the postprandial state, increased levels of glucose in plasma can initiate pancreatic β-cells to secrete insulin, consequently suppressing hepatic glucose output and increasing peripheral tissue glucose uptake [2]. However, impairment of glucose-stimulated insulin secretion as a result of oxidative stress and inflammation can result in β-cell dysfunction and insulin resistance, subsequently leading to the pathogenesis of type 2 diabetes mellitus (T2DM) [3]. There are several essential genes involved in insulin secretion pathways that are specifically expressed in pancreatic β-cells. They are known to be involved in the processes leading to insulin release from the initial glucose entry into the β-cells followed by mitochondrial adenosine triphosphate (ATP) generation and potassium and calcium membrane depolarization leading to exocytosis events [4].

They include, glucose transporter 2 (*Glut2*) [5], pancreatic and duodenal homeobox 1 (*Pdx1*) [6], sirtuin 1 (*Sirt1*) [7], mitochondrial transcription factor A (*Tfam*) [8], and insulin 1 (*Ins1*) [9].

The *Glut2* gene is located in the pancreatic plasma membrane and functions as a glucose transporter as part of the glucose-sensing mechanism for the stimulation of insulin secretion [2]. The *Pdx1* gene plays an important role in mitochondrial embryonic development and β-cell differentiation and is known to regulate the expression of a variety of different pancreatic endocrine genes, including *Glut2* [10]. The *Sirt1* gene is known to serve as a key energy redox sensor involved in generating ATP that helps promote glucose-stimulated insulin secretion in pancreatic β-cells and potentially contribute to β-cell adaptation in response to insulin resistance [1]. In the liver, skeletal muscles, and white adipose tissues, the *Sirt1* gene has key functions that include regulation of glucose production, improvement in insulin sensitivity via fatty acid oxidation, and control of the production of adipokines [7]. The *Tfam* gene plays an essential role in the maintenance of mitochondrial DNA (mtDNA) and replication [11]. Altered mitochondrial function is known to result in a defective oxidative metabolism, which seems to be involved in visceral fat gain and the development of insulin resistance [12]. Moreover, the *Tfam* gene is also involved in insulin exocytosis events by maintaining appropriate ADP/ATP ratio [4]. The *Ins1* gene and its transcription factors are regulated by the circulating levels of glucose [9]. It encodes the production of insulin that plays a vital role in the regulation of carbohydrate and lipid metabolism [13]. Therefore, a disruption in the function of these genes (*Glut2*, *Pdx1*, *Sirt1*, *Tfam*, and *Ins1*) in the pancreatic β-cells is known to impair insulin secretion and result in the development of T2DM.

Recent studies have shown the potential of plant-derived phenolic compounds in ameliorating β-cell dysfunction via their antioxidant and free radical scavenging properties [14–16]. Exposure of polyphenols to β-cells has also been responsible for the modulation of several signalling proteins, including transcription factors, protein kinase, and ion channels [17].

Rice bran (RB), a by-product of the rice milling process, is usually discarded or used as animal feed [18]. However, the bran layer is composed of several bioactive phytochemicals, including polyphenols and phenolic acids [19]. Although RB phenolic extracts are believed to target metabolic pathways associated with T2DM, the mechanisms behind its effect on gene expression under normal and diabetic conditions have not been investigated. This study aimed to determine the effect of RB phenolic extracts on the expression of genes (*Glut2*, *Pdx1*, *Sirt1*, *Tfam*, and *Ins1*) associated with insulin secretion pathways and on glucose-stimulated insulin secretion under normal and high glucose conditions.

2. Materials and Methods

2.1. Chemicals and Reagents

All chemicals and reagents used in this study were purchased from Promega Corporation (Madison, WI, USA), Bio-Rad (Hercules, CA, USA), or Sigma-Aldrich (St Louis, MO, USA).

2.2. Rice Bran Phenolic Extract Preparation

Commercially stabilized RB (drum-dried), from an Australian grown Reiziq rice variety, was obtained from SunRice Australia, courtesy of their milling plant in Leeton, NSW, Australia and subsequently stored at 4 °C until further analysis. Phenolic compounds were extracted from stabilized RB using an acetone/water/acetic acid (70:29.5:0.5, v/v) mixture, the characterization of which has been described elsewhere [18]. It is known to contain several bioactive compounds including ferulic acid, p-coumaric acid, caffeic acid, vanillic acid, syringic acid, sinapic acid, feruloyl glycoside, shikimic acid, ethyl vanillate, tricin, and their isomers. The extract was reconstituted in 50% dimethyl sulfoxide (DMSO) and stored at −20 °C before starting cell culture studies.

2.3. Cell Culture Conditions

INS-1E cells were maintained in RPMI 1640 media containing 11.1 mM glucose and supplemented with 2 mM L-Glutamine, 1 mM sodium pyruvate, 10 mM HEPES, 0.05 mM β-mercaptoethanol, 10% Fetal Bovine Serum, and 1% 10,000 U/mL Penicillin–10 mg/mL Streptomycin from Sigma-Aldrich (St Louis, MO, USA) at 37 °C in 5% CO_2 and used before reaching passage 45.

2.4. Cytotoxicity Assay

The cytotoxicity of RB phenolic extracts was examined using a resazurin red cytotoxicity assay wherein INS-1E cells were seeded into 96-well plates at a density of 50,000 cells per well and incubated for 24 h in the RPMI 1640 complete media. The cell count for experimental seeding was achieved with a Muse® Cell Analyzer from Luminex Corporation (Austin, TX, USA). INS-1E cells were then treated with 200 μL of freshly prepared RB phenolic extracts at various concentrations (25, 50, 100, 250, 500, 750, and 1000 μg/mL) for 6 h. Hydrogen peroxide (5 mM) was used as a positive control and 0.25% DMSO served as a negative control. Subsequently, all the treatment wells were emptied before adding 200 μL of resazurin red solution (14 mg/L) to each well and incubated for an additional 4 h at 37 °C in 5% CO_2. The absorbance was measured on a microplate reader (FLUOstar Omega microplate reader, BMG Labtech, Offenburg, Germany) at 570 and 600 nm against a resazurin red blank. The percentage of cell viability was calculated as described by Saji, Francis [20]. Each treatment was measured in octuplicate.

2.5. Expression of Genes Associated with β-Cell Function

2.5.1. Experimental Design

Two experimental conditions simultaneously tested were normal glucose treatment (11.1 mM) to represent a normal β-cell function and high glucose treatment (25 mM) to represent β-cell dysfunction under glucotoxic stress [4,15]. INS-1E cells were seeded at a density of 500,000 cells per well into 6-well plates and incubated for 24 h. To induce glucotoxicity, INS-1E cells were further subjected to 48 h incubation in RPMI 1640 complete media containing 25 mM glucose. Cells under both normal and high glucose conditions were treated for 6 h with RB phenolic extracts (25, 50, 100, and 250 μg/mL) and 0.125% DMSO served as the negative control. Each treatment was measured in quintuplicate.

2.5.2. Gene Expression Analysis

Total ribonucleic acid (RNA) extraction was conducted using the SV Total RNA Isolation System according to the manufacturer's instructions (Promega, Madison, WI, USA). RNA quality was determined using a NanoDrop™ 2000 c Spectrophotometer from Thermo Fisher Scientific (Waltham, MA, USA). Then, cDNA synthesis was conducted using a GoScript™ Reverse Transcriptase, according to the manufacturer's instructions (Promega, Madison, WI, USA).

Primers used for quantitative real-time polymerase chain reaction (qPCR) examinations are listed in Table 1. All of the qPCR primers were adapted from [21], designed using Primer3 software, and synthesized by Sigma-Aldrich (St Louis, MO, USA). The amplification efficiency was determined to be between 90–110% for all the primers before starting qPCR.

Gene expression was conducted in the CFX96 Touch™ Real-Time PCR Detection System (Bio-Rad) using SsoAdvanced™ Universal SYBR® Green Supermix (Bio-Rad) detection according to the manufacturer's instructions. The cycling conditions comprised 95 °C for 3 min, 95 °C for 10 s, and 60 °C for 30 s repeated for 39 cycles. The melt curve was generated at 65 °C for 5 s and 95 °C for 50 s. The endpoint or cycle threshold (Ct) values were obtained for all genes tested. The mean normalized expression of genes was determined using the Q-gene software application, as described by Muller, Janovjak [22]. *TfIIβ* served as the reference gene.

Table 1. The nucleotide sequences of the PCR primers used to assay gene expression by qPCR.

Gene	Forward Primer	Reverse Primer
Glut2	TCAGCCAGCCTGTGTATGCA	TCCACAAGCAGCACAGAGACA
Pdx1	CCGCGTTCATCTCCCTTT C	CTCCTGCCCACTGGCTTT T
Sirt1	CAGTGTCATGGTTCCTTTGC	CACCGAGGAACTACCTGA T
Tfam	GGGAAGAGCAAATGGCTGAA	TCACACTGCGACGGATGA GA
Ins1	TGCTCACCCGCGACCTT	GTTCATATGCACCACTGGACTGAA
TfIIβ	GTTCTGCTCCAACCTTTGCCT	TGTGTAGCTGCCATCTGCACT T

2.6. Glucose-Stimulated Insulin Secretion

The preparation of supernatant for the glucose-stimulated insulin secretion assay was adapted from a previous study conducted by Bhattacharya, Oksbjerg [15] with slight modifications. Briefly, INS-1E cells were seeded into a 24-well plate at a density of 1×10^5 cells/well and incubated for 24 h or until 70–80% confluency was reached. The cells were treated with DMSO control and RB extracts at different concentrations (25–250 µg/mL) and incubated for 6 h. Cells were then starved with a Krebs-Ringer bicarbonate buffer (125 mM NaCl, 5.9 mM KCl, 1.28 mM $CaCl_2$, 1.2 mM $MgCl_2$, 25 mM HEPES, and 0.1% BSA at pH 7.4) containing 5 mM glucose for 1 h. Glucose-stimulated insulin secretion was then induced by treating cells with a Krebs-Ringer bicarbonate buffer containing either 11.1 mM or 25 mM glucose for 1 h. The supernatant containing secreted insulin was collected and stored at −20 °C until further analysis. Insulin secretion was measured using a Rat *Ins1*/Insulin ELISA Kit purchased from Sigma-Aldrich (St Louis, MO, USA) according to the manufacturer's instructions. Each treatment was measured in sextuplicate.

2.7. Statistical Analysis

Statistical analysis was performed by one-way analysis of variance (ANOVA), followed by post-hoc Tukey's multiple comparisons test using GraphPad Prism 7 software (GraphPad Software Inc, San Diego, CA, USA) at a level of $p < 0.05$. The results are reported as mean ± standard deviation (SD).

3. Results

3.1. Cytotoxicity of RB Phenolic Extracts on INS-1E Cells

The cell viability of INS-1E cells 6 h post-exposure (Figure 1) to various concentrations of RB phenolic extracts did not display any cytotoxic effect on the INS-1E cells at the lower concentrations tested (25–250 µg/mL). However, higher concentrations (500–1000 µg/mL) displayed a reduction in cell viability. Optimal, non-toxic concentrations of RB extract were determined to be between 25–250 µg/mL under both normal and high glucose conditions.

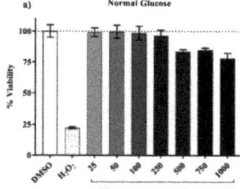
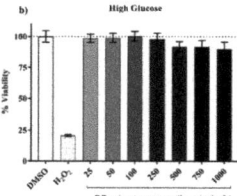

Figure 1. INS-1E cell viability 6 h post-exposure to various concentrations of RB phenolic extracts. (**a**) Normal glucose conditions, (**b**) High glucose conditions ($n = 8$). Data are presented as Mean ± SD. Dimethyl sulfoxide, DMSO; Hydrogen Peroxide, H_2O_2; Insulin-secreting rat insulinoma cell, INS-1E; Rice bran, RB.

3.2. Effect of RB Phenolic Extracts on Expression of Genes Associated with β-Cell Function

3.2.1. Expression of the *Glut2* Gene

Under normal glucose conditions, a significant increase ($p < 0.01$) in the expression of the *Glut2* gene was observed after treatment with 50 and 100 μg/mL of RB phenolic extracts when compared to that of the control. Under high glucose conditions, a significant increase ($p < 0.0001$) in the expression of the *Glut2* gene was also observed after treatment with 25–250 μg/mL of RB phenolic extracts when compared to that of the control (Figure 2).

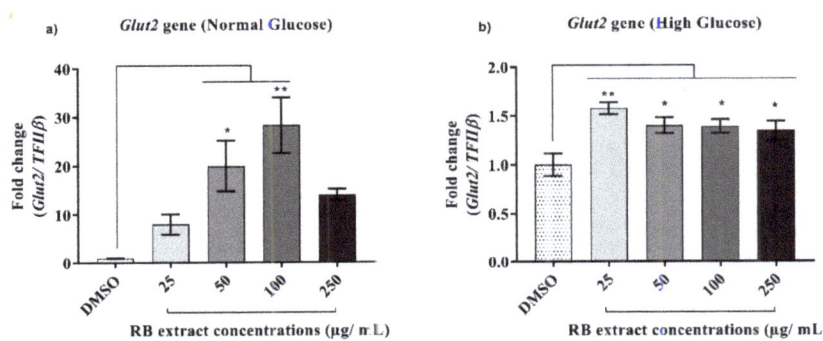

Figure 2. Effect of RB phenolic extracts on the expression of the *Glut2* gene under normal and high glucose conditions in INS-1E cells. (**a**) Normal glucose conditions, (**b**) High glucose conditions ($n = 5$). The level of significance is indicated by the asterisks, whereby * $p < 0.05$, ** $p < 0.01$. Data are presented as Mean ± SD. Dimethyl sulfoxide, DMSO; Insulin-secreting rat insulinoma cell, INS-1E; Glucose transporter 2, *Glut2*; Rice bran, RB.

3.2.2. Expression of the *Pdx1* Gene

A significant increase ($p < 0.05$) in the expression of the *Pdx1* gene was observed after treatment with 50 and 100 μg/mL of RB phenolic extracts under normal glucose conditions when compared to that of the control. A significant increase ($p < 0.001$) in the expression of the *Pdx1* gene was also observed after treatment with 25–250 μg/mL of RB phenolic extracts under high glucose conditions when compared to that of the control (Figure 3).

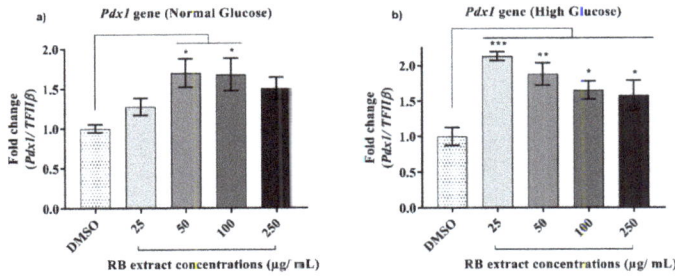

Figure 3. Effect of RB phenolic extracts on the expression of the *Pdx1* gene under normal and high glucose conditions in INS-1E cells. (**a**) Normal glucose conditions, (**b**) High glucose conditions ($n = 5$). The level of significance is indicated by the asterisks, whereby * $p < 0.05$, ** $p < 0.01$, *** $p < 0.001$. Data are presented as Mean ± SD. Dimethyl sulfoxide, DMSO; Insulin promoter factor 1, *Pdx1*; Insulin-secreting rat insulinoma cell, INS-1E; Rice bran, RB.

3.2.3. Expression of the *Sirt1* Gene

There was no significant increase in the expression of the *Sirt1* gene observed under normal glucose conditions when compared to that of the control. However, under high glucose conditions, a significant increase ($p < 0.0001$) in the expression of the *Sirt1* gene was observed after treatment with 25–250 µg/mL of RB phenolic extracts when compared to that of the control (Figure 4).

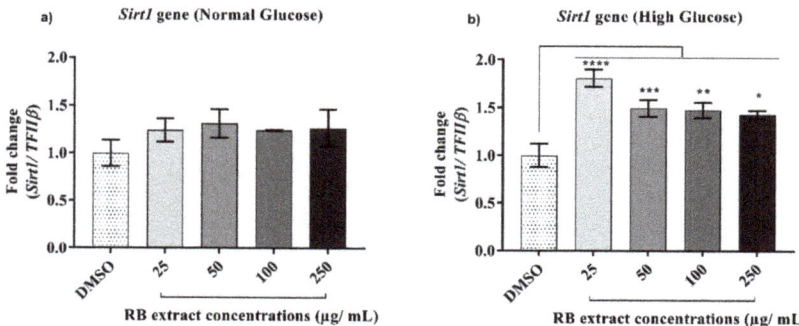

Figure 4. Effect of RB phenolic extracts on the expression of the *Sirt1* gene under normal and high glucose conditions in INS-1E cells. (**a**) Normal glucose conditions, (**b**) High glucose conditions ($n = 5$). The level of significance is indicated by the asterisks, whereby * $p < 0.05$, ** $p < 0.01$, *** $p < 0.001$, **** $p < 0.0001$. Data are presented as Mean ± SD. Dimethyl sulfoxide, DMSO; Insulin-secreting rat insulinoma cell, INS-1E; Rice bran, RB; Sirtuin 1, *Sirt1*.

3.2.4. Expression of the *Tfam* Gene

Under normal glucose conditions, a significant increase ($p < 0.001$) in the expression of the *Tfam* gene was observed after treatment with 25–250 µg/mL of RB phenolic extracts when compared to that of the control. However, under high glucose conditions, a significant increase ($p < 0.05$) in the expression of the *Tfam* gene was only observed after treatment with 25 µg/mL of RB phenolic extracts when compared to that of the control (Figure 5).

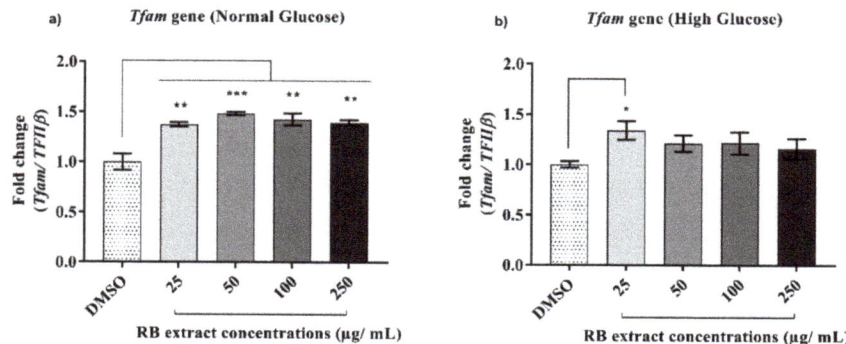

Figure 5. Effect of RB phenolic extracts on the expression of the *Tfam* gene under normal and high glucose conditions in INS-1E cells. (**a**) Normal glucose conditions, (**b**) High glucose conditions ($n = 5$). The level of significance is indicated by the asterisks, whereby * $p < 0.05$, ** $p < 0.01$, *** $p < 0.001$. Data are presented as Mean ± SD. Dimethyl sulfoxide, DMSO; Insulin-secreting rat insulinoma cell, INS-1E; Mitochondrial transcription factor A, *Tfam*; Rice bran, RB.

3.2.5. Expression of the *Ins1* Gene

RB extract did not alter the expression of the *Ins1* gene under normal glucose treatment. However, under high glucose conditions, a significant increase in the expression of the *Ins1* gene was observed after treatment with 50 µg/mL ($p < 0.01$) and 100 µg/mL ($p < 0.001$) of RB phenolic extracts when compared to that of the control (Figure 6).

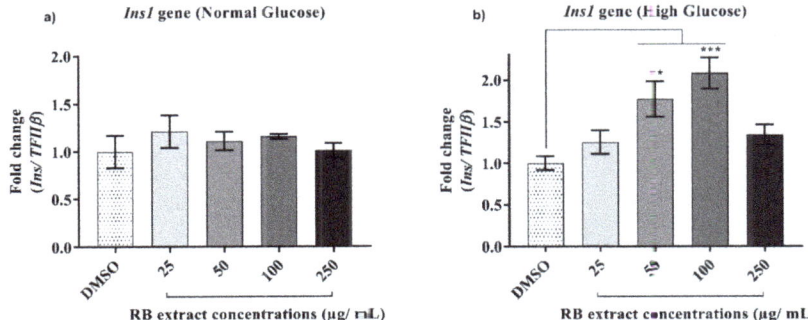

Figure 6. Effect of RB phenolic extracts on the expression of the *Ins1* gene under normal and high glucose conditions in INS-1E cells. (**a**) Normal glucose conditions, (**b**) High glucose conditions ($n = 5$). The level of significance is indicated by the asterisks, whereby ** $p < 0.01$, *** $p < 0.001$. Data are presented as Mean ± SD. Dimethyl sulfoxide, DMSO; Insulin 1, *Ins1*; Insulin-secreting rat insulinoma cell, INS-1E; Rice bran, RB.

3.3. Glucose-Stimulated Insulin Secretion

Glucose-stimulated insulin secretion was observed to significantly increase after treatment with 25 ($p < 0.0001$), 50 ($p < 0.0001$), 100 ($p < 0.0001$), and 250 ($p < 0.05$) µg/mL of RB phenolic extracts under normal glucose conditions when compared to that of the control. Similarly, under high glucose conditions, a significant increase in glucose-stimulated insulin secretion was also observed after treatment with 25 ($p < 0.0001$), 50 ($p < 0.05$), and 100 ($p < 0.05$) µg/mL of RB phenolic extracts when compared to that of the control (Figure 7).

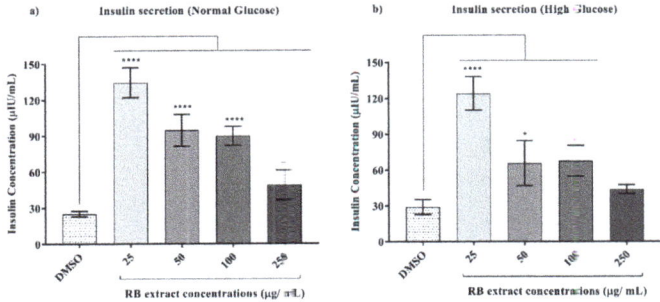

Figure 7. Effect of RB phenolic extracts on glucose-stimulated insulin secretion under normal and high glucose conditions in INS-1E cells. (**a**) Normal glucose conditions, (**b**) High glucose conditions ($n = 6$). The level of significance is indicated by the asterisks, whereby * $p < 0.05$, **** $p < 0.0001$. Data are presented as Mean ± SD. Dimethyl sulfoxide, DMSO; Insulin-secreting rat insulinoma cell, INS-1E; Rice bran, RB.

4. Discussion

Prolonged exposure of pancreatic β-cells to a high glucose environment is known to result in oxidative stress, consequently leading to the downregulation of pancreatic genes, in turn causing impaired β-cell function and insulin secretion [16]. Plant-derived phenolic compounds via their antioxidant, free radical scavenging and metal chelating properties have been observed to target metabolic pathways associated with the pathogenesis of T2DM [14]. The present study demonstrated that RB phenolic extracts effectively alter β-cell function in insulin-secreting cells by modulating the expression of genes and insulin secretion. It was observed that RB phenolic extracts upregulated the expression of key genes associated with β-cell function, including *Glut2*, *Pdx1*, *Sirt1*, *Tfam*, and *Ins1* both under normal and high glucose-induced stress conditions (Figures 2–6).

The *Glut2* gene primarily acts as a glucose transporter and the decreased expression of the *Glut2* gene is directly proportional to the loss of glucose-stimulated insulin secretion [5]. In this study, a significant increase in the expression of the *Glut2* gene was observed under normal conditions compared to that in high glucose conditions. This may have been caused by the increase in glucotoxic stress created by the high glucose environment, resulting in a reduced ability to maintain normal functioning as a glucose transporter. Nevertheless, a significant up-regulation of the *Glut2* gene was observed under both conditions compared to those of the respective controls after treatment with varying concentrations of RB extract (Figure 2). Similarly, studies in which phenolic compounds derived from *M. pumilum var. alata* extracts and purified phenolic compounds such as resveratrol were tested improved β-cell function, and insulin signalling was observed as a result of increased expression of the *Glut2* gene in the pancreas [21,23]. This is most likely due to the polyphenols targeting the exchange of calcium ions resulting in the exocytosis of insulin-containing granules, thereby favourably modulating β-cell function [5,24].

Pdx1 gene expression is essential for the homeostatic regulation of the glucose-sensing system in β-cells [6]. It is also essential for survival and differentiation of β-cells as it primarily acts by upregulating the transcription of several β-cell-specific genes, including the *Ins* and *Glut2* genes [25]. Results obtained from this study show that under both normal and high glucose conditions, a significant upregulation of the *Pdx1* gene was evident after treatment with RB phenolic extracts (Figure 3). Upregulation of the *Pdx1* gene has been observed elsewhere, in which administration of *Teucrium polium* extract, known to contain phenolic compounds with strong antioxidant and anti-inflammatory effects, was found to reverse the symptoms of streptozotocin-induced diabetes in rats [26]. Another study, wherein the effect of gallic acid against glucolipotoxicity and insulin secretion was examined, showed that pre-treatment with different concentrations of gallic acid was found to increase insulin secretion and resulted in the upregulation of the *Pdx1* gene in RINm5F β-cells [27]. Reduction in insulin secretion has been attributed to the c-Jun N-terminal kinase (JNK) pathway activation under oxidative stress conditions. JNK activation as a result of oxidative stress results in forkhead box protein O1 (FOXO1) phosphorylation, and the nuclear localization of the FOXO1 protein leads to a reduction in the expression of the *Pdx1* gene [28]. As an adequate expression of the pancreatic *Pdx1* gene is essential to maintain the proper function of insulin-producing β-cells, inhibition of the JNK pathway is crucial. As phenolic compounds are recognized to modulate the regulation of the JNK pathway [26], it is likely that the observed upregulation of the *Pdx1* gene by RB-derived phenolic extracts resulted from an inhibition of the JNK pathway.

The *Sirt1* gene is known to be a major contributor to the metabolic regulation of a cell via lipid metabolism and insulin secretion [7]. In the current study, under high glucose conditions, a significant increase in the expression of the *Sirt1* gene was observed after treatment with RB phenolic extracts (Figure 4). Sun, Zhang [29] demonstrated that resveratrol improved insulin sensitivity by repressing the protein tyrosine phosphatase (PTP) constitute and PTP_1B transcription at the chromatin level (on the *Sirt1* gene) under normal versus insulin-resistant conditions. Hence, it is believed that upregulation of the *Sirt1* gene as a result of treatment with RB phenolics can potentially target PTP_1B transcription consequently improving insulin sensitivity.

Any disruption to the *Tfam* gene in the pancreatic β-cell is known to result in impaired insulin secretion, reduced β-cell mass, and, consequently, the development of T2DM [8]. The current study shows a significant increase in the expression of the *Tfam* gene under normal and high glucose conditions post-treatment with RB phenolic extracts (Figure 5). In an in vivo study where rats were gavaged with pterostilbene, *Tfam* gene expression was significantly increased in addition to improvements to glycaemic control and insulin resistance [30]. Furthermore, the treatment of INS-1E cells with resveratrol also displayed marked potentiation of glucose-stimulated insulin secretion as a result of the up-regulation of *Tfam* [21]. From the above studies, it is believed that RB phenolics have the potential to enhance the efficiency of mitochondrial function via interaction with transcription factors such as *Tfam*.

Appropriate regulation of the *Ins1* gene is essential for central insulin signalling as it is an anorectic gene that encodes for the production of the insulin hormone that plays a vital role in the regulation of carbohydrate and lipid metabolism [31]. Chronic exposure to high glucose conditions can reduce the expression of the *Ins1* gene in β-cells and is often accompanied by the decreased binding activity of the β-cell-specific transcription factor, *Pdx1* [32]. In the current study, although there was no significant increase in *Ins1* gene expression after RB extract treatment under normal glucose conditions, the expression of the *Ins1* gene was significantly upregulated under high glucose conditions (Figure 6). Similarly, an in vivo study by the author of [33] also demonstrated blueberry-leaf extract rich in chlorogenic acid and flavonol glycosides attenuates glucose homeostasis and improves pancreatic β-cell function by increasing the expression of several genes including *Ins1*. Polyphenols present in common spices, such as cinnamon, cloves, turmeric, and bay leaves, due to their doubly-linked procyanidin type-A polymers, have also shown an insulin-like activity in vitro [34]. The mechanism of cinnamon's insulin-like activity may be in part due to increases in the amounts of insulin receptor β and *Glut4* expression [34]. Some of the polyphenols present in cinnamon include caffeic, ferulic, *p*-coumaric, protocatechuic, and vanillic acids [35], a similar phenolic profile observed in the RB samples used in this study [18]. Therefore, it is likely that the effects observed in this study may be due to the insulin-like activity displayed by the polyphenols present in RB individually or via synergistic bioactivity.

Hormones such as insulin and amylin are co-secreted by β-cells in a fixed molecular ratio that provides circulating energy in the form of glucose and stored energy in the form of visceral adipose tissue [36]. However, conditions such as obesity, T2DM, and pancreatic cancer result in an increase in the amount of amylin relative to the insulin, which can disturb the regulation of energy homeostasis [36]. It was observed that under normal and high glucose-induced conditions, RB phenolic extracts significantly increased glucose-stimulated insulin secretion (Figure 7). Bhattacharya, Oksbjerg [15] also observed a similar trend where caffeic acid, naringenin, and quercetin significantly increased glucose-stimulated insulin secretion under hyperglycaemic and glucotoxic conditions in INS-1E cells. Similarly, several other phenolic compounds such as ferulic acid [37] and *p*-coumaric acid [38] have also been shown to increase insulin secretion both in vitro and in vivo, respectively. In this study, it was observed that RB phenolic compounds increase the expression of both the *Ins1* gene and the secretion of insulin in INS-1E cells under high glucose conditions. Since the *Ins1* gene is known to encode for the production of insulin hormone, this may indicate that there may be a correlation between insulin secretion and the expression of the *Ins1* gene.

Furthermore, it was observed that lower doses of the RB extract used in this study favourably modulated β-cell function associated gene expression and insulin secretion when compared to the higher doses in vitro. This phenomenon may be explained through the effect of hormesis, a biphasic dose-response to an environmental agent, wherein glucose-stimulated insulin secretion was observed to have a stimulatory or beneficial effect at low doses and an inhibitory or toxic effect at high doses of RB extract [39]. Dietary polyphenols are known to have strong cytoprotective effects, however, the hormetic role of dietary antioxidants in free radical-related diseases have demonstrated that under uncontrolled nutritional supplementation, gene induction effects and the interaction with detoxification responses can result in a negative response by generating more reactive and harmful intermediates [40].

As a result of hindrance by cereal matrices, most of the bound phenolic compounds present in cereal grains are usually not readily accessible by digestive enzymes, leading to low bioavailability [41]. Studies have demonstrated that this could be improved by increasing their accessibility through suitable processing techniques, for example, thermal treatments [18,41]. The RB sample examined in this study was previously studied with respect to several thermal treatments. Of the treatments studied, drum drying resulted in the optimal antioxidant activity and was therefore selected for the current investigation [18]. The drum-dried RB samples resulted in a total free phenolic content of 362.17 ± 34.16 gallic acid equivalent (GAE)/100 g of RB with antioxidant activity of 975.33 ± 20.24 Fe^{2+}/100 g of RB and a total bound phenolic content of 160.65 ± 5.52 GAE/100 g of RB with antioxidant activity of 551.91 ± 8.82 Fe^{2+}/100 g of RB. This was much higher compared to that of a non-treated sample that had a total free phenolic content of 238.26 ± 30.34 GAE/100 g of RB with antioxidant activity of 621.76 ± 26.76 Fe^{2+}/100 g of RB and a total bound phenolic content of 222.94 ± 3.74 GAE/100 g of RB with antioxidant activity of 712.37 ± 14.57 Fe^{2+}/100 g of RB [18].

5. Conclusions

This study has demonstrated that RB phenolic compounds, under both normal and glucotoxic conditions, significantly increase the expression of genes associated with β-cell function, in addition to increasing glucose-stimulated insulin secretion. RB phenolic compounds could play an important role in modulating the expression of genes involved in β-cell dysfunction and insulin secretion via several mechanisms, including (1) Synergistic action of polyphenols and phenolic acids by targeting signalling molecules, including transcription factors, consequently modulating mitochondrial potential; (2) Reducing free radical damage related to β-cell dysfunction via their antioxidant activity; and (3) Stimulation of effectors or survival factors of insulin secretion. RB phenolic extracts present as a promising preventive/therapeutic target in the treatment of glucotoxicity induced β-cell dysfunction. More in vivo studies are warranted to confirm the bioactivity of RB phenolic compounds.

Author Contributions: N.S. performed the experiments outlined in this study and drafted the manuscript. N.F., L.J.S., C.L.B., and A.B.S. were involved in the experimental study design, preparation, and review of this manuscript. All authors have read and agreed to the published version of the manuscript.

Funding: This study was funded by the Australian Research Council Industrial Transformation Training Centre for Functional Grains (Project ID 100737) and from AgriFutures, Australia (PRJ-011503). We would like to acknowledge the Faculty of Science, Charles Sturt University, for providing funding towards the publication cost of this article.

Acknowledgments: The authors acknowledge SunRice, Australia, for providing the rice bran samples used in this study. We would like to acknowledge Kathryn Aston-Mourey, Head of Islet Biology Laboratory at Deakin University, Australia, for kindly donating the INS-1E cells.

Conflicts of Interest: The authors declare no conflicts of interest.

Abbreviations

c-Jun N-terminal kinase (JNK), Dimethyl sulfoxide (DMSO), Forkhead box protein O1 (FOXO1), Gallic acid equivalent (GAE), Glucose transporter 2 (*Glut2*), Insulin 1 (*Ins1*), Insulin-secreting rat insulinoma cell (INS-1E), Mitochondrial DNA (mtDNA), Mitochondrial transcription factor A (*Tfam*), One-way analysis of variance (ANOVA), Pancreatic and Duodenal Homeobox 1 (*Pdx1*), Protein tyrosine phosphatase (PTP), Quantitative real-time polymerase chain reaction (qPCR), Ribonucleic acid (RNA), Rice bran (RB), Sirtuin 1 (*Sirt1*), Standard deviation (SD), Type 2 diabetes mellitus (T2DM).

References

1. Leko, V.; Varnum-Finney, B.; Li, H.; Gu, Y.; Flowers, D.; Nourigat, C.; Bernstein, I.D.; Bedalov, A. SIRT1 is dispensable for function of hematopoietic stem cells in adult mice. *Blood J. Am. Soc. Hematol.* **2012**, *119*, 1856–1860. [CrossRef] [PubMed]
2. Hou, J.C.; Williams, D.; Vicogne, J.; Pessin, J.E. The glucose transporter 2 undergoes plasma membrane endocytosis and lysosomal degradation in a secretagogue-dependent manner. *Endocrinology* **2009**, *150*, 4056–4064. [CrossRef] [PubMed]
3. Keane, K.N.; Cruzat, V.F.; Carlessi, R.; de Bittencourt, P.I.H.; Newsholme, P. Molecular events linking oxidative stress and inflammation to insulin resistance and β-cell dysfunction. *Oxidative Med. Cell. Longev.* **2015**, *2015*. [CrossRef] [PubMed]
4. Kang, G.G.; Francis, N.; Hill, R.; LE Waters, D.; Blanchard, C.L.; Santhakumar, A.B. Coloured rice phenolic extracts increase expression of genes associated with insulin secretion in rat pancreatic insulinoma β-cells. *Int. J. Mol. Sci.* **2020**, *21*, 3314. [CrossRef] [PubMed]
5. Thorens, B. GLUT2, glucose sensing and glucose homeostasis. *Diabetologia* **2015**, *58*, 221–232. [CrossRef]
6. Gao, N.; LeLay, J.; Vatamaniuk, M.Z.; Rieck, S.; Friedman, J.R.; Kaestner, K.H. Dynamic regulation of Pdx1 enhancers by Foxa1 and Foxa2 is essential for pancreas development. *Genes Dev.* **2008**, *22*, 3435–3448. [CrossRef]
7. Imai, S.-i.; Kiess, W. Therapeutic potential of SIRT1 and NAMPT-mediated NAD biosynthesis in type 2 diabetes. *Front. Biosci. J. Virtual Libr.* **2009**, *14*, 2983. [CrossRef]
8. Lezza, A.M. Mitochondrial transcription factor A (TFAM): One actor for different roles. *Front. Biol.* **2012**, *7*, 30–39. [CrossRef]
9. Kataoka, K.; Han, S.-i.; Shioda, S.; Hirai, M.; Nishizawa, M.; Handa, H. MafA is a glucose-regulated and pancreatic β-cell-specific transcriptional activator for the insulin gene. *J. Biol. Chem.* **2002**, *277*, 49903–49910. [CrossRef]
10. Campbell, S.C.; Macfarlane, W.M. Regulation of the pdx1 gene promoter in pancreatic β-cells. *Biochem. Biophys. Res. Commun.* **2002**, *299*, 277–284. [CrossRef]
11. Gemma, C.; Sookoian, S.; Dieuzeide, G.; García, S.I.; Gianotti, T.F.; González, C.D.; Pirola, C.J. Methylation of TFAM gene promoter in peripheral white blood cells is associated with insulin resistance in adolescents. *Mol. Genet. Metab.* **2010**, *100*, 83–87. [CrossRef] [PubMed]
12. Gianotti, T.F.; Sookoian, S.; Dieuzeide, G.; García, S.I.; Gemma, C.; González, C.D.; Pirola, C.J. A decreased mitochondrial DNA content is related to insulin resistance in adolescents. *Obesity* **2008**, *16*, 1591–1595. [CrossRef] [PubMed]
13. Mehran, A.E.; Templeman, N.M.; Brigidi, G.S.; Lim, G.E.; Chu, K.-Y.; Hu, X.; Botezelli, J.D.; Asadi, A.; Hoffman, B.G.; Kieffer, T.J. Hyperinsulinemia drives diet-induced obesity independently of brain insulin production. *Cell Metab.* **2012**, *16*, 723–737. [CrossRef] [PubMed]
14. Kaup, R.M.; Khayyal, M.T.; Verspohl, E.J. Antidiabetic effects of a standardized egyptian rice bran extract. *Phytother. Res.* **2013**. [CrossRef]
15. Bhattacharya, S.; Oksbjerg, N.; Young, J.; Jeppesen, P. Caffeic acid, naringenin and quercetin enhance glucose-stimulated insulin secretion and glucose sensitivity in INS-1E cells. *Diabetes Obes. Metab.* **2014**, *16*, 602–612. [CrossRef]
16. Cheng, A.-S.; Cheng, Y.-H.; Chang, T.-L. Resveratrol protects RINm5F pancreatic cells from methylglyoxal-induced apoptosis. *J. Funct. Foods* **2013**, *5*, 1774–1783. [CrossRef]
17. Dall'Asta, M.; Bayle, M.; Neasta, J.; Scazzina, F.; Bruni, R.; Cros, G.; Del Rio, D.; Oiry, C. Protection of pancreatic β-cell function by dietary polyphenols. *Phytochem. Rev.* **2015**, *14*, 933–959. [CrossRef]
18. Saji, N.; Schwarz, L.J.; Santhakumar, A.B.; Blanchard, C.L. Stabilization treatment of rice bran alters phenolic content and antioxidant activity. *Cereal Chem.* **2020**, *97*, 281–292. [CrossRef]
19. Saji, N.; Francis, N.; Schwarz, L.J.; Blanchard, C.L.; Santhakumar, A.B. Rice bran derived bioactive compounds modulate risk factors of cardiovascular disease and type 2 diabetes mellitus: An updated review. *Nutrients* **2019**, *11*, 2736. [CrossRef]
20. Saji, N.; Francis, N.; Blanchard, C.L.; Schwarz, L.J.; Santhakumar, A.B. Rice Bran phenolic compounds regulate genes associated with antioxidant and anti-inflammatory activity in human umbilical vein endothelial cells with induced oxidative stress. *Int. J. Mol. Sci.* **2019**, *20*, 4715. [CrossRef]

21. Vetterli, L.; Brun, T.; Giovannoni, L.; Bosco, D.; Maechler, P. Resveratrol potentiates glucose-stimulated insulin secretion in INS-1E β-cells and human islets through a SIRT1-dependent mechanism. *J. Biol. Chem.* **2011**, *286*, 6049–6060. [CrossRef] [PubMed]
22. Muller, P.; Janovjak, H.; Miserez, A.; Dobbie, Z. Processing of gene expression data generated by quantitative real-time RT PCR (vol 32, pg 1378, 2002). *Biotechniques* **2002**, *33*, 514.
23. Dharmani, M.; Kamarulzaman, K.; Giribabu, N.; Choy, K.; Zuhaida, M.; Aladdin, N.; Jamal, J.; Mustafa, M. Effect of Marantodes pumilum Blume (Kuntze) var. alata on β-cell function and insulin signaling in ovariectomised diabetic rats. *Phytomedicine* **2019**, *65*, 153101. [CrossRef] [PubMed]
24. Henquin, J.-C. Triggering and amplifying pathways of regulation of insulin secretion by glucose. *Diabetes* **2000**, *49*, 1751–1760. [CrossRef] [PubMed]
25. Grondin, M.; Robinson, I.; Do Carmo, S.; Ali-Benali, M.A.; Ouellet, F.; Mounier, C.; Sarhan, F.; Averill-Bates, D.A. Cryopreservation of insulin-secreting INS832/13 cells using a wheat protein formulation. *Cryobiology* **2013**, *66*, 136–143. [CrossRef]
26. Tabatabaie, P.S.; Yazdanparast, R. Teucrium polium extract reverses symptoms of streptozotocin-induced diabetes in rats via rebalancing the Pdx1 and FoxO1 expressions. *Biomed. Pharmacother.* **2017**, *93*, 1033–1039. [CrossRef] [PubMed]
27. Sameermahmood, Z.; Raji, L.; Saravanan, T.; Vaidya, A.; Mohan, V.; Balasubramanyam, M. Gallic acid protects RINm5F β-cells from glucolipotoxicity by its antiapoptotic and insulin-secretagogue actions. *Phytother. Res.* **2010**, *24*, S83–S94. [CrossRef] [PubMed]
28. Kawamori, D.; Kaneto, H.; Nakatani, Y.; Matsuoka, T.-a.; Matsuhisa, M.; Hori, M.; Yamasaki, Y. The forkhead transcription factor Foxo1 bridges the JNK pathway and the transcription factor PDX-1 through its intracellular translocation. *J. Biol. Chem.* **2006**, *281*, 1091–1098. [CrossRef]
29. Sun, C.; Zhang, F.; Ge, X.; Yan, T.; Chen, X.; Shi, X.; Zhai, Q. SIRT1 improves insulin sensitivity under insulin-resistant conditions by repressing PTP1B. *Cell Metab.* **2007**, *6*, 307–319. [CrossRef]
30. Gómez-Zorita, S.; Fernández-Quintela, A.; Aguirre, L.; Macarulla, M.; Rimando, A.; Portillo, M. Pterostilbene improves glycaemic control in rats fed an obesogenic diet: Involvement of skeletal muscle and liver. *Food Funct.* **2015**, *6*, 1968–1976. [CrossRef]
31. Lu, C.; Zhu, W.; Shen, C.-L.; Gao, W. Green tea polyphenols reduce body weight in rats by modulating obesity-related genes. *PLoS ONE* **2012**, *7*, e38332. [CrossRef] [PubMed]
32. Puddu, A.; Storace, D.; Odetti, P.; Viviani, G. Advanced glycation end-products affect transcription factors regulating insulin gene expression. *Biochem. Biophys. Res. Commun.* **2010**, *395*, 122–125. [CrossRef] [PubMed]
33. Li, H.; Park, H.-M.; Ji, H.-S.; Han, J.; Kim, S.-K.; Park, H.-Y.; Jeong, T.-S. Phenolic-enriched blueberry-leaf extract attenuates glucose homeostasis, pancreatic β-cell function, and insulin sensitivity in high-fat diet–induced diabetic mice. *Nutr. Res.* **2020**, *73*, 83–96. [CrossRef] [PubMed]
34. Hanhineva, K.; Törrönen, R.; Bondia-Pons, I.; Pekkinen, J.; Kolehmainen, M.; Mykkänen, H.; Poutanen, K. Impact of dietary polyphenols on carbohydrate metabolism. *Int. J. Mol. Sci.* **2010**, *11*, 1365–1402. [CrossRef]
35. Pramote, K.; Nucha, S.; Suched, S.; Parinda, P.; Prasong, S.; Shuji, A. Subcritical water extraction of flavoring and phenolic compounds from cinnamon bark (Cinnamomum zeylanicum). *J. Oleo Sci.* **2012**, *61*, 349–355.
36. Woods, S.C.; Lutz, T.A.; Geary, N.; Langhans, W. Pancreatic signals controlling food intake; insulin, glucagon and amylin. *Philos. Trans. R. Soc. B Biol. Sci.* **2006**, *361*, 1219–1235. [CrossRef]
37. Nomura, E.; Kashiwada, A.; Hosoda, A.; Nakamura, K.; Morishita, H.; Tsuno, T.; Taniguchi, H. Synthesis of amide compounds of ferulic acid, and their stimulatory effects on insulin secretion In vitro. *Bioorganic Med. Chem.* **2003**, *11*, 3807–3813. [CrossRef]
38. Zabad, O.M.; Samra, Y.A.; Eissa, L.A. P-Coumaric acid alleviates experimental diabetic nephropathy through modulation of Toll like receptor-4 in rats. *Life Sci.* **2019**, *238*, 116965. [CrossRef]
39. Mattson, M.P. Hormesis defined. *Ageing Res. Rev.* **2008**, *7*, 1–7. [CrossRef]

40. Calabrese, V.; Cornelius, C.; Trovato-Salinaro, A.; Cambria, M.T.; Locascio, M.; Rienzo, L.; Condorelli, D.; Mancuso, C.; De Lorenzo, A.; Calabrese, E. The hormetic role of dietary antioxidants in free radical-related diseases. *Curr. Pharm. Des.* **2010**, *16*, 877–883. [CrossRef]
41. Karakaya, S. Bioavailability of phenolic compounds. *Crit. Rev. Food Sci. Nutr.* **2004**, *44*, 453–464. [CrossRef] [PubMed]

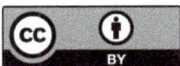

© 2020 by the authors. Licensee MDPI, Basel, Switzerland. This article is an open access article distributed under the terms and conditions of the Creative Commons Attribution (CC BY) license (http://creativecommons.org/licenses/by/4.0/).

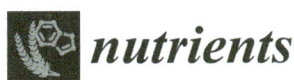

Article

Black Sorghum Phenolic Extract Modulates Platelet Activation and Platelet Microparticle Release

Borkwei Ed Nignpense [1], Kenneth A Chinkwo [1,2], Christopher L Blanchard [1,2] and Abishek B Santhakumar [1,2,*]

[1] School of Biomedical Sciences, Charles Sturt University, Locked Bag 588, Wagga Wagga, NSW 2678, Australia; bednignpense@csu.edu.au (B.E.D.); kchinkwo@csu.edu.au (K.A.C.); CBlanchard@csu.edu.au (C.L.B.)
[2] Australian Research Council (ARC) Industrial Transformation Training Centre (ITTC) for Functional Grains, Graham Centre for Agricultural Innovation, Charles Sturt University, Wagga Wagga, NSW 2650, Australia
* Correspondence: asanthakumar@csu.edu.au; Tel.: +61-2-6933-2678

Received: 20 May 2020; Accepted: 10 June 2020; Published: 12 June 2020

Abstract: Platelet hyper-activation and platelet microparticles (PMPs) play a key role in the pathogenesis of cardiovascular diseases. Dietary polyphenols are believed to mimic antiplatelet agents by blunting platelet activation receptors via its antioxidant phenomenon. However, there is limited information on the anti-platelet activity of grain-derived polyphenols. The aim of the study is to evaluate the effects of sorghum extract (Shawaya short black 1 variety), an extract previously characterised for its high antioxidant activity and reduction of oxidative stress-related endothelial dysfunction, on platelet aggregation, platelet activation and PMP release. Whole blood samples collected from 18 healthy volunteers were treated with varying non-cytotoxic concentrations of polyphenol-rich black sorghum extract (BSE). Platelet aggregation study utilised 5 µg/mL collagen to target the GPVI pathway of thrombus formation whereas adenine phosphate (ADP) was used to stimulate the P2Y1/P2Y12 pathway of platelet activation assessed by flow cytometry. Procaspase-activating compound 1 (PAC-1) and P-selectin/CD62P were used to evaluate platelet activation- related conformational changes and degranulation respectively. PMPs were isolated from unstimulated platelets and quantified by size distribution and binding to CD42b. BSE treatment significantly reduced both collagen-induced platelet aggregation and circulatory PMP release at 40 µg/mL ($p < 0.001$) when compared to control. However, there was no significant impact of BSE on ADP-induced activation-dependent conformational change and degranulation of platelets. Results of this study suggest that phenolic rich BSE may confer cardio-protection by modulating specific signalling pathways involved in platelet activation and PMP release.

Keywords: black sorghum; polyphenols; platelets; platelet microparticles; atherosclerosis

1. Introduction

According to a World Health Organisation report, cardiovascular diseases accounted for an estimated 31% of deaths globally with majority being a result of stroke or heart attack [1,2]. In clinical settings, treatment involves blunting the activity of platelets using antiplatelet drugs. These drugs interfere with the thrombotic pathophysiology—wherein a rupture of an atherosclerotic plaque triggers platelet hyper-activation resulting in unwanted clot formation and occlusion of the blood vessel. Macrovesicles referred to as platelet microparticles (PMPs) are released following platelet activation and can contribute to the thrombotic situation [3,4].

The several signalling pathways involved in platelet activation and thrombus formation include receptor-agonist pathways such as P2Y1/P2Y12-ADP, GPVI-collagen, PAR1-thrombin and the COX-1-thromboxane [5]. An agonist such as collagen when exposed by atherosclerotic plaque may activate nearby platelets by binding to their GPVI receptor resulting in complex intracellular signalling that produce a conformational change (indicated by GPIIb/IIIa receptor expression), degranulation (indicated by P-selectin secretion) and subsequent formation of platelet aggregates [5]. In addition, PMP released upon activation possess adhesive and pro-coagulant platelet-derived receptors that further enhance thrombus formation, thereby acting as biomarkers of platelet activation [3]. The common antiplatelet agents, clopidogrel and aspirin, used in clinical treatments inhibit platelet activation and its circulating biomarkers by selectively targeting P2Y1/P2Y12-ADP and COX-1-thromboxane respectively [6]. Unfortunately, because of the unresponsiveness and side effects associated with administration there have been considerable research in dietary bioactive agents known as polyphenols [7].

One such example of a polyphenol-rich functional food is sorghum whole grain. Although mainly used as animal feed, studies have demonstrated that it possesses anti-inflammatory, anti-cancer and antioxidant properties which add value to it as a food for human consumption [8]. Sorghum of different types exist that are classified based on the pigmentation of the pericarp and vary in their phenolic content [9]. The polyphenols found in sorghum that contribute to its bioactivity include flavonoids, hydroxybenzoic acids and hydroxycinnamic acid [8]. Furthermore Francis et al. [10] recently demonstrated that black sorghum rich in catechins and their derivatives may confer cardioprotective properties. The treatment of human umbilical vein cells with flavonoid-rich extract was found to prevent oxidative stress-related endothelial dysfunction through the modulation of gene expression.

Furthermore, these cardio-protective benefits of polyphenols apply in the context of platelet function. Several studies have demonstrated that polyphenols may inhibit platelet activation, adhesion, degranulation and aggregation by targeting specific thrombogenic pathways for example $P2Y_1/P2Y_{12}$-ADP, GPVI-collagen, PAR1-thrombin and the COX-1-thromboxane. As reviewed by Ed Nignpense et al. [11] many of the studies that investigate the polyphenol impact on platelet function and PMP generation utilise aggregometry and flow cytometry. However there is limited research on sorghum-derived polyphenols in modulating biomarkers of platelet activation. This study aims to investigate the impact of black sorghum derived polyphenol extracts on collagen-induced platelet aggregation, ADP-induced platelet activation and PMP generation.

2. Materials and Methods

2.1. Research Ethics

The study protocol was approved by the Charles Sturt University Human Research Ethics Committee (HR17012) and the Institutional Biosafety Committee (19HB02). The study was performed in compliance with relevant laws and institutional guidelines.

2.2. Volunteer Recruitment

Eighteen healthy volunteers between 18–65 years of age (9 males and 9 females) were recruited from Charles Sturt University and the local community. Informed consent was obtained from all participants prior to commencement of the study. The criteria for recruitment involved normal health status with no history of conditions such as cardiovascular, metabolic, liver or lung disease. Other parameters that could affect the integrity of the analysis such as alcohol consumption, smoking, pregnancy, allergies or venepuncture difficulty were considered during the recruitment process. A health screening questionnaire was used to assess the already mentioned parameters. A dietary questionnaire (adapted from WINTEC and NZ academy of sport) was used to assess the usual dietary intake of volunteers and to avoid recruitment of participants on a high antioxidant diet. The cut-off figure for each type of food listed in the questionnaire was based on nutrient reference ranges for Australia and New Zealand—recommended daily nutrient intake values.

2.3. Blood Collection and Processing

After fasting for at least 8 h, whole blood was collected from each participant by a trained phlebotomist into a tri-potassium ethylene diamine tetra-acetic acid (EDTA-1.8 mg/mL concentration) anticoagulant tube (Vacuette Greiner Bio-one, Interpath Services, Heidelberg West, VIC, Australia) and a tri-sodium citrate (28.12 g/L concentration) anticoagulant tube (Becton, Dickson and Company, North Ryde, NSW, Australia). A 20-mL syringe (Becton, Dickson and Company, North Ryde, NSW, Australia) and 21-gauge 1.5-inch needle (Terumo Medical Corporation, Macquarie Park, Australia) were used to draw blood from the median cubital vein. The purpose of choosing a larger gauge was to avoid the activation of platelets while drawing or dispensing blood. Utmost care was taken to ensure samples were not obtained through a traumatic collection and that none contained obvious clots. In addition, care was taken to ensure minimal specimen handling and agitation in order to prevent artefactual platelet activation. The first 2 mL of blood was discarded before drawing into the tri-sodium citrate tubes in order to avoid the risk of collecting platelets activated by venepuncture. Tri-sodium tubes were used for aggregometry and flow cytometry assays whereas the EDTA was used to perform full blood examinations.

2.4. Full Blood Examination

Using an Abbott CELL-DYN Emerald 22 Haematology Analyser (Abbott Diagnostics, Illinois, USA), a full blood examination (FBE) was performed on all samples. The FBE results of volunteers indicated that the blood cell parameters were within normal reference ranges as determined by the Royal College of pathologists of Australia. Individuals with cell counts, especially platelet counts, outside of the reference range were excluded from the study. Quality control validation and maintenance were all performed according to the Abbott CELL-DYN Emerald 22 Haematology Analyser manual.

2.5. Extraction of Black Sorghum Polyphenols

Sorghum (*Sorghum bicolor*) samples of six different pericarp varieties were obtained from glasshouse trials conducted by Curtin University, Perth, Western Australia. Six pigmented varieties of sorghum were cultivated under the same conditions, grown in a glasshouse equipped with Lumisol Clear AF cover (200 μm thick, at a transparency of ca UV-A 94%, UV-B 84% and photosynthetic active radiation (PAR, 400-700 nm) 93% [8]. Extraction and analysis of phenolic composition and antioxidant activity were performed previously using methods described by Rao et al. [8]. Among the different sorghum varieties, the black pericarp variety (Shawaya short black 1) was selected for this study because of its relatively high antioxidant activity when analysed with ferric reducing antioxidant power (FRAP; 20.19 ± 2.69 mg/g TE) and 2,2-dipheny-1-picrylhydrazyl (DPPH; 18.04 ± 3.53 mg/g TE) antioxidant assays (Supplementary Figure S1, Tables S1 and S2). The highest level of polyphenols found in the BSE included catechin derivatives, catechins and pentahydroxyflavanone-(3->4)-catechin-7-O- glucoside (Supplementary Table S2). Stock concentrations of BSE (20 mg/mL in 50% DMSO) were diluted in phosphate buffered saline (PBS) to achieve desired concentrations (5 μg/mL, 20 μg/mL and 40 μg/mL) in whole blood. Desired concentrations were selected based on viability studies done by Francis et al. [10].

2.6. Whole Blood Platelet Aggregometry

Platelets in whole blood were stimulated for aggregation using 5 μg/mL collagen exogenous platelet agonists (DSKH Australia Pty. Ltd., Hallam, VIC, Australia) to investigate the effect of BSE treatment on the platelet aggregation. Five hundred microliters of citrated whole blood were added to 100 μL of 0.1% DMSO control (Sigma-Aldrich, Castle Hill, NSW, Australia) or BSE stock concentrations (5 μg/mL, 20 μg/mL and 40 μg/mL) and mixed with 400 μL of saline. The sample was then incubated at 37 °C for 20 min. Using a Chrono-log model 700 lumi-aggregometer (DKSH Australia Pty. Ltd., Hallam, VIC, Australia) the samples were analysed by means of electrical impedance (ohms) to determine the amount of platelet aggregation occurring in the sample over a 6-min time period (Supplementary Figure S2).

2.7. Flow Cytometry

2.7.1. Standardisation

Flow-check fluorospheres were run as quality control for optimal laser alignments. Antibody capture beads (Anti-Mouse Ig, K CompBeads, BD Biosciences, North Ryde, NSW, Australia) were used for single colour compensation controls in order to achieve optimal compensation. Megamix beads (0.1 µm, 0.3 µm, 0.5 µm, 1 µm) from Biocytex, Marseille, France were used as per manufacturer's instructions to set up an appropriate gating to detecting microparticles. They were run before each PMP analysis.

2.7.2. Measurement of Platelet Activation-Dependent Conformational Change and Degranulation

The effects of BSE on ADP-induced platelet activation were analysed and interpreted using a Gallios flow cytometer (Beckman Coulter, Inc., Lane Cove NSW, Australia). The protocols were adopted from the method described by Santhakumar et al. [12] with some modifications. Platelet activation and thrombogenic indicators were assessed via activation-dependent platelet monoclonal antibodies (mAbs) purchased from Becton, Dickinson and Company, North Ryde, NSW, Australia. Procaspase activating compound-1 (PAC-1)-fluorescein isothiocyanate-fluorescein isothiocyanate was used to detect platelet activation-related conformational change and P-selectin/CD62P-allophycocyanin highlighted activation dependent degranulation. CD42b-phycoerythrin identified the GPIb-IX-V receptor, a common receptor found on the surface of all platelets, activated and resting included. A decreased expression of mAb exhibits alleviation of thrombogenesis. Within 5 min of collection tri-sodium citrated whole blood was used for assay preparation to avoid artefactual activation of platelets. A volume of 40 µL of blood was incubated with DMSO control or the various BSE concentration for 20 min at 37 °C in the dark. A 10-µL mixture of all three monoclonal antibodies (3.33 µL each of PAC-1, CD62P and CD42b) was added to blood samples and incubated for 20 min at room temperature in the dark. To induce platelet activation, 10 µM ADP (Helena laboratories Pty. Ltd., Mt Waverly, VIC, Australia) was added, and samples were incubated for a further 15 min in the dark at room temperature, after which erythrocytes were lysed (575 µL of 10 % lysing solution). Samples were thoroughly vortexed to ensure homogeneity and incubated in the dark at room temperature for a further 15 min and then analysed. In all, 10,000 platelet events were acquired, gated based on light scatter and CD42b mAb expression and activated platelets were articulated as mean fluorescence intensity (MFI) (Supplementary Figure S3).

2.7.3. Measurement of Circulatory PMPs

Using the microparticle gating established with Megamix beads, PMPs were identified and quantified by size distribution and binding to CD42b (Supplementary Figure S4). The protocol for circulatory PMP analysis was adapted from Lu et al. [13]. A volume of 1 mL whole blood was added to micro-centrifuge tubes in the presence of PGE1 (120 nmol/L; Sigma-Aldrich, Castle Hill, NSW, Australia). PGE1 was added to prevent artefactual activation during centrifugation. The blood samples were incubated with the respective 100 µL BSE concentrations and DMSO control for 20 min at 37 °C in the dark. Each sample was then centrifuged for 15 min at a 1000 rpm and the resultant platelet rich plasma (PRP) was discarded. The remaining blood was spun a further 15 min at 3000 rpm. The supernatant rich in PMPs (40 µL) was collected into flow tubes and incubated with 4 µL of CD42b and 6 µL of stain buffer (Becton, Dickson and Company, North Ryde, NSW, Australia) in dark room for 15 min. Four percent formaldehyde was used to fix any activation of platelets left in the supernatant. After a 10-min incubation period the samples were run for PMP analysis on the flow cytometer.

2.8. Statistical Analysis

A two-way ANOVA following Tukey's post comparison test was performed using GraphPad Prism version 8.0 for Windows (GraphPad Software, La Jolla, California, USA). A minimum sample size of 14 participants in total was required for 80% power to detect a 5% variation in the laboratory parameters measured where a 3–5% standard deviation exists in the population, assuming an alpha error of 0.05. All the data were expressed as mean ± standard deviation (SD). Differences between the groups were significant when $p < 0.05$. Any significant statistical interactions were included in the analysis where applicable.

3. Results

The baseline parameters including full blood counts for all 18 participants were within normal reference ranges set by the Royal College of Pathologists of Australasia (Table 1) [14].

Table 1. Baseline full blood counts of participants.

Parameters	Mean ± SD
Age (years)	26 ± 8
WBC ($\times 10^9$/L)	5.5 ± 1.3
Neutrophil (%)	48.6 ± 9.5
Lymphocytes (%)	37.8 ± 9.2
Monocytes (%)	10.6 ± 2.3
Eosinophils (%)	2.8 ± 1.3
Basophils (%)	0.1 ± 0.1
RBC ($\times 10^{12}$/L)	4.6 ± 0.5
Haemoglobin (g/L)	147.9 ± 16.1
PCV (%)	0.41 ± 0.04
MCV (fL)	90.0 ± 3.5
MCH (pg)	35.8 ± 15.2
MCHC (g/dL)	360.1 ± 6.0
RDW (%)	14.9 ± 0.8
Platelet count ($\times 10^9$/L)	248.3 ± 50.0
MPV	8.41 ± 0.89

Values are represented as mean ± Standard deviation (SD). RBC, red blood cell, PCV, packed cell volume, MCV, mean cell volume, MCH, mean cell haemoglobin, MCHC, mean cell haemoglobin concentration, RDW, red cell distribution width, MPV, mean platelet volume.

3.1. Effect of BSE on Whole Blood Platelet Aggregation and Platelet Activation

BSE at 40 µg/mL concentration significantly reduced platelet aggregation stimulated by collagen by 19 % ($p = 0.0004$) (Figure 1). BSE at lower concentrations did not exhibit any significant reduction in aggregation.

It was observed that whole blood treatment with the varying concentrations of BSE did not significantly affect ADP-induced platelet conformational change and degranulation indicated by PAC-1 and P-selectin expression respectively (Supplementary Figures S5 and S6).

3.2. Effect of BSE on Circulatory PMPs

BSE at a concentration of 40 µg/mL significantly reduced the amount of circulatory PMPs in whole blood by 47% ($p = 0.0008$). Lower concentrations of BSE did not exhibit any significant reduction to the amount circulatory PMPs (Figure 2).

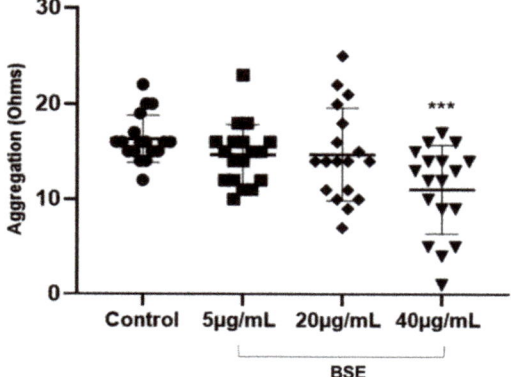

Figure 1. The effect of varying concentrations of BSE on collagen-induced aggregation. BSE at 40 µg/mL significantly reduced platelet aggregation (5.3 ± 1.3; p value = 0.0004). BSE at 5 µg/mL and 20 µg/mL did not reduce platelet aggregation when compared to control (p value > 0.1). N = 18 and data is represented in aggregation (Ohms) versus BSE concentrations. *** signifies statistical significance $p < 0.001$ compared to control. Error bars expressed as mean ± SD.

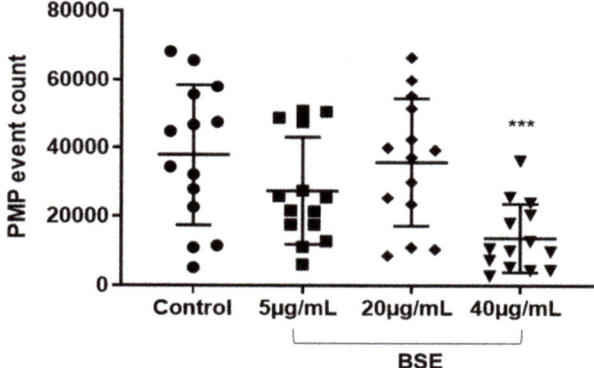

Figure 2. The effect of varying concentrations of BSE on circulatory PMP production in vitro. BSE at 40 µg/mL significantly reduced the amount of circulatory PMPs (<24190 ± 4935, p = 0.0008). BSE at 5 µg/mL and 20 µg/mL did not reduce platelet aggregation when compared to control (p value > 0.1). N = 14 and data are represented in number of PMP events versus BSE concentrations. *** signifies statistical significance $p < 0.001$ compared to control. Error bars expressed as mean ± SD.

4. Discussion

There is growing interest in understanding the therapeutic benefits of functional foods. Sorghum for example is one of the functional foods that is showing promise in this area. With sorghum-derived polyphenols already having demonstrated anti-inflammatory, anti-cancer and antioxidant properties, the current study aimed to evaluate the effects of polyphenol-rich BSE on platelet function in terms of aggregation, conformational change, degranulation and circulatory PMP production [8–10]. It was observed that BSE significantly inhibited collagen-induced platelet aggregation and decreased the release of circulatory PMPs but did not have a significant effect on ADP-induced platelet conformational change or degranulation. Although these results do not reflect a typical dose-dependent inhibition, they suggest a potential role of BSE polyphenols at optimum concentrations to interfere with pathways in the GPVI-collagen signalling and the release of circulatory PMPs but little or no effect on $F2Y_1$/$P2Y_{12}$-ADP pathway.

To the best of our knowledge only a few studies have investigated the antiplatelet effects of sorghum extracts. Li, Yu and Fan et al. [15] extracted alditols and monosaccharides from sorghum vinegar to evaluate their anti-aggregation activity using the turbidimetric method. Results from their study indicated a significant dose-dependent inhibition of aggregation via multiple agonists, arachidonic acid, collagen, ADP and thrombin. Furthermore, a different study by Fan et al. [16] reported in vitro inhibition of ADP- and thrombin- induced rabbit platelet aggregation by methanolic extracts of aged sorghum vinegar with the half maximal inhibitory concentrations (IC_{50}) of 1.7 ± 0.3 and 8.9 ± 1.9 mg/mL respectively. When rats were orally administered the extracts (>100 mg/kg), both collagen- and epinephrine-induced pulmonary thrombosis were inhibited. In comparison with the present study it is to be noted that these studies employed platelet-rich plasma rather than whole blood hence not accounting for the possible involvement of other blood cells and extracellular mediators involved in thrombus formation. In addition, sorghum vinegar extracts were used at higher concentrations; milligrams compared to micrograms used in this study. This raises the question of bioavailability and the importance of employing physiological concentrations of extracts.

Although the BSE concentration of 40 μg/mL at which antiplatelet effect were observed is relatively lesser in concentration than used in the other studies, the most bioactive compounds with respect to antioxidant activity were catechins and other flavonoids which are usually considered to have low bioavailability [8]. It has been suggested that the total plasma polyphenol concentration rarely exceeds 1 μM and that their antiplatelet effects are only found at high non-physiological concentrations (greater than 50 μM) [17,18]. However, it is likely that these plasma concentrations are underestimations due to the ability of polyphenols to bind to the surface of red blood cells and thereby exert their bioactivity [19]. Furthermore polyphenols (structurally related to catechin) and their metabolites have been shown to inhibit platelet function in vitro [20]. This highlights the possibility of sorghum catechins and their metabolites having antiplatelet effects in vivo despite bioavailability concern. Interestingly, an in vivo human dietary intervention trial compared consumption of red and white wholegrain sorghum-based pasta to a control pasta in order to investigate its acute effect on the total phenol content and antioxidant activity in the plasma of healthy subjects [21]. Results showed that when compared to the control pasta, the red sorghum pasta showed significantly increased net plasma phenolic content and antioxidant activity post consumption (from 216.90 ± 2.62 at baseline to 269.40 ± 2.33 at 2 h; $p < 0.001$), thus demonstrating a plausible correlation between antioxidant activity and sorghum polyphenol consumption—which in turn may contribute to antiplatelet effects.

The antiplatelet effects was observed with BSE-included inhibition of collagen-induced aggregation and circulatory PMP production but no effect on ADP-induced platelet activation. The absence of antiplatelet effects on the $P2Y_1$/ $P2Y_{12}$-ADP activation pathway suggests that BSE polyphenols are not mimicking the action of drugs such as clopidogrel that antagonise $P2Y_{12}$ receptor activation [22]. However, the inhibition of collagen-induced aggregation suggest that BSE polyphenols interfere with GPVI-collagen signalling pathways by either blunting the GPVI receptor directly or by other mechanisms [5]. Previous studies have demonstrated that flavonoids, specifically quercetin and catechin, can act synergistically to inhibit collagen-induced aggregation by blunting the associated burst of H_2O_2 and subsequent PLC activation [23,24]. Thus, a possible mechanism of inhibition BSE flavonoids may be a synergistic antagonism of the positive feedback activation of intracellular signals triggered by H_2O_2. Moreover, it has been shown that the phosphorylation cascade initiated by collagen can be inhibited by flavonoids [25,26]. Flavones, especially apigenin and luteolin, by virtue of a double bond in the C2-C3 and the keto group in C4 can also inhibit collagen-induced activation by antagonizing the TxA_2 receptor activation which is also involved in the positive feedback loop [27]. Besides inhibition of the GPVI-collagen signalling, BSE polyphenols showed inhibition of the circulatory PMP production.

To the best of our knowledge, this is the first study investigating the effect of sorghum-derived polyphenols on PMP production. In contrast to this study, other PMP studies have employed the use of Annexin V as well as the platelet specific antibody CD42b, to identify pro-coagulant PMPs by their phosphatidylserine expression and to limit background noise [28]. However, because of the heterogeneity of PMPs, not all PMPs express phosphatidylserine [29]. Moreover, the measurement of CD42b-positive PMPs alone is significant as its increase has been associated with an increased risk of coronary heart disease [30]. From the current study, the significant inhibition of CD42b-positive circulatory PMPs observed in vitro may be attributed to the antioxidant properties of BSE polyphenols. It is believed that the inhibition of PMP generation may be the result of neutralisation of H_2O_2, scavenging of other free radicals or interaction with intracellular signalling leading to PMP release.

The juxtaposition of both the present study and that of an earlier study by Francis et al. [10] highlights the multifaceted role of BSE polyphenols in cardio-protection. The group investigated the effects of BSE polyphenols on the expression of antioxidant- and inflammatory-linked genes involved in endothelial dysfunction under oxidative stress. Results indicated that BSE polyphenols alleviate oxidative stress–induced damage to endothelial cells. Since vascular dysfunction is a precursor to cardiovascular diseases, the current study builds upon earlier findings by exhibiting the antiplatelet effects of BSE. In the context of endothelial dysfunction, platelet activation and circulatory PMPs play central roles in the pathogenesis of atherothrombosis. The disruption of the plaque exposes collagen that binds to the GPVI receptor resulting in platelet activation and subsequent thrombus formation [31]. Circulatory PMPs may contribute to thrombosis via GPIb-IX-V receptor binding and have a pro-inflammatory effect to promote the development of the plaque [32]. Therefore, by reducing collagen-induced platelet aggregation and circulatory PMP generation, BSE polyphenols may be displaying the potential to augment thrombosis.

5. Conclusion and Future Considerations

In summary, the present study contributes to the growing body of literature on bioactivity of sorghum polyphenols and highlights possible mechanisms of antiplatelet action that may result in cardiovascular health benefits. Because of the ability to reduce collagen-induced platelet activation and circulatory PMP generation, BSE polyphenols demonstrate the potential to interfere with pathological processes involved in vascular disorders and thrombotic complications. However, a larger panel of agonist for the flow cytometry and aggregometry studies will aid to further elucidate antiplatelet mechanisms. Because of the bioavailability concerns, well-controlled dietary intervention trials using larger sample sizes to evaluate the antiplatelet effects of sorghum consumption in healthy and pro-thrombotic populations are warranted to justify our findings. Because of the varied phenolic profiles of the different sorghum varieties, further research comparing the antiplatelet therapeutic potential of different grains is also warranted. Furthermore, this study attest to the measurement of circulatory PMPs as a biomarker of platelet activation to assess the bioactivity of functional foods.

Supplementary Materials: The following are available online at http://www.mdpi.com/2072-6643/12/6/1760/s1, Figure S1: Characterisation of phenolic compounds in BSE. Ultra-high-performance liquid chromatography (UHPLC) was employed to quantify the different phenolic compounds identified by the peak (on top). An online 2,2′-azino-bis(3-ethylbenzothiazoline-6-sulfonic acid) (ABTS) was coupled with UHPLC to quantify the relative antioxidant activity (peaks below) of each compound identified, Figure S2: A report derived from the collagen induced platelet aggregation study using the Chrono-log model 700 lumi-aggregometer (DKSH Australia Pty. Ltd, Hallam, VIC, Australia). The blue tracing represents the control (whole blood with no BSE) and the black tracing represents the whole blood pre-treated with 5 µg/mL BSE. The addition of BSE reduced the maximum platelet aggregation expressed in Ohms from 15 ohms to 11 ohms, Figure S3: A report from the ADP-induced platelet activation analysis using Kaluza Flow Cytometry Software (Beckman Coulter, Brea, CA, USA). Results indicate the gating of whole platelet population (CD42b positive events) and the proportion of activated platelets indicated by PAC-1 and P-selectin expression, Figure S4: A report from the PMP analysis using Kaluza Flow Cytometry Software (Beckman Coulter, Brea, CA, USA). Microparticle gating was established using Megamix beads of standard sizes. PMPs were distinguished from other microparticles by size (0.5 µm - 0.9 µm) and expression of CD42b. The number of CD42b positive events in the microparticle gate was used to quantify the PMPs, Figure S5: The effect of varying concentrations of BSE on PAC-1 expression. BSE did not significantly reduce ADP-induced platelet conformational change detected by PAC-1 expression (p values > 0.1 compared to control) N=14 and data is represented in mean fluorescence intensity (MFI) versus BSE concentrations. Error bars expressed as mean ± SD, Figure S6: The effect of varying concentrations of BSE on P-selectin expression. BSE did not significantly reduce ADP-induced platelet degranulation detected by P-selectin expression (p values > 0.1 compared to control) N=14 and data is represented in mean fluorescence intensity (MFI) versus BSE concentrations Error bars expressed as mean ± SD, Table S1: Phenolic composition and antioxidant activity of sorghum varieties on as is basis, Table S2: List of top ten phenolic compounds identified in the black sorghum phenolic rich extracts by Q-TOF LC/MS and quantified using UHPLC-Online ABTS system (Adapted from Rao et al., 2018).

Author Contributions: B.E.N. conducted the experiments outlined in this study and drafted the manuscript. K.A.C., C.L.B. and A.B.S. were involved in the designing and critical reviewing of the manuscript. All authors have read and agreed to the published version of the manuscript.

Funding: This study was funded by the Australian Research Council Industrial Transformations Training Centre for Functional Grains (Project ID 100737).

Acknowledgments: The authors would like to acknowledge Graham Centre for Agricultural Innovation for providing funding towards open access publication of this article. Borkwei Ed Nignpense is a recipient of a PhD Scholarship from the Australian Government Research Training Program and also a recipient of a top-up scholarship by the Graham Centre.

Conflicts of Interest: The authors declare no conflict of interest.

Abbreviations

ADP	Adenosine diphosphate
ATP	Adenosine triphosphate
BSE	Black sorghum extract
COX-1	Cyclooxygenase-1
DMSO	Dimethyl sulfoxide
EDTA	Ethylene diamine tetra-acetic acid
FBE	Full blood examination
GAE	Gallic acid equivalents
MCH	Mean cell haemoglobin
MCHC	Mean cell haemoglobin concentration
MCV	Mean cell haemoglobin
MFI	Mean fluorescence intensity
MPV	Mean platelet volume
PAR	Protease-activated receptor
PAC-1	Procaspase activating compound-1
PBS	Phosphate buffered saline
PCV	Packed cell volume
PGE1	Prostaglandin E1
PMP	Platelet microparticle
RBC	Red blood cell
SD	Standard deviation
WBC	White blood cell

References

1. Waters, A.M.; Trinh, T.; Chau, M.B.; Moon, L. Latest Statistics on Cardiovascular Disease in Australia. *Clin. Exp. Pharm. Physiol.* **2013**, *40*, 347–356. [CrossRef] [PubMed]
2. Organization World Health. *Cardiovascular Diseases (Cvds) Fact. Sheet*; Organization World Health: Geneva, Switzerland, 2017.
3. Zaldivia, M.T.K.; McFadyen, J.D.; Lim, B.; Wang, X.; Peter, K. Platelet-Derived Microvesicles in Cardiovascular Diseases. *Front. Cardiovasc. Med.* **2017**, *4*, 74. [CrossRef] [PubMed]
4. Wolf, P. The Nature and Significance of Platelet Products in Human Plasma. *Br. J Haematol.* **1967**, *13*, 269–288. [CrossRef] [PubMed]
5. Santhakumar, B.A.; Bulmer, A.C.; Singh, I. A Review of the Mechanisms and Effectiveness of Dietary Polyphenols in Reducing Oxidative Stress and Thrombotic Risk. *J. Hum. Nutr. Diet.* **2014**, *27*, 1–21. [CrossRef]
6. Sambu, N.; Curzen, N. Monitoring the Effectiveness of Antiplatelet Therapy: Opportunities and Limitations. *Br. J. Clin. Pharmacol.* **2011**, *72*, 683–696. [CrossRef]

7. Sharma, R.; Reddy, V.; Singh, R.S.; Bhatt, G. Aspirin and Clopidogrel Hyporesponsiveness and Nonresponsiveness in Patients with Coronary Artery Stenting. *Vasc. Health Risk Manag.* **2009**, *5*, 965–972. [CrossRef]
8. Rao, S.; Santhakumar, A.B.; Chinkwo, K.A.; Wu, G.; Johnson, S.K.; Blanchard, C.L. Characterization of phenolic compounds and antioxidant activity in sorghum grains. *J. Cereal Sci.* **2018**, *84*, 103–111. [CrossRef]
9. Dykes, L.; Rooney, L.W.; Waniska, R.D.; Rooney, W.L. Phenolic compounds and antioxidant activity of sorghum grains of varying genotypes. *J. Agric. Food Chem.* **2005**, *53*, 6813–6818. [CrossRef]
10. Francis, N.; Rao, S.; Blanchard, C.; Santhakumar, A. Black Sorghum Phenolic Extract Regulates Expression of Genes Associated with Oxidative Stress and Inflammation in Human Endothelial Cells. *Molecules* **2019**, *24*, 3321. [CrossRef]
11. Ed Nignpense, B.; Chinkwo, K.A.; Blanchard, C.L.; Santhakumar, A.B. Polyphenols: Modulators of Platelet Function and Platelet Microparticle Generation? *Int. J. Mol. Sci.* **2020**, *21*, 146. [CrossRef]
12. Santhakumar, A.B.; Stanley, R.; Singh, I. The ex vivo antiplatelet activation potential of fruit phenolic metabolite hippuric acid. *Food Funct.* **2015**, *6*, 2679–2683. [CrossRef] [PubMed]
13. Lu, G.Y.; Xu, R.J.; Zhang, S.H.; Qiao, Q.; Shen, L.; Li, M.; Xu, D.Y.; Wang, Z.Y. Alteration of circulatory platelet microparticles and endothelial microparticles in patients with chronic kidney disease. *Int. J. Clin. Exp. Med.* **2015**, *8*, 16704–16708. [PubMed]
14. Royal College of Pathologists of Australasia. RCPA manual. 2004.
15. Li, J.; Yu, G.; Fan, J. Alditols and monosaccharides from sorghum vinegar can attenuate platelet aggregation by inhibiting cyclooxygenase-1 and thromboxane-A2 synthase. *J. Ethnopharmacol.* **2014**, *155*, 285–292. [CrossRef]
16. Fan, J.; Zhang, Y.; Chang, X.; Bolin, Z.; Jiang, D.; Saito, M.; Zaigui, L. Antithrombotic and fibrinolytic activities of methanolic extract of aged sorghum vinegar. *J. Agric. Food Chem.* **2009**, *57*, 8683–8687. [CrossRef]
17. Scalbert, A.; Williamson, G. Dietary Intake and Bioavailability of Polyphenols. *J. Nutr.* **2000**, *130*, 2073S–2085S. [CrossRef]
18. Ostertag, L.M.; O'Kennedy, N.G.W.; Horgan, P.A.; Kroon, G.G.D.; de Roos, B. In Vitro Anti-Platelet Effects of Simple Plant-Derived Phenolic Compounds Are Only Found at High, Non-Physiological Concentrations. *Mol. Nutr. Food Res.* **2011**, *55*, 1624–1636. [CrossRef] [PubMed]
19. Koren, E.; Kohen, R.; Ginsburg, I. Polyphenols enhance total oxidant-scavenging capacities of human blood by binding to red blood cells. *Exp. Biol. Med.* **2010**, *235*, 689–699. [CrossRef]
20. Wright, B.; Moraes, C.; Kemp, W.M.; Jonathan, M.G. A Structural Basis for the Inhibition of Collagen-Stimulated Platelet Function by Quercetin and Structurally Related Flavonoids. *Br. J. Pharmacol.* **2010**, *159*, 1312–1325. [CrossRef] [PubMed]
21. Khan, I.; Yousif, A.M.; Johnson, S.K.; Gamlath, S. Acute effect of sorghum flour-containing pasta on plasma total polyphenols, antioxidant capacity and oxidative stress markers in healthy subjects: A randomised controlled trial. *Clin. Nutr.* **2015**, *34*, 415–421. [CrossRef]
22. Damman, P.; Kuijt, R.; Stefan, K.J. P2y12 Platelet Inhibition in Clinical Practice. *J. Thromb. Thrombolysis* **2012**, *33*, 143–153. [CrossRef]
23. Pignatelli, P.; Pulcinelli, F.M.; Celestini, A.; Lenti, L.; Ghiselli, A.; Gazzaniga, P.P.; Violi, F. The flavonoids quercetin and catechin synergistically inhibit platelet function by antagonizing the intracellular production of hydrogen peroxide. *Am. J. Clin. Nutr.* **2000**, *72*, 1150–1155. [CrossRef] [PubMed]
24. Pignatelli, P.; Pulcinelli, F.M.; Lenti, L.; Gazzaniga, P.P.; Violi, F. Hydrogen peroxide is involved in collagen-induced platelet activation. *Blood* **1998**, *91*, 484–490. [CrossRef] [PubMed]
25. Jang, J.Y.; Min, J.; Chae, Y.H.; Baek, J.Y.; Wang, S.B.; Park, S.J.; Oh, G.T.; Lee, S.; Ho, Y.; Chang, T. Reactive oxygen species play a critical role in collagen-induced platelet activation via SHP-2 oxidation. *Antioxid. Redox Signal.* **2014**, *20*, 2528–2540. [CrossRef] [PubMed]
26. Yao, Y.; Chen, Y.; Adili, R.; McKeown, T.; Chen, P.; Zhu, G.; Li, D.; Ling, W.; Ni, H.; Yang, Y. Plant-Based Food Cyanidin-3-Glucoside Modulates Human Platelet Glycoprotein Vi Signaling and Inhibits Platelet Activation and Thrombus Formation. *J. Nutr.* **2017**, *147*, 1917–1925. [CrossRef]
27. Guerrero, J.A.; Lozano, M.L.; Castillo, J.; Benavente-Garcia, O.; Vicente, V.; Rivera, J. Flavonoids inhibit platelet function through binding to the thromboxane A2 receptor. *J. Thromb. Haemost.* **2005**, *3*, 369–376. [CrossRef]

28. Poncelet, P.; Robert, S.; Bailly, N.; Garnache-Ottou, F.; Bouriche, T.; Devalet B.; Seghatchian, J.; Saas, P.; Mullier, F. Tips and tricks for flow cytometry-based analysis and counting of microparticles. *Transfus. Apher. Sci.* **2015**, *53*, 110–126. [CrossRef]
29. Connor, D.E.; Exner, T.; Ma, D.D.; Joseph, J.E. The majority of circulating platelet-derived microparticles fail to bind annexin V, lack phospholipid-dependent procoagulant activity and demonstrate greater expression of glycoprotein Ib. *Thromb. Haemost.* **2010**, *103*, 1044–1052.
30. Ueba, T.; Nomura, S.; Inami, N.; Nishikawa, T.; Kajiwara, M.; Iwata, R.; Yamashita, K. Plasma level of platelet-derived microparticles is associated with coronary heart disease risk score in healthy men. *J. Atheroscler. Thromb.* **2010**, *17*, 342–349. [CrossRef]
31. Badimon, L.; Padró, T.; Vilahur, G. Atherosclerosis, platelets and thrombosis in acute ischaemic heart disease. *Eur. Heart J. Acute Cardiovasc. Care* **2012**, *1*, 60–74. [CrossRef]
32. Merten, M.; Pakala, R.; Thiagarajan, P.; Benedict, C.R. Platelet microparticles promote platelet interaction with subendothelial matrix in a glycoprotein IIb/IIIa-dependent mechanism. *Circulation* **1999**, *99*, 2577–2582. [CrossRef]

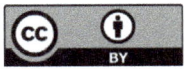

© 2020 by the authors. Licensee MDPI, Basel, Switzerland. This article is an open access article distributed under the terms and conditions of the Creative Commons Attribution (CC BY) license (http://creativecommons.org/licenses/by/4.0/).

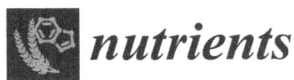

Article

Dietary Polyphenol Intake is Associated with HDL-Cholesterol and A Better Profile of Other Components of the Metabolic Syndrome: A PREDIMED-Plus Sub-Study

Sara Castro-Barquero [1,2,†], Anna Tresserra-Rimbau [2,3,4,5,†], Facundo Vitelli-Storelli [6], Mónica Doménech [1,2], Jordi Salas-Salvadó [2,3,4,5], Vicente Martín-Sánchez [6,7], María Rubín-García [6], Pilar Buil-Cosiales [2,8,9], Dolores Corella [2,10], Montserrat Fitó [2,11], Dora Romaguera [2,12], Jesús Vioque [7,13], Ángel María Alonso-Gómez [2,14], Julia Wärnberg [2,15], José Alfredo Martínez [2,16,17], Luís Serra-Majem [2,18], Francisco José Tinahones [2,19], José Lapetra [2,20], Xavier Pintó [2,21], Josep Antonio Tur [2,12,22], Antonio Garcia-Rios [23], Laura García-Molina [7,24], Miguel Delgado-Rodriguez [13,25], Pilar Matía-Martín [26], Lidia Daimiel [17], Josep Vidal [27,28], Clotilde Vázquez [2,29], Montserrat Cofán [2,30], Andrea Romanos-Nanclares [8], Nerea Becerra-Tomas [2,3,4,5], Rocio Barragan [2,10], Olga Castañer [2,11], Jadwiga Konieczna [2,12], Sandra González-Palacios [7,13], Carolina Sorto-Sánchez [2,14], Jessica Pérez-López [2,15], María Angeles Zulet [2,16,17], Inmaculada Bautista-Castaño [2,18], Rosa Casas [1,2], Ana María Gómez-Perez [2,19], José Manuel Santos-Lozano [2,20], María Ángeles Rodríguez-Sanchez [21], Alicia Julibert [2,12,22], Nerea Martín-Calvo [2,8], Pablo Hernández-Alonso [2,3,4,5,31], José V Sorlí [2,10], Albert Sanllorente [2,11], Aina María Galmés-Panadés [2,12], Eugenio Cases-Pérez [32], Leire Goicolea-Güemez [2,14], Miguel Ruiz-Canela [2,8], Nancy Babio [2,3,4,5], Álvaro Hernáez [1,2], Rosa María Lamuela-Raventós [2,33] and Ramon Estruch [1,2,34,*]

1. Department of Medicine, Faculty of Medicine and Life Sciences, University of Barcelona, Barcelona, Spain. Institut d'Investigacions Biomèdiques August Pi I Sunyer (IDIBAPS), 08036 Barcelona, Spain; sara.castro@ub.edu (S.C.-B.); mdomen@clinic.cat (M.D.); rcasas1@clinic.cat (R.C.); alvaro.hernaez1@gmail.com (Á.H.)
2. Centro de Investigación Biomédica en Red Fisiopatología de la Obesidad y la Nutrición (CIBEROBN), Instituto de Salud Carlos III, 28029 Madrid, Spain; anna.tresserra@iispv.cat (A.T.-R.); jordi.salas@urv.cat (J.S.-S.); pilarbuilc@gmail.com (P.B.-C.); dolores.corella@uv.es (D.C.); mfito@imim.es (M.F.); mariaadoracion.romaguera@ssib.es (D.R.); angelmaria.alonsogomez@osakidetza.eus (Á.M.A.-G.); jwarnberg@uma.es (J.W); jalfmtz@unav.es (J.A.M.); lluis.serra@ulpgc.es (L.S.-M.); fjtinahones@uma.es (F.J.T.); jose.lapetra.sspa@juntadeandalucia.es (J.L.); xpinto@bellvitgehospital.cat (X.P.); pep.tur@uib.es (J.A.T.); clotilde.vazquez@fjc.es (C.V.); mcofan@clinic.cat (M.C.); nerea.becerra@urv.cat (N.B.-T.); rocio.barragan@uv.es (R.B.); ocastaner@imim.es (O.C.); jadwiga.konieczna@ssib.es (J.K.); daisysorto2@yahoo.com (C.S.-S.); jessicaperezlopez@uma.es (J.P.-L.); mazulet@unav.es (M.A.Z.); inmaculada.bautista@ulpgc.es (I.B.-C.); anamgp86@gmail.com (A.M.G.-P.); josem.santos.lozano.sspa@juntadeandalucia.es (J.M.S.-L.); alicia.julibert@uib.es (A.J.); nmartincalvo@unav.es (N.M.-C.); pablo1280@gmail.com (P.H.-A.); Sorli@uv.es (J.V.S.); albertsanllorente@gmail.com (A.S.); aina.galmes@uib.es (A.M.G.-P.); leiregoiko@gmail.com (L.G.-G.); mcanela@unav.es (M.R.-C.); nancy.babio@urv.cat (N.B.); lamuela@ub.edu (R.M.L.-R.)
3. Universitat Rovira i Virgili, Departament de Bioquímica i Biotecnologia, Unitat de Nutrició, 43204 Reus, Spain
4. University Hospital of Sant Joan de Reus, Nutrition Unit, 43201 Reus, Spain
5. Institut d'Investigació Sanitària Pere Virgili (IISPV), 43201 Reus, Spain
6. Institute of Biomedicine (IBIOMED), University of León, 24071 León, Spain; fvits@unileon.es (F.V.-S.); vicente.martin@unileon.es (V.M.-S.); mrubig@estudiantes.unileon.es (M.R.-G.)
7. CIBER de Epidemiología y Salud Pública (CIBERESP), Instituto de Salud Carlos III, 28029 Madrid, Spain; vioque@umh.es (J.V.); lgarmol@ugr.es (L.G.-M.); sandra.gonzalezp@umh.es (S.G.-P.)

8   University of Navarra, Department of Preventive Medicine and Public Health, Instituto de Investigación Sanitaria de Navarra (IdiSNA), 31008 Pamplona, Spain; aromanos@unav.es
9   Servicio Navarro de Salud-Osasunbidea-Instituto de Investigación Sanitaria de Navarra (IdiSNA), 31008 Pamplona, Spain
10   Department of Preventive Medicine, University of Valencia, 46010 Valencia, Spain
11   Cardiovascular Risk and Nutrition Research group, Institut Hospital del Mar de Investigaciones Médicas (IMIM), 08007 Barcelona, Spain
12   Health Research Institute of the Balearic Islands (IdISBa), University Hospital Son Espases (Research Unit), 07120 Palma de Mallorca, Spain
13   Miguel Hernandez University, ISABIAL-FISABIO, 03010 Alicante, Spain; mdelgado@ujaen.es
14   Bioaraba Health Research Institute; Osakidetza Basque Health Service, Araba University Hospital; University of the Basque Country UPV/EHU, 01009 Vitoria-Gasteiz, Spain
15   Department of Nursing. University of Málaga, Instituto de Investigación Biomédica de Málaga (IBIMA), 29010 Málaga, Spain
16   Department of Nutrition, Food Sciences, and Physiology, Center for Nutrition Research, University of Navarra, 31008 Pamplona, Spain
17   Precision Nutrition Program, IMDEA Food, CEI UAM + CSIC, 28049 Madrid, Spain; lidia.daimiel@imdea.org
18   Research Institute of Biomedical and Health Sciences (IUIBS), University of Las Palmas de Gran Canaria & Centro Hospitalario Universitario Insular Materno Infantil (CHUIMI), Canarian Health Service, 35016 Las Palmas de Gran Canaria, Spain
19   Virgen de la Victoria Hospital, Department of Endocrinology, Instituto de Investigación Biomédica de Málaga (IBIMA). University of Málaga, 29010 Málaga, Spain
20   Department of Family Medicine, Research Unit, Distrito Sanitario Atención Primaria Sevilla, 41010 Sevilla, Spain
21   Lipids and Vascular Risk Unit, Internal Medicine, Hospital Universitario de Bellvitge, IDIBELL, Hospitalet de Llobregat, 08908 Barcelona, Spain; mrodriguezsa@bellvitgehospital.cat
22   Research Group on Community Nutrition & Oxidative Stress, University of Balearic Islands, 07122 Palma de Mallorca, Spain
23   Department of Internal Medicine, Maimonides Biomedical Research Institute of Cordoba (IMIBIC), Reina Sofia University Hospital, University of Cordoba, 14004 Cordoba, Spain; angarios2004@yahoo.es
24   Department of Preventive Medicine and Public Health, University of Granada, 18016 Granada, Spain
25   Division of Preventive Medicine, Faculty of Medicine, University of Jaén, 23071 Jaén, Spain
26   Department of Endocrinology and Nutrition, Instituto de Investigación Sanitaria Hospital Clínico San Carlos (IdISSC), 28040 Madrid, Spain; mmatia@ucm.es
27   CIBER Diabetes y Enfermedades Metabólicas (CIBERDEM), Instituto de Salud Carlos III (ISCIII), 28029 Madrid, Spain; jovidal@clinic.cat
28   Department of Endocrinology, Institut d'Investigacions Biomédiques August Pi Sunyer (IDIBAPS), Hospital Clinic, University of Barcelona, 08036 Barcelona, Spain
29   Department of Endocrinology and Nutrition, Hospital Fundación Jimenez Díaz, Instituto de Investigaciones Biomédicas IISFJD. University Autonoma, 28040 Madrid, Spain
30   Lipid Clinic, Department of Endocrinology and Nutrition, Institut d'Investigacions Biomèdiques August Pi Sunyer (IDIBAPS), Hospital Clínic, 08036 Barcelona, Spain
31   Unidad de Gestión Clínica de Endocrinología y Nutrición del Hospital Virgen de la Victoria, Instituto de Investigación Biomédica de Málaga (IBIMA), 29010 Málaga, Spain
32   Centro de Salud Raval, 03203 Alicante, Spain; ecases@coma.es
33   Department of Nutrition, Food Science and Gastronomy, XaRTA, INSA, School of Pharmacy and Food Sciences, University of Barcelona, 08028 Barcelona, Spain
34   Department of Internal Medicine, Hospital Clinic de Barcelona, 08036 Barcelona, Spain
*   Correspondence: restruch@clinic.cat; Tel.: +34-932-279-935
†   These authors contributed equally to this work.

Received: 7 February 2020; Accepted: 29 February 2020; Published: 4 March 2020

Abstract: Dietary polyphenol intake is associated with improvement of metabolic disturbances. The aims of the present study are to describe dietary polyphenol intake in a population with metabolic syndrome (MetS) and to examine the association between polyphenol intake and the components of MetS. This cross-sectional analysis involved 6633 men and women included in the PREDIMED (PREvención con DIeta MEDiterranea-Plus) study. The polyphenol content of foods was estimated from the Phenol-Explorer 3.6 database. The mean of total polyphenol intake was 846 ± 318 mg/day. Except for stilbenes, women had higher polyphenol intake than men. Total polyphenol intake was higher in older participants (>70 years of age) compared to their younger counterparts. Participants with body mass index (BMI) >35 kg/m^2 reported lower total polyphenol, flavonoid, and stilbene intake than those with lower BMI. Total polyphenol intake was not associated with a better profile concerning MetS components, except for high-density lipoprotein cholesterol (HDL-c), although stilbenes, lignans, and other polyphenols showed an inverse association with blood pressure, fasting plasma glucose, and triglycerides. A direct association with HDL-c was found for all subclasses except lignans and phenolic acids. To conclude, in participants with MetS, higher intake of several polyphenol subclasses was associated with a better profile of MetS components, especially HDL-c.

Keywords: polyphenols; metabolic syndrome; Mediterranean diet; glignans; stilbenes; HDL-cholesterol

1. Introduction

Polyphenols are plant-derived molecules characterized by the presence of one or more aromatic rings and attached hydroxyl groups [1]. They are classified into five subclasses according to their chemical structure, including flavonoids and nonflavonoids subclasses defined as phenolic acids, stilbenes, lignans, and other polyphenols. These bioactive compounds are responsible for some health and sensory properties of foods, such as bitterness, astringency, and antioxidant capacity. The intake of phenolic compounds and their food sources is highly variable and depends on dietary patterns, sex, socioeconomic factors, and the native foods of each region [2]. The Mediterranean diet (MedDiet) is characterized by a high intake of phenolic compounds because MedDiet interventions promote the intake of phenolic rich and plant-based products, such as legumes, vegetables, fruits, nuts and wholegrain cereals, and promote the use of extra virgin olive oil as the main source of fat. It has been suggested that phenolic compounds are partly responsible for the beneficial effects attributed to the MedDiet [3].

The metabolic syndrome (MetS) is defined as a cluster of metabolic disturbances, which include impaired glucose metabolism, elevated blood pressure, and low level of HDL-c, dyslipidemia, and abdominal obesity [4]. Sedentary lifestyle, smoking, and unbalanced diets are well-known modifiable risk factors for MetS, and lifestyle interventions in those areas, especially dietary interventions based on the MedDiet [3–6], might improve this condition. Considering the chronic low-grade inflammation and oxidative stress observed in MetS, polyphenols are good candidates to improve the condition because of their antioxidant and anti-inflammatory properties [7]. Moreover, several epidemiological studies have observed a negative association between polyphenol intake and MetS rates [8]. Regarding MetS components, an adequate intake of phenolic compounds has been shown to improve lipid profile and insulin resistance, and decrease blood pressure levels and body weight [8,9].

Despite the fact that phenol-rich dietary patterns are effective in improving some MetS components, there is no single phenolic compound or extract able to improve all the components of MetS [10]. Nevertheless, given the complexity of MetS and the heterogeneity of polyphenols, more large randomized trials with MetS patients are needed to evaluate the effect of polyphenol intake in reducing MetS complications, and whether intake of the different polyphenol subclasses could be associated with improvements in MetS components, because each subtype has different absorption and metabolism [11].

Therefore, the aims of our study were firstly to describe polyphenol intake in 6633 participants with MetS from the PREvención con DIeta MEDiterranea-Plus (PREDIMED-Plus) trial and to identify the main food sources of polyphenols in those participants, and secondly to examine whether higher intakes of some polyphenol sub-classes are associated with MetS components in this population.

2. Materials and Methods

2.1. Design of the Study

A cross-sectional analysis of the baseline data of participants included in the PREvención con DIeta MEDiterranea-Plus (PREDIMED-Plus) study was performed. The profile of the cohort, recruiting methods, and data collection processes have been described elsewhere [12] and on the website http://predimedplus.com. The study protocol was approved by the 23 recruiting centers Institutional Review Boards and registered in 2014 at the International Standard Randomized Controlled Trial Number registry (http://www.isrctn.com/ISRCTN89898870). All participants provided written informed consent before joining the study.

2.2. Participants

A total of 6874 subjects were recruited and randomized in the 23 recruiting centers between September 2013 and December 2016. Primary care medical doctors from primary care centers of the National Health System assessed potential participants for eligibility. Eligible participants were men (aged 55–75 years) and women (aged 60–75 years) with overweight or obesity (body mass index [BMI] ≥27 and <40 kg/m^2) and at least three components of MetS according to the comprehensive definition of the International Diabetes Federation; National Heart, Lung, and Blood Institute; and American Heart Association (2009) [4]. Exclusion criteria were documented history of cardiovascular diseases (CVD), having a long-term illness, drug or alcohol use disorder, a BMI of 40 or higher, a history of allergy or intolerance to extra virgin olive oil or nuts, malignant cancer, inability to follow the recommended diet or physical activity program, history of surgical procedures for weight loss, and obesity of known endocrine disease (except for treated hypothyroidism). Of the total sample of 6874 randomized participants, 241 participants were excluded from the current analysis (Figure 1): 53 without food-frequency questionnaire (FFQ) data at baseline, and 188 participants who reported energy intake values outside the predefined limits (<3347 kJ [800 kcal]/day or >17,573 kJ [4000 kcal]/day for men; <2510 kJ [500 kcal]/day or >14,644 kJ [3500 kcal]/day for women) [13].

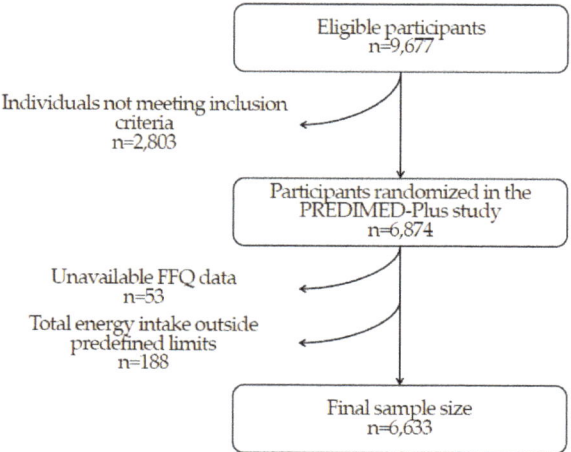

Figure 1. Flowchart of the participants.

2.3. Estimation of Dietary Polyphenol Intake

The total dietary polyphenol intake and polyphenol subclasses were obtained at baseline by the 143-item FFQs used in the PREDIMED-Plus study. As described elsewhere [14], dietary polyphenol intake was estimated following these steps: (1) All foods from the FFQ with no polyphenol content, or only traces, were excluded; (2) recipes were calculated according to their ingredients and portions using traditional MedDiet recipes; (3) when an item from the FFQ included several foods (e.g., oranges and tangerines), the proportion of intake was calculated according to data available in the national survey; (4) no retention or yield factors were used to correct weight changes during cooking because this was already taken into account in the FFQ; (5) the polyphenol content in 100 g of each food item was obtained from the Phenol-Explorer database (version 3.6) [15]; (6) finally, the individual polyphenol intake from each food was calculated by multiplying the content of each polyphenol by the daily consumption of each food. Total polyphenol intake was calculated as the sum of all individual polyphenol intakes from the food sources reported in the FFQ.

The data used to calculate polyphenol intake was obtained by chromatography of all the phenolic compounds, except proanthocyanidins, the content of which was obtained by normal-phase high-performance liquid chromatography. In the case of lignans and phenolic acids in certain foods (i.e., swiss chard, chickpeas, plums, and strawberry jam), data corresponding to chromatography after hydrolysis was also collected, since these treatments are needed to release phenolic compounds that could otherwise not be analyzed. Total and polyphenol subclass intakes were adjusted for energy intake (kcal/day) using the residual method [13].

2.4. Measurements and Outcome Assessment

Data on age, sex, educational levels, anthropometric measurements, dietary habits and lifestyle were collected at baseline. Anthropometric measurements were measured according to the PREDIMED-Plus protocol. Weight was recorded with participants in light clothing without shoes or accessories using a high-quality calibrated scale. Height was measured with a wall-mounted stadiometer. Waist circumference was measured midway between the lowest rib and the iliac crest. The BMI was calculated as weight (kg) divided by the square of height (m^2).

Physical activity and sedentary behaviors were evaluated using the validated Regicor Short Physical Activity Questionnaire [16] and the validated Spanish version of the Nurses' Health Study questionnaire [17], respectively.

Information related to sociodemographic and lifestyle habits, individual and family medical history, smoking status, medical conditions, and medication use was evaluated using self-reported questionnaires. Sociodemographic and lifestyle variables were categorized as follows: age (three categories: <65, 65–70, or >70 years), educational level (three categories: primary, secondary, or high school), physical activity level (three categories: low, moderate, or high), BMI (three categories: 27.0–29.9, 30.0–34.9, or ≥35 kg/m^2), and smoking status (three categories: never, former, or current smoker).

Blood samples were collected after overnight fasting. Biochemical analyses were performed to determine plasma glucose (mg/dL), glycated hemoglobin (%), HDL-c (mg/dL), and triglyceride (mg/dL) levels using standard laboratory enzymatic methods. Low-density lipoprotein cholesterol (LDL-c; mg/dL) was calculated using the Friedewald formula whenever triglyceride levels were less than 300 mg/dL. Blood pressure measurements were obtained after the participant had rested for five minutes. Each measurement was obtained with a validated semiautomatic oscillometer (Omron HEM-705CP), ensuring the use of the proper cuff size for each participant.

2.5. Statistical Analysis

Descriptive statistics were used to define the baseline characteristics of the participants. The database used was the PREDIMED-Plus baseline database generated in September 2018.

Continuous variables are expressed as mean ± SD. Categorical variables are expressed as number (n) and percentage (%). Comparisons among quartiles of dietary polyphenol intake used the Pearson chi square test (χ^2) for categorical variables or one-way ANOVA for continuous variables. The associations between dietary polyphenol intake and MetS components were analyzed by linear regression models to determine differences between quartiles of polyphenol subclass intake. The results of the regression models are expressed as unstandardized β-coefficients. For regression models, polyphenol and polyphenol subclasses are expressed as quartiles of energy-adjusted dietary intake. We used robust variance estimators to account for intra-cluster correlation in all linear models, considering members of the same household as a cluster. All regression models were adjusted for potential confounders. Model 1 was adjusted for sex, age, recruiting center, and members of the same household. Model 2 was additionally adjusted for physical activity level, BMI (except for waist circumference criteria), smoking status, and educational level. We additionally adjusted for anti-diabetic treatment when assessing glycemia and antihypertensive treatments when assessing blood pressure. Lastly, model 3 was additionally adjusted for total energy intake (continuous, kcal/day), saturated fatty acids (g/day), and distilled drinks alcohol intake (g/day). In model 3, the analysis of glycemia was additionally adjusted for dietary simple sugar intake (g/day), whereas the analysis of systolic and diastolic blood pressures was also adjusted for dietary sodium intake (mg/day). The normality of the continuous outcomes and standardized residuals was assessed with the Shapiro–Wilk test. Values are shown as 95% confidence interval (CI) and significance for all statistical tests was based on bilateral contrast set at $p < 0.05$. The P value for linear trends was computed by fitting a continuous variable that assigned the median value for each quartile in regression models. The descriptive analyses shown in Tables 1–3 were performed using SPSS software version 22.0 (Chicago, IL, USA) and the regression analysis was performed using Stata software version 16 (StataCorp LP, College Station, TX, USA).

Table 1. Baseline characteristic of participants by quartiles of total polyphenol intake.

	Q1 (<623.3 mg/d)	Q2 (623.4–799.4 mg/d)	Q3 (799.5–1019.2 mg/d)	Q4 (>1019.3 mg/d)	p	p for Linear Trend
n	1658	1658	1660	1657		
Age, years	65.2 ± 4.90	64.8 ± 4.87	65.0 ± 4.87	64.9 ± 4.98	0.10	0.19
Women, n (%)	894 (53.9)	845 (51.0)	785 (47.3)	685 (41.3)	<0.001	<0.001
Family history of CVD [1], n (%)	659 (39.7)	698 (42.1)	662 (39.9)	678 (40.9)	0.48	0.81
Current smokers, n (%)	197 (11.9)	205 (12.4)	203 (12.2)	216 (13.0)	0.78	0.36
Former smokers, n (%)	647 (39.0)	695 (41.9)	728 (43.9)	800 (48.3)	<0.001	<0.001
BMI, kg/m²	32.6 ± 3.46	32.6 ± 3.49	32.6 ± 3.51	32.3 ± 3.31	0.03	0.02
Waist circumference, cm	107.0 ± 9.76	107.4 ± 9.70	107.8 ± 9.75	107.8 ± 9.36	0.06	0.01
Body weight, kg	85.2 ± 12.8	86.2 ± 12.8	87.3 ± 13.3	87.5 ± 12.8	<0.001	<0.001
Glucose, mg/dL	113.4 ± 28.9	113.9 ± 31.0	113.9 ± 29.0	113.0 ± 27.6	0.78	0.71
Glycated hemoglobin, %	6.10 ± 0.88	6.22 ± 2.58	6.25 ± 3.53	6.10 ± 0.88	0.15	0.85
Total cholesterol, mg/dL	196 ± 38.4	197 ± 37.7	196 ± 37.0	198 ± 42.8	0.59	0.57
HDL-cholesterol, mg/dL	47.6 ± 11.5	48.2 ± 11.7	48.7 ± 12.2	47.9 ± 11.9	0.06	0.32
Medications, n (%)						
Antihypertensive agents	1272 (76.7)	1285 (77.5)	1294 (77.9)	1304 (78.7)	0.48	0.46
Colesterol-lowering agents	862 (52.0)	846 (51.0)	858 (51.7)	842 (50.8)	0.97	0.52
Insulin	84 (5.07)	98 (5.91)	67 (4.04)	63 (3.80)	0.01	0.01
Metformin	380 (22.9)	404 (24.4)	383 (23.1)	347 (20.9)	0.13	0.12
Other hypoglycemic drugs	324 (19.5)	331 (20.0)	327 (19.7)	303 (18.3)	0.62	0.35
Aspirin or antiplatelet drugs	246 (14.8)	272 (16.4)	249 (15.0)	271 (16.3)	0.26	0.61
NSAIDs	534 (32.2)	469 (28.3)	484 (29.2)	446 (26.9)	0.01	0.01
Vitamins and minerals	210 (12.7)	184 (11.1)	220 (13.3)	183 (11.0)	0.19	0.11
Sedative or tranquilliser agents	417 (25.1)	416 (25.1)	389 (23.4)	392 (23.7)	0.85	0.31
Hormonal treatment (only women)	42 (2.50)	41 (2.47)	33 (1.99)	38 (2.29)	0.924	0.935
Educational level, n (%)					<0.001	<0.001
Primary school	887 (53.6)	854 (51.5)	805 (48.5)	719 (43.4)		
Secondary school	468 (28.3)	467 (28.2)	497 (30.0)	481 (29.0)		
University and other studies	301 (18.2)	337 (20.3)	356 (21.5)	456 (27.5)		

[1] Cardiovascular diseases (CVD), body mass index (BMI), high-density lipoprotein-cholesterol (HDL-c) and nonsteroidal anti-inflammatory drugs (NSAIDs). Continue variables are expressed as mean (± SD). Categorical variables are expressed as number (n) and percentage (%). Comparisons among quartiles of dietary polyphenol intake with Pearson's chi square test for categorical variables or one-way ANOVA for continuous variables. For glycated hemoglobine parameter, 9% of participants had no values available. The P value for linear trend was computed by fitting a continuous variable that assigned the median value for each quartile in regression models.

Table 2. Contribution (%) of polyphenol subclasses to total polyphenol intake and food sources.

Polyphenol Subclasses	Contribution, Mean (mg/d) ± SD, (%)	Polyphenol Contribution as Aglycones, Mean (mg/d) ± SD, (%)	Food Sources (% of Contribution)
Total polyphenols	846 ± 318	620.9 ± 273.5	
Flavonoids	491 ± 253, (58.0)	406.3 ± 237.2 (65.44)	
• Anthocyanins	43.5 ± 37.8, (5.14)	24.7 ± 21.7 (3.98)	Cherries (42.2), red wine (24.1), olives (10.5), strawberries (10.1), grape (9.30), other foods (3.8)
• Chalcones	0.009 ± 0.18, (<0.01)	0.006 ± 0.01 (<0.01)	Beer (100)
• Dihydrochalcones	1.72 ± 1.59, (0.20)	0.98 ± 0.91 (0.16)	Apples (93.2), fruit juices from concentrate (6.77)
• Dihydroflavonols	2.62 ± 4.92, (0.31)	1.81 ± 3.43 (0.29)	Red wine (97.6), white wine (1.80), rosé wine (0.59)
• Catechins	28.1 ± 22.4, (3.32)	27.1 ± 20.7 (4.36)	Tea (23.0), red wine (19.2), apples (18.6), chocolate (11.6), peaches (6.0), cocoa powder (3.18), fruit juices from concentrate (2.83), other foods (15.6)
• Proanthocyanidins	204± 185, (24.1)	200.7 ± 189.4 (32.32)	Chocolate (42.7), apples (20.4), plums (9.53), red wine (7.09), cocoa powder (5.68), strawberries (4.20), other foods (10.4)
• Theaflavin	0.70 ± 1.81, (0.08)	0.57 ± 1.46 (0.09)	Tea (100)
• Flavanones	83.2 ± 76.6, (9.83)	58.1 ± 55.0 (9.35)	Oranges (71.3), natural orange juice (23.0), fruit juices from concentrate (3.22), other foods (2.09)
• Flavones	73.2 ± 47.4, (8.65)	54.7 ± 32.9 (8.81)	Whole-grain bread (30.0), bread (23.6), oranges (21.6), natural orange juice (8.53), artichoke (3.80), other foods (12.5).
• Flavonols	54.0 ± 22.3, (6.40)	35.6 ± 15.3 (5.73)	Onions (27.8), spinach (26.7), lettuce (11.9), red wine (6.02), olives (5.10), asparagus (4.93), other foods (17.55)
• Isoflavonoids	0.002 ± 0.004, (<0.01)	0.002 ± 0.003 (<0.01)	Beer (100)
Phenolic acids	280 ± 131, (33.1)	164.2 ± 70.8 (26.44)	
• Hydroxybenzoic acids	15.5 ± 10.3, (1.83)	20.5 ± 12.4 (3.30)	Red wine (21.2), olives (19.9), walnuts (18.1), tea (9.46), swiss chard leaves (6.15), white wine (1.34), other foods (23.8)
• Hydroxycinnamic acids	264 ± 129, (30.9)	141.6 ± 66.8 (22.80)	Decaffeinated coffee (37.7), coffee (26.1), plums (5.66), potatoes (5.50), olives (4.21), red wine (1.79), other foods (19.0)
• Hydroxyphenylacetic acids	0.90 ± 1.04, (0.10)	1.16 ± 1.40 (0.19)	Olives (87.2), red wine (6.57), beer (3.86), extra virgin olive oil (1.52), white wine (0.65)
• Hydroxyphenylpropanoic acids	0.48 ± 0.65, (0.06)	0.91 ± 1.23 (0.14)	Olives (100)
Stilbenes	2.13 ± 3.92, (0.25)	1.78 ± 3.19 (0.29)	Red wine (91.9), white wine (3.94), grapes (1.60), rosé wine (1.21), other foods (0.07)
Lignans	1.53 ± 0.56, (0.18)	1.33 ± 0.55 (0.21)	Extra virgin olive oil (16.7), seeds (9.84), oranges (9.73), green bean (5.42), pepper (5.32), peaches (4.97), broccoli (4.71), bread (4.48), red wine (4.16), cabbage (2.77), other foods (31.9)
Other polyphenols	70.8 ± 41.5, (8.37)	45.6 ± 27.8 (7.34)	
• Alkylmethoxyphenols	0.93 ± 0.87, (0.11)	0.93 ± 0.87 (0.15)	Decaffeinated coffee (74.1), coffee (16.2), beers (9.77)
• Alkylphenols	13.7 ± 17.8, (1.62)	13.8 ± 18.5 (2.23)	Whole-grain bread (69.1), whole-grain pastries (14.8), breakfast cereals (8.40), pasta (3.29), other foods (4.41)
• Furanocoumarins	0.37 ± 0.38, (0.04)	0.37 ± 0.39 (0.06)	Celery stalks (98.3), grapefruit juice (1.7)
• Hydroxybenzaldehydes	0.42 ± 0.65, (0.05)	0.42 ± 0.66 (<0.01)	Red wine (78.9), walnuts (14.5), beer (2.61), white wine (1.95), other foods (2.04)
• Hydroxybenzoketones	0.002 ± 0.004, (<0.01)	0.002 ± 0.003 (<0.01)	Beer (100)
• Hydroxycoumarins	0.10 ± 0.19, (0.01)	0.09 ±0.18 (<0.01)	Beer (73.6), white wine (26.3), cocoa powder (0.10)
• Methoxyphenols	0.13 ± 0.12, (0.01)	0.11 ± 0.12 (0.01)	Decaffeinated coffee (81.3), coffee (18.7)
• Naphtoquinones	0.82 ± 1.12, (0.09)	0.84 ± 1.14 (0.14)	Walnuts (100)
• Tyrosols	52.4 ± 37.8, (6.19)	30.0 ± 21.2 (4.83)	Olives (50.0), extra virgin olive oil (34.8), refined olive oil (5.17), red wine (3.29), other foods (6.74)
• Other	1.96 ± 2.30, (0.23)	0.66 ± 0.54 (0.11)	Orange juice (45.4), pears (18.2), coffee (16.0), other fruit juices (9.98), olives (5.86), other foods (4.56)

Table 3. Energy-adjusted intake of total polyphenol and their main subclasses according to sociodemographic and lifestyle characteristics.

	n	Total Polyphenols (mg/d)	p	Flavonoids (mg/d)	p	Phenolic Acids (mg/d)	p	Stilbenes (mg/d)	p	Lignans (mg/d)	p	Other Polyphenols (mg/d)	p
Total population	6633	846 ± 275 [1]		491 ± 229		290 ± 127		2.13 ± 3.81		1.53 ± 0.54		70.8 ± 38.5	
Men	3424	830 ± 288	<0.001	469 ± 234	<0.001	285 ± 134	0.003	3.00 ± 4.74	<0.001	1.53 ± 0.54	0.933	72.1 ± 42.5	0.006
Women	3209	863 ± 259		515 ± 220		276 ± 118		1.21 ± 2.12		1.53 ± 0.53		69.5 ± 33.7	
Age (years)													
<65	3530	835 ± 275		476 ± 230		285 ± 128		2.15 ± 4.03		1.51 ± 0.54		70.7 ± 39.2	
65-70	2122	854 ± 271	0.002	503 ± 225	<0.001	276 ± 123	0.014	2.07 ± 3.62	0.605	1.55 ± 0.52	0.006	71.0 ± 38.3	0.967
>70	981	866 ± 281		517 ± 228		275 ± 127		2.21 ± 3.40		1.55 ± 0.54		70.8 ± 36.4	
BMI (Kg/m²)													
<29.9	1762	847 ± 268		501 ± 225		272 ± 124		2.26 ± 3.85		1.52 ± 0.49		69.9 ± 36.8	
30-34.9	3258	852 ± 280	0.042	493 ± 232	0.004	284 ± 129	0.006	2.24 ± 3.90	<0.001	1.53 ± 0.54	0.679	71.5 ± 39.7	0.353
>35	1613	831 ± 270		475 ± 226		282 ± 124		1.77 ± 3.57		1.54 ± 0.57		70.5 ± 37.9	
Physical activity level													
Low	3953	833 ± 278		480 ± 231		280 ± 129		1.85 ± 3.48		1.51 ± 0.54		70.0 ± 38.5	
Moderate	1253	841 ± 267	<0.001	503 ± 217	<0.001	282 ± 123	0.884	2.30 ± 3.79	<0.001	1.57 ± 0.54	<0.001	71.7 ± 36.6	0.034
Active	1408	867 ± 271		510 ± 230		280 ± 123		2.76 ± 4.55		1.58 ± 0.53		72.8 ± 40.0	
Educational level													
Primary school	3266	834 ± 259		482 ± 213		278 ± 121		1.80 ± 3.38		1.54 ± 0.55		70.9 ± 40.2	
Secondary school	1913	840 ± 270	<0.001	487 ± 227	<0.001	279 ± 125	0.070	2.27 ± 3.98	<0.001	1.51 ± 0.53	0.093	69.9 ± 38.1	0.290
University	1450	880 ± 311		517 ± 260		287 ± 139		2.70 ± 4.40		1.55 ± 0.52		72.0 ± 35.0	
Smoking status													
Current smokers	821	841 ± 296	0.581	455 ± 243	<0.001	311 ± 143	<0.001	2.33 ± 4.43	0.114	1.47 ± 0.53	<0.001	70.5 ± 46.3	0.768
Non-smokers	5812	847 ± 272		496 ± 226		276 ± 123		2.10 ± 3.72		1.54 ± 0.54		70.9 ± 37.3	

[1] Mean ± Standard deviation. BMI: body mass index. Total and polyphenol subclasses were adjusted for total energy intake using the residual method. Comparison between subcategories was performed using ANOVA.

3. Results

The present study was conducted on 6633 participants from the PREDIMED-Plus study. The mean age was 65.0 ± 4.9 years, and mean BMI was 32.5 ± 3.44 kg/m^2. Table 1 shows the main characteristics of the participants according to quartiles of dietary total polyphenol intake. We observed that participants included in the highest quartile of polyphenol intake (>1019.3 mg/day) were mainly men and former smokers with a higher educational level (all three $p < 0.001$). We observed an inverse trend in the relationship between polyphenol intake and BMI ($p = 0.02$), whereas this trend was direct for waist circumference ($p = 0.01$) and body weight ($p < 0.001$). Moreover, fewer participants with insulin and nonsteroidal anti-inflammatory drug treatment were observed in the highest quartile of polyphenol intake (both $p = 0.01$).

Total polyphenol intake was 846 ± 318 mg/day, of which 58.0% were flavonoids (491 ± 253 mg/day), 33.1% phenolic acids (280 ± 131 mg/day), and the rest other polyphenols, stilbenes, and lignans (70.8 ± 41.5, 2.13 ± 3.92, and 1.53 ± 0.56 mg/day, respectively). The mean of the total polyphenol aglycone intake was 620.9 ± 273.5 mg/day. Table 2 shows the contribution (%) of each polyphenol subclass and polyphenol aglycones. The highest contributor to total polyphenol intake was hydroxycinnamic acids (30.9%). Regarding flavonoids, flavanols were the main contributors (24.1% from proanthocyanidins, 3.32% catechins, and 0.08% of theaflavins), followed by flavanones (9.83%), flavones (8.65%), flavonols (6.40%), and anthocyanins (5.14%). Additionally, tyrosols represented 6.19% of the total polyphenol intake, being the most abundant polyphenol classified within the group of other polyphenols.

The main food sources for each polyphenol subclass are also shown in Table 2. In the case of flavonoids, the most important contributors to the intake of proanthocyanidins were fruits and chocolate and its derivatives. Fruits (mainly oranges and orange juice) were the greatest contributors of flavanones, while vegetables (mainly onion, spinach, and lettuce) were the greatest contributors of flavones. Red wine, olives, tea, and wholegrain cereals were also important contributors to the remaining subclasses. Coffee was the most significant contributor of phenolic acids, especially of hydroxycinnamic acids, followed by olives and red wine. Stilbenes were mainly provided by red wine (91.9%). Lignans were widely distributed among foods, with extra virgin olive oil, fruits, and vegetables the main contributors. The main contributors of other polyphenols were olives, olive oil, cereals, coffee, and alcoholic beverages (mainly beer and red wine).

Table 3 shows the energy-adjusted intake of total polyphenols and the main subclasses by sex, age, BMI, level of physical activity, educational level, and smoking status. Total polyphenol intake was significantly higher in women due to their high intake of flavonoids ($p < 0.001$), whereas men consumed more phenolic acids ($p = 0.003$), stilbenes, and other polyphenols. The intake of total polyphenols, flavonoids, and lignans increased with age ($p = 0.002$, $p < 0.001$, and $p = 0.006$, respectively). Interestingly, participants with the highest BMI (>35 kg/m^2) showed the lowest total polyphenol ($p = 0.042$), flavonoid ($p = 0.004$), and stilbene intake ($p < 0.001$), whereas phenolic acid intake was significantly higher in this group ($p = 0.006$). The level of physical activity was directly associated with total polyphenol intake ($p < 0.001$) and with all polyphenol classes except for phenolic acids ($p < 0.001$ in all cases except $p = 0.03$ for other polyphenols). Participants with a higher educational level (high school) showed higher total polyphenol, flavonoid, and stilbene intake ($p < 0.001$ in all cases). Current smokers reported a significantly higher intake of coffee than non-smokers ($p < 0.001$) and, consequently, showed a significantly higher intake of phenolic acids ($p < 0.001$). Otherwise, the smokers group showed significantly lower intake of flavonoids and lignans than their counterparts ($p < 0.001$, both).

The associations between dietary polyphenol intake and MetS components after full adjustment are shown in Figure 2. High flavonoid and low phenolic acid intake were associated with lower waist circumference ($p = 0.02$ and $p < 0.001$, respectively). The highest intake of other polyphenols was significantly and inversely associated with systolic ($p = 0.001$) and diastolic blood pressure levels ($p = 0.002$). An inverse association was found between fasting plasma glucose levels and lignans ($p = 0.04$). Positive associations were found between HDL-c levels and all polyphenol classes except for phenolic acid and lignan intake. Lastly, triglyceride concentration was inversely associated with lignans and stilbenes ($p = 0.006$ and $p = 0.004$, respectively). Changes in the linear regression models after adjustment are shown in the Supplementary Table (Supplementary Table S1).

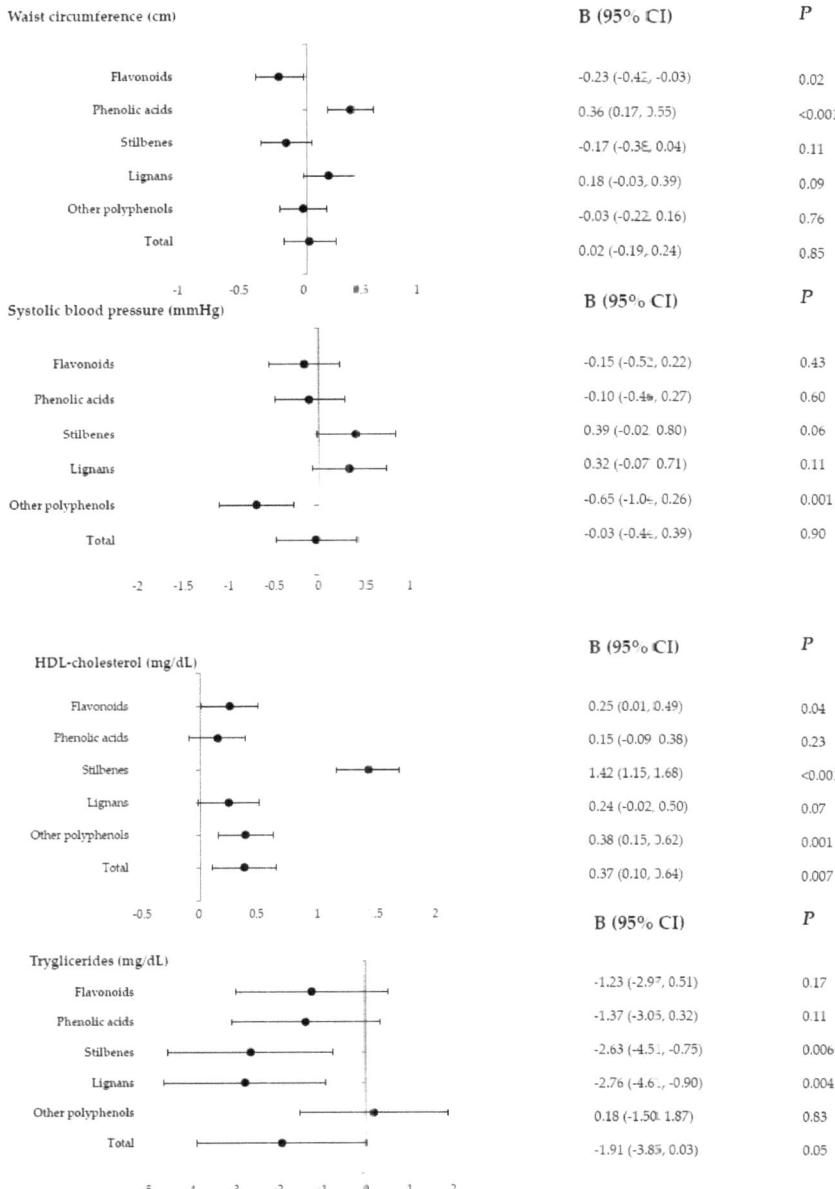

Figure 2. Energy-adjusted subclasses of dietary polyphenol intake by metabolic syndrome components (standardized β-coefficients [95% Confidence Intervals]).

4. Discussion

In this cross-sectional study of the PREDIMED-Plus study, we showed that high intake of some polyphenol subclasses was inversely associated with levels of the MetS components. These associations were especially observed for the subclasses whose contribution to total polyphenol intake was lower, such as other polyphenols, lignans, and stilbenes. Previous epidemiological studies have investigated the association between dietary polyphenol intake and MetS components in healthy populations or those at high risk of CVD, but to our knowledge there are no previous studies on these associations in subjects previously diagnosed with MetS.

In our study, the polyphenol intake was 846 ± 318 mg/day, and the intake was highest for flavonoids (58% of total), followed by phenolic acids (33.1%), similar to results of other Spanish cohorts [14,18]. By contrast, the total polyphenol intake was considerably lower than the intake observed in Mediterranean countries of the EPIC Study (1011 mg/day) [19], the SU.VI.MAX cohort study (1193 mg/day) [20], and the data from other studies conducted in non-Mediterranean countries, such as the UK National Diet and Nutrition Survey Rolling Programme for participants of similar age (1053 mg/day) [21]. The main noteworthy difference between our results and those of other countries was the relevant contribution of seeds, olives and olive oil, and red wine [14,20], while coffee, tea, and cocoa products are the foods most commonly observed in non-Mediterranean countries [22–24].

In addition to the differences observed according to geographical location and dietary habits, sociodemographic and lifestyle habits significantly influence the quantity and profile of intake of polyphenol subclasses. The intake of total polyphenols, particularly flavonoids and lignans, increased with age compared to younger participants (<65 years), although Grosso et al. reported the opposite observation [23]. In addition, BMI was inversely associated with total polyphenol intake, mainly with lower flavonoid and stilbene intake. This finding was also reported in the TOSCA.IT and EPIC studies [19,25].

The intake of polyphenol subclasses has been reported to have an impact on MetS components [26,27]. Even though flavonoids were the principal contributors of total polyphenol intake in our study, no associations were found with any of the MetS components, except for an inverse association with waist circumference. Similar findings were described in the HELENA study [28], where flavonoid intake was associated with lower BMI. Research on the mechanisms of action involved in the anti-obesogenic properties of flavonoids suggests that the improvements in glucose homeostasis are promoted by reducing insulin resistance and decreasing oxidative stress levels [29]. Phenolic acid intake was associated with higher fasting plasma glucose levels and waist circumference. These results are opposite from those observed in the HAPIEE cohort study, which described the beneficial effects of phenolic acid on the overall risk of developing MetS and lowering blood pressure [30]. Nevertheless, it must be taken into account that the dietary intake of phenolic acids and total polyphenol in the mentioned study doubled the amount estimated in our results, probably because of the higher intake of tea and its contribution to phenolic acid intake compared to our study population [23]. In Mediterranean countries, dietary intake of stilbenes is relatively high compared to other countries [19], with red wine being their main source (>90%). In this setting, higher stilbene intake was associated with higher HDL-c levels, but since HDL-c is the best-established cardiovascular protective factor by alcohol consumption, we cannot exclude that the alcohol content of red wine may interfere with this result [31]. In the PREDIMED study, the intake of red wine was associated with improvements in four out of five MetS criteria (i.e., elevated abdominal obesity, low HDL-c levels, high blood pressure, and high fasting plasma glucose levels) [32]. Other studies also found an inverse association between abdominal adiposity and stilbene intake, BMI, and waist circumference [30,33]. As a mechanistic pathway for stilbenes, resveratrol has shown potential anti-obesogenic effects decreasing adipocyte proliferation while activating lipolysis and β-oxidation [34]. However, the association with lower body weight and waist circumference observed in the present study and the promising effects against obesity associated with polyphenol intake observed in other studies were not clinically relevant [35]. Our results showed an inverse association between fasting glucose and lignans, and an increase in HDL-c levels and lower levels of systolic and diastolic blood pressure measurements for other polyphenols. The same finding was described in a Brazilian cohort for hypertension and other polyphenols [36]. In contrast with our results, flavonoids, mainly anthocyanins, showed greater antihypertensive effects in another study [37]. Finally, the association between lignan intake and fasting glucose levels was not demonstrated to be linked with the diagnosis of type 2 diabetes (T2D) in the EPIC study [38], but this inverse association aligned with the results observed in the PREDIMED cohort and PREDIMED-Plus study [39,40]. The potential mechanism of action underlying this association might be explained by the improvements observed in gut microbiota. This assumption was also observed in a study of US women [41], showing an inverse association between levels of gut microbiota metabolites from dietary lignan intake and T2D incidence.

Interestingly, in our study we found an association between intake of all polyphenol subclasses except phenolic acids and lignans and higher HDL-c levels. These associations were also found with total polyphenol intake in the TOSCA.IT study in T2D subjects [25] and in a similar cohort of participants at high cardiovascular risk [42]. We also observed that triglyceride levels were inversely associated with stilbene and lignan intake. Despite the fact that the antioxidant properties of polyphenols for the prevention of LDL-c oxidation are well described, the effects of dietary polyphenols on the reduction of total cholesterol levels or triglycerides are controverted [43].

The major strengths of the present study are its large sample size, the multicenter design, and the use of the Phenol-Explorer as the most comprehensive food composition database on dietary polyphenols [15]. In prior studies, the FFQ was validated to evaluate total polyphenol intake in both clinical and cross-sectional studies [44]. Our study has also some limitations. First, it used a cross-sectional design which does not allow attributing conclusions to plausible causes. In order to establish causality, a randomized controlled trial based on the intake of different polyphenol subclasses should be performed. Second, potential residual confounding and the lack of generalizability of the results to other populations than middle-aged to elderly people with higher BMI and MetS are limitations. Third, the use of the FFQ may have led to a misclassification of the exposure due to self-reported information of food intake and to the fact that some polyphenol-rich foods are grouped in the same item (e.g., spices). Nevertheless, the FFQ used has been validated in the adult Spanish population and showed good reproducibility and validity [45]. Fourth, other factors that affect food polyphenol content, such as bioavailability, variety, ripeness, culinary technique, storage, region, and environmental conditions, were not collected.

Even though recent research postulates that polyphenols are effective in improving MetS, no single phenolic compound or food has an impact on all the MetS components, suggesting that healthy and polyphenol-rich dietary patterns such as the MedDiet may be an adequate strategy for MetS management. This research might be useful for setting dietary and health counseling for MetS patients, especially those with low HDL-c levels. The use of a consensus methodology and polyphenol database might facilitate this in future studies. Future large-scale clinical trials are needed to clarify the underlying mechanisms of action and establish safe doses for the potential health effects described.

5. Conclusions

This study provides detailed information about the relationship between polyphenol intake and the components of MetS in a population of overweight or obese adults. Higher intake of all the subclasses of polyphenols was associated with a better profile of the components of MetS, especially with HDL-c levels.

Supplementary Materials: The following are available online at http://www.mdpi.com/2072-6643/12/3/689/s1, Table S1: Energy-adjusted sub-classes of dietary polyphenol intake by metabolic syndrome criterias.

Author Contributions: Conceptualization, J.S.-S., D.C., M.F., D.R., J.V. (Jesús Vioque), J.W., J.A.M., L.S.-M., F.J.T., J.L., X.P., J.A.T., L.G.-M., M.D.-R., P.M.-M., L.D., J.V. (Josep Vidal), C.V., and R.E.; methodology, J.S-S, D.C., M.F., D.R., J.V. (Jesús Vioque), J.W., J.A.M., L.S.-M., F.J.T., J.L., X.P., J.A.T., L.G.-M., M.D.-R., P.M.-M., L.D., J.V. (Josep Vidal), C.V., and R.E.; validation, R.E.; formal analysis, S.C.-B. and A.T.-R.; investigation, J.S.-S.; funding acquisition,

J.S-S, D.C., M.F., D.R., J.V. (Jesús Vioque), J.W., J.A.M., L.S.-M., F.J.T., J.L., X.P., J.A.T., L.G.-M., M.D.-R., P.M.-M., L.D., J.V. (Josep Vidal), C.V., and R.E.; data curation, S.C.-B., A.T.-R. and F.V.-S.; writing—original draft preparation, S.C.-B. and A.T.-R.; writing—review and editing, F.V.-S., M.D., J.S.-S., V.M.-S., M.R.-G., P.B.-C., D.C., M.F., D.R., J.V. (Jesús Vioque), Á.M.A.-G., J.W., J.A.M., L.S.-M., F.J.T., J.L., X.P., J.A.T., A.G.-R., L.G.-M., M.D.-R., P.M.-M., L.D., J.V.(Josep Vidal), C.V., M.C., A.R.-N., N.B.-T., R.B., O.C., J.K., S.G.-P., C.S.-S., J.P.-L., M.A.Z., I.B.-C., R.C., A.M.G.-P., J.M.S.-L., M.Á.R.-S., A.J., N.M.-C., P.H.-A., J.V.S., A.S., A.M.G.-P., E.C.-P., L.G.-G., M.R.-C., N.B., Á.H., R.M.L.-R. and R.E.; visualization, S.C.-B. and R.E.; supervision, R.E.; project administration, J.S.-S. All authors have read and agreed to the published version of the manuscript.

Funding: The PREDIMED-Plus trial was supported by official Spanish institutions for funding scientific biomedical research, CIBER Fisiopatología de la Obesidad y Nutrición (CIBERobn) and Instituto de Salud Carlos III (ISCIII), through the Fondo de Investigación para la Salud (FIS), which is co-funded by the European Regional Development Fund (four coordinated FIS projects led by J.S.-S. and J.Vi., including the following projects: PI13/00673, PI13/00492, PI13/00272, PI13/01123, PI13/00462, PI13/00233, PI13/02184, PI13/00728, PI13/01090, PI13/01056, PI14/01722, PI14/00636, PI14/00618, PI14/00696, PI14/01206, PI14/01919, PI14/00853, PI14/01374, PI14/00972, PI14/00728, PI14/01471, PI16/00473, PI16/00662, PI16/01873, PI16/01094, PI16/00501, PI16/00533, PI16/00381, PI16/00366, PI16/01522, PI16/01120, PI17/00764, PI17/01183, PI17/00855, PI17/01347, PI17/00525, PI17/01827, PI17/00532, PI17/00215, PI17/01441, PI17/00508, PI17/01732, and PI17/00926), the Special Action Project entitled: Implementación y evaluación de una intervención intensiva sobre la actividad física Cohorte PREDIMED-Plus grant to J.S.-S., the Recercaixa grant to J.S.-S. (2013ACUP00194), a grant from the Fundació la Marató de TV3 (PI044003), grants from the Consejería de Salud de la Junta de Andalucía (PI0458/2013, PS0358/2016, and PI0137/2018),grants from the Generalitat Valenciana (PROMETEO/2017/017, APOSTD/2019/136), a SEMERGEN grant, a CICYT grant provided by the Ministerio de Ciencia, Innovación y Universidades (AGL2016-75329-R) and funds from the European Regional Development Fund (CB06/03). The Spanish Ministry of Science Innovation and Universities for the Formación de Profesorado Universitario (FPU17/00785) contract. Food companies Hojiblanca (Lucena, Spain) and Patrimonio Comunal Olivarero (Madrid, Spain) donated extra virgin olive oil, and the Almond Board of California (Modesto, CA), American Pistachio Growers (Fresno, CA), and Paramount Farms (Wonderful Company, LLC, Los Angeles, CA) donated nuts. This call is co-financed at 50% with charge to the Operational Program FSE 2014-2020 of the Balearic Islands.

Acknowledgments: We thank all the volunteers for their participation and medical professionals for their contribution to the PREDIMED-Plus trial. CIBEROBN, CIBERESP, and CIBERDEM are initiatives of the Instituto de Salud Carlos III (ISCIII), Madrid, Spain. A.T.R. and P.H.A. thanks the Ministry of Science Innovation and Universities for the Juan de la Cierva-formación contract. J.K. is grateful to the Fundación Instituto de Investigación Sanitaria Illes Balears (call financed by 2017annual plan of the sustainable tourism tax and at 50% with charge to the ESF Operational Program 2014–2020 of the Balearic Islands) for the postdoctoral contract for the 'FOLIUM' programme within the FUTURMed.

Conflicts of Interest: R.E. reported receiving grants from Instituto de Salud Carlos III and olive oil for the trial from Fundacion Patrimonio Comunal Olivarero during the conduct of the study and personal fees from Brewers of Europe, Fundación Cerveza y Salud, Interprofesional del Aceite de Oliva, Instituto Cervantes, Instituto Cervantes, Pernaud Richar, Fundación Dieta Mediterránea, Wine and Culinary International Forum; nonfinancial support from Sociedad Española de Nutrición and Fundación Bosch y Gimpera; and grants from Uriach Laboratories outside the submitted work.. R.M.L.-R. reports personal fees from Cerveceros de España, personal fees and other from Adventia, other from Ecoveritas, S.A., outside the submitted work. The rest of authors have no conflict of interest. None of the funding sources took part in the design, collection, analysis, or interpretation of the data or in the decision to submit the manuscript for publication.

References

1. Del Rio, D.; Rodriguez-Mateos, A.; Spencer, J.P.; Tognolini, M.; Borges, G.; Crozier, A. Dietary (poly)phenolics in human health: Structures, bioavailability, and evidence of protective effects against chronic diseases. *Antioxid. Redox Signal.* **2013**, *18*, 1818–1892. [CrossRef] [PubMed]
2. Barreca, D.; Gattuso, G.; Bellocco, E.; Calderaro, A.; Trombetta, D.; Smeriglio, A.; Laganà, G.; Daglia, M.; Meneghini, S.; Nabavi, S.M. Flavanones: Citrus phytochemical with health-promoting properties. *BioFactors* **2017**, *43*, 495–506. [CrossRef] [PubMed]
3. Godos, J.; Zappalà, G.; Bernardini, S.; Giambini, I.; Bes-Rastrollo, M.; Martínez-González, M.A. Adherence to the Mediterranean diet is inversely associated with metabolic syndrome occurrence: A meta-analysis of observational studies. *Int. J. Food Sci. Nutr.* **2017**, *68*, 138–148. [CrossRef] [PubMed]
4. Alberti, K.G.M.M.; Eckel, R.H.; Grundy, S.M.; Zimmet, P.Z.; Cleeman, J.I.; Donato, K.A.; Fruchart, J.C.; James, W.P.; Loria, C.M.; Smith, S.C., Jr.; et al. Harmonizing the metabolic syndrome: A joint interim statement of the international diabetes federation task force on epidemiology and prevention; national heart, lung, and blood institute; American heart association; world heart federation; international atherosclerosis society; and international association for the study of obesity. *Circulation* **2009**, *120*, 1640–1645. [CrossRef]

5. Koloverou, E.; Esposito, K.; Giugliano, D.; Panagiotakos, D. The effect of Mediterranean diet on the development of type 2 diabetes mellitus: A meta-analysis of 10 prospective studies and 136,846 participants. *Metabolism* **2014**, *63*, 903–911. [CrossRef]
6. Grosso, G.; Stepaniak, U.; Micek, A.; Topor-Madry, R.; Stefler, D.; Szafraniec, K.; Bobak, M.; Pajak, A. A Mediterranean-type diet is associated with better metabolic profile in urban Polish adults: Results from the HAPIEE study. *Metabolism* **2015**, *64*, 738–746. [CrossRef]
7. Giglio, R.V.; Patti, A.M.; Cicero, A.F.G.; Lippi, G.; Rizzo, M.; Toth, P.P.; Banach, M. Polyphenols: Potential use in the prevention and treatment of cardiovascular diseases. *Curr. Pharm. Des.* **2018**, *24*, 239–258. [CrossRef]
8. Chiva-Blanch, G.; Badimon, L. Effects of polyphenol intake on metabolic syndrome: Current evidence from human trials. *Oxid. Med. Cell. Longev.* **2017**, *2017*, 5812401. [CrossRef]
9. Patti, A.M.; Al-Rasadi, K.; Giglio, R.V.; Nikolic, D.; Mannina, C.; Castellino, G.; Chianetta, R.; Banach, M.; Cicero, A.F.G.; Lippi, G.; et al. Natural approaches in metabolic syndrome management. *Arch. Med. Sci.* **2018**, *14*, 422–441. [CrossRef]
10. Amiot, M.J.; Riva, C.; Vinet, A. Effects of dietary polyphenols on metabolic syndrome features in humans: A systematic review. *Obes. Rev.* **2016**, *17*, 573–586. [CrossRef]
11. Manach, C.; Scalbert, A.; Morand, C.; Rémésy, C.; Jiménez, L. Polyphenols: Food sources and bioavailability. *Am. J. Clin. Nutr.* **2004**, *79*, 727–747. [CrossRef] [PubMed]
12. Martínez-González, M.A.; Buil-Cosiales, P.; Corella, D.; Bulló, M.; Fitó, M.; Vioque, J.; Romaguera, D.; Martínez, J.A.; Wärnberg, J.; López-Miranda, J.; et al. Cohort profile: Design and methods of the PREDIMED-Plus randomized trial. *Int. J. Epidemiol.* **2019**, *48*, 387–388. [CrossRef]
13. Willett, W.C.; Howe, G.R.; Kushi, L.H. Adjustment for total energy intake in epidemiologic studies. *Am. J. Clin. Nutr.* **1997**, *65*, 1220S–1228S. [CrossRef] [PubMed]
14. Tresserra-Rimbau, A.; Medina-Remón, A.; Pérez-Jiménez, J.; Martínez-González, M.A.; Covas, M.I.; Corella, D.; Salas-Salvadó, J.; Gómez-Garcia, E.; Lapetra, J.; Arós, F.; et al. Dietary intake and major food sources of polyphenols in a Spanish population at high cardiovascular risk: The PREDIMED study. *Nutr. Metab. Cardiovasc. Dis.* **2013**, *23*, 953–959. [CrossRef] [PubMed]
15. Rothwell, J.A.; Pérez-Jiménez, J.; Neveu, V.; Medina-Ramon, A.; M'Hiri, N.; Garcia Lobato, P.; Manach, C.; Knox, K.; Eisner, R.; Wishart, D.; et al. Phenol-Explorer 3.0: A major update of the Phenol-Explorer database to incorporate data on the effects of food processing on polyphenol content. *Database* **2013**. [CrossRef]
16. Molina, L.; Sarmiento, M.; Peñafiel, J.; Donaire, D.; Garcia-Aymerich, J.; Gomez, M.; Bie, M.; Ruiz, S.; Frances, A.; Schröder, H.; et al. Validation of the regicor short physical activity questionnaire for the adult population. *PLoS ONE* **2017**, *12*, e0168148. [CrossRef]
17. Martínez-González, M.A.; López-Fontana, C.; Varo, J.J.; Sánchez-Villegas, A.; Martinez, J.A. Validation of the Spanish version of the physical activity questionnaire used in the nurses' health study and the health professionals' follow-up study. *Public Health Nutr.* **2005**, *8*, 920–927. [CrossRef]
18. Mendonça, R.D.; Carvalho, N.C.; Martin-Moreno, J.M.; Pimenta, A.M.; Lopes, A.C.S.; Gea, A.; Martine-González, M.A.; Bes-Rastrollo, M. Total polyphenol intake, polyphenol subtypes and incidence of cardiovascular disease: The SUN cohort study. *Nutr. Metab. Cardiovasc. Dis.* **2019**, *29*, 69–78. [CrossRef]
19. Zamora-Ros, E.; Knaze, V.; Rothwell, J.; Hémon, B.; Moskal, A.; Overvad, K.; Tjonneland, A.; Kyro, C.; Fagherazzi, G.; Boutron-Ruault, M.C. Dietary polyphenol intake in Europe: The European Prospective Investigation into Cancer and Nutrition (EPIC) study. *Eur. J. Nutr.* **2016**, *55*, 1359–1375. [CrossRef]
20. Pérez-Jiménez, J.; Fezeu, L.; Touvier, M.; Arnault, N.; Manach, C.; Hercberg, S.; Galan, P.; Scalbert, A. Dietary intake of 337 polyphenols in French adults. *Am. J. Clin. Nutr.* **2011**, *93*, 1220–1228. [CrossRef]
21. Ziauddeen, N.; Rosi, A.; Del Rio, D.; Amoutzopoulos, B.; Nicholson, S.; Page, P.; Scazzina, F.; Brighenti, F.; Ray, S.; Mena, P. Dietary intake of (poly)phenols in children and adults: Cross-sectional analysis of the UK national diet and nutrition survey rolling programme (2008–2014). *Eur. J. Nutr.* **2019**, *58*, 3183–3198. [CrossRef] [PubMed]
22. Pinto, P.; Santos, C.N. Worldwide (poly)phenol intake: Assessment methods and identified gaps. *Eur. J. Nutr.* **2017**, *59*, 1393–1408. [CrossRef] [PubMed]
23. Grosso, G.; Stepaniak, U.; Topor-Madry, R.; Szafraniec, K.; Pajak, A. Estimated dietary intake and major food sources of polyphenols in the Polish arm of the HAPIEE study. *Nutrition* **2014**, *30*, 1398–1403. [CrossRef] [PubMed]

24. Ovaskainen, M.L.; Torronen, R.; Koponen, J.M.; Sinkko, H.; Hellstrom, J.; Reinivuo, H.; Mattila, P. Dietary intake and major food sources of polyphenols in Finnish adults. *J. Nutr.* **2008**, *138*, 562–566. [CrossRef]
25. Vitale, M.; Masulli, M.; Rivellese, A.A.; Bonora, E.; Cappellini, F.; Nicolucci, A.; Squatrito, S.; Antenucci, D.; Barrea, A.; Bianchi, C.; et al. Dietary intake and major food sources of polyphenols in people with type 2 diabetes: The TOSCA.IT study. *Eur. J. Nutr.* **2018**, *57*, 679–688. [CrossRef]
26. Vetrani, C.; Vitale, M.; Bozzetto, L.; Della Pepa, G.; Cocozza, S.; Costabile, G.; Mangione, A.; Cipriano, P.; Annuzzi, G.; Rivellese, A.A. Association between different dietary polyphenol subclases and the improvement in cardiometabolic risk factors: Evidence from a randomized controlled clinical trial. *Acta Diabetol.* **2018**, *55*, 149–153. [CrossRef]
27. Marseglia, L.; Manti, S.; D'Angelo, G.; Nicotera, A.; Parisi, E.; Di Rosa, G.; Gitto, E.; Arrigo, T. Oxidative stress in obesity: A critical component in human diseases. *Int. J. Mol. Sci.* **2015**, *16*, 378–400. [CrossRef] [PubMed]
28. Wisnuwardani, R.W.; De Henauw, S.; Androutsos, O.; Forsner, M.; Gottrand, F.; Huybrechts, I.; Knaze, V.; Le Donne, C.; Marcos, A.; Molnár, D.; et al. Estimated dietary intake of polyphenols in European adolescents: The HELENA study. *Eur. J. Nutr.* **2019**, *58*, 2345–2363. [CrossRef] [PubMed]
29. Hossain, M.K.; Dayem, A.A.; Han, J.; Yin, K.; Kim, K.; Saha, S.K.; Yang, G.M.; Choi, H.Y.; Cho, S.G. Molecular mechanisms of the anti-obesity and anti-diabetic properties of flavonoids. *Int. J. Mol. Sci.* **2016**, *17*, 569. [CrossRef] [PubMed]
30. Grosso, G.; Stepanlak, U.; Micek, A.; Stefler, D.; Bobak, M.; Pajak, A. Dietary polyphenols are inversely associated with metabolic syndrome in Polish adults of the HAPIEE study. *Eur. J. Nutr.* **2017**, *56*, 1709–1720. [CrossRef]
31. Ellison, R.C.; Zhang, Y.; Qureshi, M.M.; Knox, S.; Arnett, D.K.; Province, M.A.; Investigators of the NHLBI Family Heart Study. Lifestyle determinants of high-density lipoprotein cholesterol: The national heart, lung, and blood institute family heart study. *Am. Heart J.* **2004**, *147*, 529–535. [CrossRef] [PubMed]
32. Tresserra-Rimbau, A.; Medina-Remón, A.; Lamuela-Raventós, R.M.; Bulló, M.; Salas-Salvadó, J.; Corella, D.; Fitó, M.; Gea, A.; Gómez-Garcia, E.; Lapetra, J.; et al. Moderate red wine consumption is associated with a lower prevalence of the metabolic syndrome in the PREDIMED population. *Br. J. Nutr.* **2015**, *113*, S121–S130. [CrossRef] [PubMed]
33. Wilsgaard, T.; Jacobsen, B.K. Lifestyle factors and incident metabolic syndrome. The Tromso study 1979–2001. *Diabetes Res. Clin. Pract.* **2007**, *78*, 217–224. [CrossRef] [PubMed]
34. Wang, S.; Moustaid-Moussa, N.; Chen, L.; Mo, H.; Shastri, A.; Su, R.; Bapat, P.; Kwun, I.; Shen, C.L. Novel insights of dietary polyphenols and obesity. *J. Nutr. Biochem.* **2014**, *25*, 1–18. [CrossRef]
35. Lee, S.H.; Mantzoros, C.; Kim, Y.B. Resveratrol: Is selectivity opening the key to therapeutic effects? *Metabolism* **2012**, *61*, 289–290. [CrossRef]
36. Miranda, A.M.; Steluti, J.; Fisberg, R.M.; Marchioni, D.M. Association between polyphenol intake and hypertension in adults and older adults: A population-based study in Brazil. *PLoS ONE* **2016**, *11*, e0165791. [CrossRef]
37. Grosso, G.; Stepaniak, U.; Micek, A.; Kozela, M.; Stefler, D.; Bobak, M.; Pajak, A. Dietary polyphenol intake and risk of hypertension in the Polish arm of the HAPIEE study. *Eur. J. Nutr.* **2018**, *57*, 1535–1544. [CrossRef]
38. Zamora-Ros, R.; Forouhi, N.G.; Sharp, S.J.; González, C.A.; Buijsse, B.; Guevara, M.; van der Schouw, Y.T.; Amiano, P.; Boeing, H.; Bredsdorff, L.; et al. The association between dietary flavonoid and lignan intakes and incident type 2 diabetes in European populations: The EPIC-InterAct study. *Diabetes Care* **2013**, *36*, 3961–3970. [CrossRef]
39. Tresserra-Rimbau, A.; Guasch-Ferré, M.; Salas-Salvadó, J.; Toledo, E.; Corella, D.; Castañer, O.; Guo, X.; Gómez-Garcia, E.; Lapetra, J.; Arós, F.; et al. Intake of total polyphenols and some clases of polyphenols is inversely associated with diabetes in elderly people at high cardiovascular disease risk. *J. Nutr.* **2016**. [CrossRef]
40. Tresserra-Rimbau, A.; Castro-Barquero, S.; Vitelli-Storelli, F.; Becerra-Tomas, N.; Vázquez-Ruiz, Z.; Díaz-López, A.; Corella, D.; Castañer, O.; Romaguera, D.; Vioque, J.; et al. Associations between dietary polyphenols and type 2 diabetes in a cross-sectional analysis of the PREDIMED-plus trial: Role of the body mass index and sex. *Antioxidants* **2019**, *8*, 537. [CrossRef]
41. Sun, Q.; Wedick, N.M.; Pan, A.; Townsend, M.K.; Cassidy, A.; Franke, A.A.; Rimm, E.B.; Hu, F.B.; van Dam, R.M. Gut microbiota metabolites of dietary lignans and risk of type 2 diabetes: A prospective investigation in two cohorts of U.S. women. *Diabetes Care* **2014**, *37*, 1287–1295. [CrossRef]

42. Guo, X.; Tresserra-Rimbau, A.; Estruch, R. Martínez-González, M.A.; Medina-Remón, A.; Castañer, O.; Corella, D.; Salas-Salvadó, J.; Lamuela-Raventós, R.M. Effects of polyphenol, measured by a biomarker of total polyphenols in urine, on cardiovascular risk factors after a long-term follow-up in the PREDIMED study. *Oxid. Med. Cell. Longev.* **2016**, *2016*, 2572606. [CrossRef] [PubMed]
43. Cicero, A.F.G.; Colletti, A. Polyphenols effect on circulating lipids and lipoproteins: From biochemistry to clinical evidence. *Curr. Pharm. Des.* **2018**, *24*, 178–190. [CrossRef] [PubMed]
44. Medina-Remón, A.; Barrionuevo-González, A.; Zamora-Ros, R.; Andres-Lacueva, C.; Estruch, R.; Martínez-González, M.A.; Diez-Espino, J.; Lamuela-Raventós, R.M. Rapid Folin-Ciocalteu method using microtiter 96-well plate cartridges for solid phase extraction to assess urinary total phenolic compounds, as a biomarker of total polyphenols intake. *Anal. Chim. Acta* **2009**, *634*, 56–60. [CrossRef] [PubMed]
45. Fernández-Ballart, J.D.; Piñol, J.L.; Zazpe, I.; Corella, D.; Carrasco, P.; Toledo, E.; Perez-Bauer, M.; Martínez-González, M.A.; Salas-Salvadó, J.; Martín-Moreno, J.M. Relative validity of a semi-quantitative food-frequency questionnaire in an elderly Mediterranean population of Spain. *Br. J. Nutr.* **2010**, *103*, 1808–1816. [CrossRef] [PubMed]

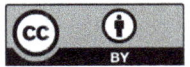

© 2020 by the authors. Licensee MDPI, Basel, Switzerland. This article is an open access article distributed under the terms and conditions of the Creative Commons Attribution (CC BY) license (http://creativecommons.org/licenses/by/4.0/).

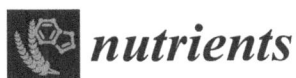

Review

Effects of Dietary Phytoestrogens on Hormones throughout a Human Lifespan: A Review

Inés Domínguez-López [1], Maria Yago-Aragón [1], Albert Salas-Huetos [2], Anna Tresserra-Rimbau [1,3,4,5,*] and Sara Hurtado-Barroso [1,3]

1. Department of Nutrition, Food Science and Gastronomy, XaRTA, INSA, School of Pharmacy and Food Sciences, University of Barcelona, 08028 Barcelona, Spain; idominlo8@alumnes.ub.edu (I.D.-L.); myagoara7@alumnes.ub.edu (M.Y.-A.); sara.hurtado_17@ub.edu (S.H.-B.)
2. Andrology and IVF Laboratory, Division of Urology, Department of Surgery, University of Utah School of Medicine, Salt Lake City, UT 84108, USA; albert.salas@utah.edu
3. Centro de Investigación Biomédica en Red Fisiopatología de la Obesidad y la Nutrición (CIBEROBN), Instituto de Salud Carlos III, 28029 Madrid, Spain
4. Unitat de Nutrició, Departament de Bioquímica i Biotecnologia, Universitat Rovira i Virgili, 43204 Reus, Spain
5. Institut d'Investigació Sanitària Pere Virgili (IISPV), 43201 Reus, Spain
* Correspondence: anna.tresserra@iispv.cat

Received: 7 July 2020; Accepted: 12 August 2020; Published: 15 August 2020

Abstract: Dietary phytoestrogens are bioactive compounds with estrogenic activity. With the growing popularity of plant-based diets, the intake of phytoestrogen-rich legumes (especially soy) and legume-derived foods has increased. Evidence from preclinical studies suggests these compounds may have an effect on hormones and health, although the results of human trials are unclear. The effects of dietary phytoestrogens depend on the exposure (phytoestrogen type, matrix, concentration, and bioavailability), ethnicity, hormone levels (related to age, sex, and physiological condition), and health status of the consumer. In this review, we have summarized the results of human studies on dietary phytoestrogens with the aim of assessing the possible hormone-dependent outcomes and health effects of their consumption throughout a lifespan, focusing on pregnancy, childhood, adulthood, and the premenopausal and postmenopausal stages. In pregnant women, an improvement of insulin metabolism has been reported in only one study. Sex hormone alterations have been found in the late stages of childhood, and goitrogenic effects in children with hypothyroidism. In premenopausal and postmenopausal women, the reported impacts on hormones are inconsistent, although beneficial goitrogenic effects and improved glycemic control and cardiovascular risk markers have been described in postmenopausal individuals. In adult men, different authors report goitrogenic effects and a reduction of insulin in non-alcoholic fatty liver patients. Further carefully designed studies are warranted to better elucidate the impact of phytoestrogen consumption on the endocrine system at different life stages.

Keywords: isoflavones; soy; dietary flavonoids; lignans; flaxseeds; endocrine; stages of life; estrogenic; polyphenols; health

---

1. Introduction

Phytoestrogens are polyphenolic molecules with a structural similarity to endogenous human hormones, hence their estrogenic activity. The main dietary source of these plant secondary metabolites is legumes (particularly soy), and to a lesser extent fruits, vegetables, and cereals [1]. Figure 1 shows the most common phytoestrogens in diet. According to their origin, lignins are classified into plant lignans (e.g., pinoresinol, secoisolariciresinol, matairesinol, and sesamin) and enterolignans (e.g., enterodiol and enterolactone), which are metabolized from plant lignans by intestinal bacteria [1]. Although ingested in lower quantities than isoflavones and lignans, prenylflavonoids from beer and coumestans from soy are also regarded as polyphenols with estrogenic activity.

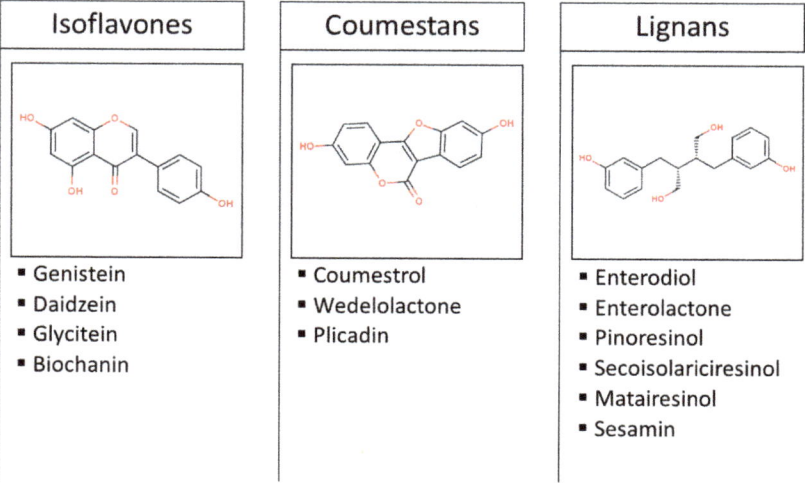

Figure 1. Classification and examples of the most common dietary phytoestrogens. Images are the chemical structures of genistein, coumestrol, and enterodiol.

The intake of phytoestrogens has increased due to the widespread use of soy products for human consumption and as cattle food [2]. In Europe, the lowest average intake of phytoestrogens occurs in Mediterranean countries, whereas consumption in Northern countries is 0.76 mg/day [3]. The highest soy-derived isoflavone intakes worldwide are still in China and Japan, where the population consumes an average of 15–50 mg per day, compared to only about 2 mg per day in Western countries [4,5]. The promising health effects of soy have driven some people in developed countries to consume it as an alternative to meat or dairy products.

Dietary phytoestrogens are digested in the small intestine, where they are poorly absorbed. Those that reach the liver are conjugated and circulate in the plasma until excretion in urine. Thos that are not absorbed are metabolized by the gut microbiota into lower weight compounds [1]. The diversity of food matrices (from pure compounds to complex foods) used in clinical studies could also lead to different results although interindividual variability seems more determinant. It has been demonstrated that phytoestrogen extraction from complex food matrices, such as those with high content of sugars and proteins, is more difficult in in vitro studies; however, no clear differences regarding food matrices were observed in humans [6]. Nevertheless, results using pure compounds must be extrapolated carefully because not only is the matrix different, but also the concentration, which is higher in pure extracts.

Results from human studies suggest that phytoestrogens may lower the risk of osteoporosis, some cardiometabolic diseases, cognitive dysfunction, breast and prostate cancer, and menopausal symptoms by modulating the endocrine system (Figure 2). However, some authors describe phytoestrogens as endocrine disruptors and believe their beneficial effects have been overestimated [2,5,7]. This ambiguity could be partially due to the variability of published studies, as the beneficial or harmful effects of phytoestrogens depend on the exposure (type, amount consumed, and bioavailability), ethnicity, hormonal status (age and sex and physiological condition), and health status of the consumer [2,5,7].

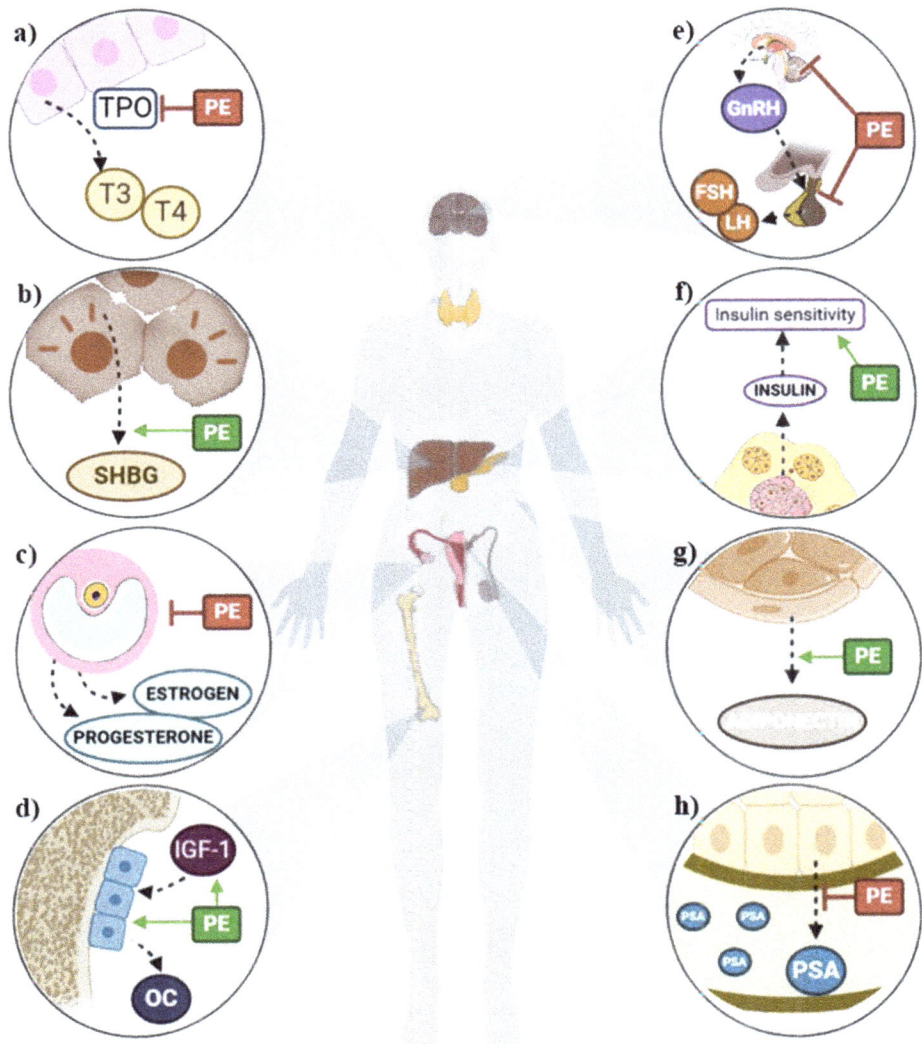

Figure 2. Summary of potential health outcomes of phytoestrogens through the modulation of the endocrine system in (**a**) thyroids, (**b**) liver, (**c**) ovaries, (**d**) bones, (**e**) hypothalamic–pituitary–gonadal axis, (**f**) pancreas, (**g**) fat tissue, (**h**) prostate. FSH: follicle-stimulating hormone; GnRH: gonadotropin-releasing hormone; IGF-1: insulin growth factor 1; LH: luteinizing hormone; OC: osteocalcin; PE: phytoestrogens; PSA: prostate-specific antigen; SHBG: stimulating hormone-binding globulin; T3: triiodothyronine; T4: thyroxine; TPO: thyroperoxidase.

A plausible mechanism of action for phytoestrogens is estrogen receptor (ER) binding. The effects of isoflavones, which have a five-fold greater affinity for β-ER than α-ER [8], on the endocrine system may be through modulation of the hypothalamic–pituitary axis [9]. However, not all the biological effects of phytoestrogens involve estrogen receptors. They can also activate serotonergic and insulin-like growth factor (IGF) receptors 1, induce free radical binding and modify tyrosine kinases, cycle adenosine monophosphate (cAMP), phosphatidylinositol-3 kinase (PI3K)/Akt, mitogen-activated protein (MAP) kinases, transcription of nuclear factor-kappa β (NF-Kβ), as well as promote DNA methylation and affect histone and RNA expression. In addition, phytoestrogens can act as intracellular regulators of the cell cycle and apoptosis. Thus, due to their antioxidant, antiproliferative, antimutagenic, and antiangiogenic roles, phytoestrogens can improve health [10]. In addition, some authors observed that estrogen and androgen seem to be involved in breast and prostate cancer regulating proliferative and migratory signaling, such as Src/PI3K. Hormonal therapy response may vary depend on interactions between estrogen or androgen receptors and proteins, according to hormone levels [11–13].

This integrative review aims to synthesize the results obtained by human studies and assess the potential hormone-related health effects of dietary phytoestrogens throughout the human lifespan.

2. Effects of Phytoestrogen Intake on Sex Hormones

The anti-estrogenic activity of phytoestrogens is due to their structural similarity with 17-β-estradiol (E2), the main female sex hormone [5]. As well as interacting with ERs, phytoestrogens can affect the secretion of gonadotropin-releasing hormone (GnRH) [14]. Phytoestrogens could disrupt the endocrine system by interfering with the hypothalamic–pituitary–gonadal axis, which controls estrogen secretion. The hypothalamus releases GnRH and stimulates the pituitary to produce follicle-stimulating hormone (FSH) and luteinizing hormone (LH), gonadotropins that promote the secretion of estrogen, progesterone, and testosterone by the ovaries or testes. Low estrogen levels are a signal for the hypothalamus to release GnRH, whereas high levels provide a negative feedback [15]. Therefore, the presence of exogenous compounds structurally similar to E2 may interfere with this system.

Some studies have focused on how phytoestrogen affects urinary estrogen metabolites, some of which may be involved in the development of breast cancer. In particular, the ratio of 2-hydroxyestrone (2-OH-E1) to 16α-hydroxyestrone (16α-OH-E1) (2:16α-OH-E1) is considered a useful biomarker of estrogen-related cancer risk. A major 2:16α-OH-E1 ratio is related to lower risk of breast cancer. Previously, it was observed that a higher concentration of 16α-OH-E1 was associated with breast and endometrial cancer, while an increase of metabolite 2-OH-E1 seems to inhibit the carcinogenesis [16].

Phytoestrogens have also been reported to affect sex hormones through ER-independent mechanisms of action, such as by altering hormone-binding globulin (SHBG) levels. Circulating estrogens and androgens are mostly bound to albumin and SHBG, with only a small fraction remaining free. As estrogens and androgens are only biologically active in their free form, SHBG affects steroidal activity. In vitro studies have shown that isoflavonoids stimulate the synthesis of SHBG by liver cancer cells [17], but available data from human studies are inconclusive [18,19]. In addition, phytoestrogens inhibit aromatase and other enzymes involved in the synthesis of steroid hormones [20].

Preclinical studies have suggested that phytoestrogens influence sexual function and the incidence of cancer associated with the reproductive system such as ovarian and breast cancer [21], but the results of cross-sectional studies and clinical trials are conflicting [22,23]. In addition to factors such as dose, type, and bioavailability, the effects of phytoestrogens on sexual function could also depend on the life stage of the consumer, as explained below.

2.1. Pregnancy

The results of a longitudinal study that measured E2, estriol (E3), testosterone, and isoflavones in urine and serum from 194 pregnant women weakly support the initial hypothesis that genistein and daidzein would reduce levels of E2 and testosterone at the 10th week of gestation. Additionally, sex hormones quantified in umbilical cord serum were not related to isoflavones (genistein, daidzein, and equol) measured at delivery [24].

2.2. Children

Dietary phytoestrogens seem to be transferred from maternal blood to the fetus, but there is no evidence that they alter sex hormones in infants [25–27]. Although isoflavone bioavailability in this sensitive period may be higher than in adults [28], no estrogenic effects were observed in infants fed with a soy formula [29–31]. Nevertheless, a cross-sectional study carried out in children aged 3–6 years reported an increase of androgens in girls and a decrease of estrogens in boys consuming higher amounts of soy and isoflavones [25]. In a crossover trial conducted in girls aged 8–14 years, the consumption of a high-soy diet for 8 weeks significantly increased dehydroepiandrosterone (DHEA) concentrations but not other sexual hormones. Although the level of all sex hormone metabolites excreted was very low, positive correlations with the intervention were found, being higher for total androgens than for estrogens and pregnanediol [32].

2.3. Men

A cross-sectional study in randomly selected Japanese men found a negative association between soy product consumption and E2 serum concentrations, but no link was observed with peripheral concentrations of androgen hormones [33]. In a randomized clinical study in Japanese healthy male volunteers consuming 60 mg per day of soy isoflavones, no changes in serum levels of E2 and total testosterone were observed compared to the baseline at the end of the 3-month intervention. However, serum levels of SHBG increased and free testosterone and dihydrotestosterone decreased [34].

There is weak evidence that phytoestrogens contribute to reducing the risk of prostate cancer (PCa). Several observational studies have found a negative association between the consumption of phytoestrogens (soy and its isoflavones) and the levels of prostate-specific antigen (PSA) in blood [35]. PSA, a protein produced by the prostate gland, is used as a marker to detect PCa, although its levels also increase with benign prostate hypertrophy. In a randomized controlled trial, a reduction in PSA levels was observed in men with PCa after consuming soy isoflavones for a mean of 23 days [36]. However, longer studies (minimum 3 weeks and maximum 12 months) did not find beneficial effects on PSA levels after a soy isoflavone intervention [37–40], nor were changes in PSA plasma levels observed in PCa patients that consumed rye bran bread for 3 weeks [41].

There is a relationship between sex hormones and the pathogenesis of PCa. High levels of androgens, which promote prostate cell growth, may contribute to the risk of PCa in some men. Some epidemiological studies suggest that low levels of testosterone are associated with a lower risk of PCa [42,43]. A meta-analysis of 32 studies published in 2010 by Hamilton-Reeves et al. reported that the consumption of isoflavones had no significant effect on circulating testosterone or free testosterone levels in men [44], in agreement with other clinical trials evaluating phytoestrogen intake in PCa patients [37,39–41]. Nor have effects on dihydrotestosterone been described [36,40]. However, in an open-labeled, non-randomized clinical trial of men with higher levels of PSA, free testosterone was depleted after 12 months of daily consumption of 141 mg of isoflavones in soy milk [38].

Recent studies have pointed to a protective role of estrogens in PCa development and progression, alone or in synergy with androgens [45]. Several studies have focused on the beneficial effect of soy isoflavones, specifically genistein and daidzein, as these components can act as weak estrogens. A 6-month randomized controlled study evaluating the effects of isoflavone on men at high risk of developing advanced PCa found an increase in concentrations of the estrogen hormones estrone (E1), E2, 2-hydroxi-estradiol (2-OH-E2), and 16α-OH-E1. An increase in the 2:16α-OH-E1 ratio was also reported, which is related to a reduced risk of estrogen-mediated cancer. No differences were observed for 2-methoxyestradiol (2-ME2), 1-methoxyestrone (2-ME1), E3 and 2-OH-E1 [46]. Conversely, Bylund A. et al. reported that levels of E2, FSH, and LH in PCa patients remained unaltered after a 3-week rye bran bread intervention [41].

2.4. Premenopausal Women

In agreement with the potential anti-estrogenic effect of phytoestrogens, some authors have observed a significant decrease in estrogen levels after the consumption of soy products [18,22,47–49]. In a randomized controlled cross-over trial conducted in 12 healthy premenopausal women, those consuming a high-soy diet for three menstrual cycles had lower urinary concentrations of total estrogens (E1, E2, E3), and some metabolites compared to individuals on a low-soy diet [22].

Although significant correlations were obtained between serum levels of unconjugated estrogens, and urinary conjugated and unconjugated estrogen metabolites, the large intra-subject variability in urinary estrogen levels limits its use as a biomarker [50]. Similarly, a fall in the circulating levels of E2 after the consumption of a soy-rich diet has been reported [47–49]. In a cross-sectional study, Kapiszewska M. et al. found an association between low salivary E2 concentrations and the intake of black tea (only or plus green tea), catechins, theaflavins, and epigallocatechin gallate (EGCG), being more pronounced in premenopausal women living in urban areas than in those living in rural areas [51]. As well as a decline in estrogens, a significant decrease in progesterone levels after phytoestrogen consumption has been observed [47–49,52]. Conversely, other clinical trials and observational studies do not report any modifications of sex hormones attributed to the consumption of dietary soy-isoflavones [14,19,23,53–58].

It has been proposed that changes in estrogen levels induced by dietary phytoestrogens could depend on the individual capacity to produce equol [59,60], mainly the S-equol enantiomer, due to its high affinity for β-ER [61]. Accordingly, Duncan et al. reported that premenopausal equol excretors had a lower risk of breast cancer compared to non-excretors [60].

In summary, it is still uncertain if a phytoestrogen-rich diet triggers an imbalance of estrogen and progesterone concentrations. In randomized controlled crossover trials, no significant changes were observed in the progesterone/E2 ratio in women who consumed a soy diet for two menstrual cycles [56], whereas the ratio increased after the intake of 10 g/day of flaxseeds for three menstrual cycles [62].

The status of sex hormones can also be an indicator of breast cancer risk. Although measuring estrogen and progesterone concentrations in nipple aspirate fluid may be better than using serum samples to detect dietary-associated changes in the breast, the correlation between dietary phytoestrogen and estrogens was poor in both matrices [58]. On the other hand, the scant evidence for an increase in the 2:16α-OH-E1 ratio after the consumption of soy and flaxseed suggests such high-phytoestrogen foods may have a protective role against breast cancer [22,48,63]. In the same vein, Xu et al. observed a decrease in the ratio of genotoxic metabolites (16α-OH-E1, 4-hydroxyestradiol (4-OH-E2), and 4-hydroxyestrone (4-OE-E1)) and total estrogens [22]. However, no effects on biomarkers related to breast cancer risk have been reported in other studies [23,56,59].

Inconclusive effects of phytoestrogen supplementation in the form of soy protein powder (low and high doses) on the concentrations of FSH and LH have been observed. Both hormones decreased after low- but not high-isoflavone diets [18], as well as after the consumption of soy products [52,64]. However, other studies found no significant changes in FSH and LH concentration after phytoestrogen supplementation [14,23,48,49,53–55].

Most authors have not found any effects of a phytoestrogen-rich diet on circulating levels of androgens [23,53,56,57,64,65]. Two clinical trials did report a decrease of DHEA-sulfate concentrations in healthy premenopausal women after 1 to 3 months on a diet high in soy and soy products [18,47]. In contrast, in a randomized controlled clinical trial (RCT) conducted in healthy premenopausal women consuming 10 g/day of flaxseeds for three menstrual cycles, an increase in serum levels of testosterone in the mid-follicular phase was observed [62]. Overall, there is no solid evidence supporting the influence of phytoestrogens on SHBG [19,23,49,52,53,55–57,62,64–66], although a weak increase has been described [18,67,68].

A prolonged menstruation after regular intake of phytoestrogens has been reported [62,68], but most studies indicate no significant changes in menstrual cycle length or concentration of prolactin [18,23,53,56,57,62,65,66].

2.5. Postmenopausal Women

Menopausal transition is caused by the depletion of ovarian follicles and their responsiveness to the pituitary gonadotropins FSH and LH. This results in low serum levels of the ovarian hormones estrogen and progesterone, and also an increase in FSH concentrations due to the disruption in the negative feedback regulating the hypothalamic–pituitary–gonadal axis [69]. These hormonal changes are responsible for several menopausal symptoms, such as vasomotor symptoms, hot flushes, and vaginal dryness, as well as long-term disorders like osteoporosis, cardiovascular diseases, and breast cancer.

In postmenopausal women there is little evidence supporting the hypothesis that phytoestrogens affect sex hormone levels. Numerous studies have reported that phytoestrogens—including isoflavones, flavonoids, and lignans—do not affect estrogen or progesterone concentrations in postmenopausal women [7,14,19,70–95]. However, other clinical studies did find that isoflavone administration produced significant changes in E2 [96,97] or progesterone concentrations [98]. Two other postmenopausal studies suggested that flaxseed lignans may reduce E2 and E1 sulfate [99] in healthy women, and E1 concentrations in obese and overweight women [100]. Tormala R. et al. (2008) also reported lower E1 concentrations after soy protein supplementation in tibolone-using postmenopausal women who were equol producers [101]. In one epidemiological study, the relationship between isoflavone intake and peripheral E2 concentrations was assessed in postmenopausal women, and urinary excretion of daidzein, genistein, and glycitein and serum levels of daidzein and glycitein were associated with lower plasma E2 levels. Interestingly, these associations were stronger in 18 postmenopausal women with the CC genotype for ESR1 $PvuII$ polymorphism, suggesting that genes influence diet effects [102].

Phytoestrogen effects on urinary estrogen metabolites have been studied in order to assess their potential protective role against breast cancer. One of the most recent studies reports an increase in the 2:16α-OH-E1 ratio after red clover-derived isoflavone supplementation in postmenopausal osteopenic women [103]. These results are consistent with prior research that found an increase in the 2:16α-OH-E1 ratio after flaxseed supplementation [104,105]. Other studies, however, did not find any difference in the ratio after phytoestrogen supplementation in postmenopausal women [81,95], and one even reports a lower ratio [106].

Other hormones affected by the disruption of the hypothalamic–pituitary–gonadal axis are the gonadotropins FSH and LH, which according to different clinical trials are not affected by phytoestrogen supplementation [14,79,82,83,107–109]. Only Crisafulli A et al. found lower gonadotropin levels after 54 mg/day of genistein supplementation for 6 months in 60 postmenopausal women compared to the control group [110].

Whereas some clinical studies found that isoflavone consumption increased SHBG levels in postmenopausal women [18,71,96,110], others concluded the opposite. Thus, Wu A.H. et al. (2012) and Uesugi S et al. report lower concentrations of SHBG in healthy postmenopausal women after supplementation with EGCG or isoflavones [91,97], but most of the studies found no association between SHBG levels and phytoestrogen intake [19,78,79,81,83,85,86,88,95,99,100,102,108,109,111–113]. Lastly, results from epidemiological studies support the hypothesis that some phytoestrogens may have a positive influence on SHBG. Monroe K.R. et al. showed that plasma enterolactone levels were associated with higher concentrations of SHBG in postmenopausal Latina women [114]. Low et al. also reported higher concentrations of SHBG in postmenopausal women with higher urinary excretion of lignans, but no association was found with the excretion of other phytoestrogens, such as isoflavones, equol, or O-desmethylangolesin (O-DMA) [115].

To date, most of the few human studies evaluating phytoestrogen effects on androgens in postmenopausal women have found no associations between phytoestrogen intake and androgen peripheral concentrations [74,82,85,86,91,109,116]. Yet Basaria S. et al. reported a decrease in testosterone levels after 12 weeks of isoflavone supplementation, results that were supported by Kapoor R. et al. only in normal-weight postmenopausal women consuming pomegranate for 3 weeks [111,113]. Bioavailable testosterone remained unchanged in both trials. Furthermore, Wu W.H. et al. also reported lower levels of DHEA-sulphate, an androgen precursor, in postmenopausal women after a 5-week intervention with sesame lignans [81].

3. Effect of Phytoestrogen Intake on Thyroid Hormones

It is not clearly established if phytoestrogen consumption alters the hypothalamic–pituitary–thyroid axis and triggers goitrogenic effects in humans [9,117]. A randomized, double-blind, and crossover trial carried out in 60 patients with subclinical hypothyroidism and an adequate iodine intake reported an advance to overt hypothyroidism in 10% of cases (6 females) after administering soy protein with isoflavones for 8 weeks [118]. Nevertheless, soy isoflavones appear not to affect euthyroid populations with an optimal iodine status [9,117]. Controversial results have been obtained by studies in healthy humans, who did not experience anti-thyroid or any other effects after consuming dietary phytoestrogens, particularly isoflavones. The evidence for the impact of phytoestrogens on thyroid function according to the life stage is provided below.

3.1. Pregnant Women

A cross-sectional study found no association between soy consumption in early pregnancy and the development of thyroid dysfunction or autoimmunity in 505 women living in areas with an optimal intake of iodine [119]. However, further studies in countries with iodine deficiency are needed.

3.2. Children

A cross-sectional study in children aged 8–15 years in an iodine-deficient region of the Czech Republic did not obtain conclusive results. Although levels of free thyroxine (free-T4) increased after a higher intake of soy, a positive correlation was observed between serum daidzein levels and thyroid stimulating hormone (TSH) [120]. In a retrospective study, children with congenital hypothyroidism fed with soy formula had a higher concentration of TSH compared to those fed with non-soy formula [121]. Nevertheless, a study in 12 hypercholesterolemic children consuming toffee candies containing isoflavone extract for 8 weeks did not find any effect on TSH, triiodothyronine (T3), or T4 levels [122].

3.3. Men

Two clinical trials showed that products with a high phytoestrogen content had anti-thyroid effects in male populations [123,124]. Hampl R. et al. observed a significant increase of serum TSH in young males after supplementation with 2 g/kg body weight/day of boiled unprocessed natural soybeans for 7 days [123]. Similarly, significant changes in TSH (increasing) and free-T4 (decreasing) were found in men with type-2 diabetes mellitus and compensated hypogonadism after consumption of 15 g/day of soy protein isoflavones for 3 months [124].

3.4. Premenopausal Women

No significant changes in thyroid function were found in healthy and obese premenopausal women consuming soy isoflavones for periods of 1 week to 6 months [53,123,125], but reduced free-T3 levels were found in healthy young females following a high-soy diet for three menstrual cycles [126].

3.5. Postmenopausal Women

A randomized, double-blind and parallel trial conducted in 120 postmenopausal women reported a significant increase in TSH and a decrease of free-T4 after the intake of 66 mg/day of soy isoflavones for 6 months [124]. Jayagopal V. et al. obtained similar results in a cross-over design trial involving 32 postmenopausal women with type-2 diabetes mellitus consuming twice the amount for half the duration [109]. Another parallel RCT conducted by Mittal et al. in oophorectomized women showed a decrease in free T3 after a 12-week intervention with 75 mg/day isoflavone [127]. Other authors found no significant differences in the level of thyroid hormones, but other thyroid-related parameters such as thyroxine-binding globulin (TBG) and the T3:T4 ratio were altered, indicating possible goitrogenic activity derived from phytoestrogen consumption [18,108]. In addition, Sosvorová et al. observed the presence of mono-iodinated derivatives of daidzein and genistein in urine after daily consumption of isoflavonoids for 3 months, which could explain the entry of genistein and daidzein in human thyroid follicles and thyroperoxidase modification [108]. However, other RCT observed no significant changes in thyroid function after isoflavone intake [84,128–130]. Nor was an effect reported in longer studies (1 to 3 years of duration) after the administration of different doses of isoflavones (2–200 mg/day) [74,93,131–133], possibly because adaptation to long-term changes in dietary isoflavone intake triggers endocrine autoregulation [95].

4. Effect of Phytoestrogen Intake on Cardiometabolic Risk-Related Hormones

Cardiometabolic diseases encompass a set of dysfunctions affecting the cardiovascular system. These are not limited to hard cardiovascular events such as coronary heart disease, myocardial infarction, and stroke, but also include cardiovascular risk factors, namely obesity, insulin resistance, endothelial dysfunction, atherosclerosis, lipid profile, or non-alcoholic fatty liver disease, among others [134].

Obesity is usually the first risk factor that triggers chronic low-grade inflammation, which plays a crucial role in systemic metabolic dysfunction. Adipose tissue and adipocytes are dysfunctional in obese individuals, causing the secretion of pro-inflammatory adipokines that contribute to chronic inflammation and subsequently to the progression of cardiometabolic disorders like insulin resistance [135–137].

Another condition that increases the odds of suffering cardiovascular diseases is type-2 diabetes mellitus, which involves alterations in intestinal sensitivity to insulin and glucagon-like peptide-1 (GLP-1), as does its previous state, insulin resistance. GLP-1 has a variety of metabolic effects, including the glucose-dependent stimulation of insulin secretion, and is also involved in cardiovascular health [138]. Insulin, an anabolic hormone secreted in the pancreas, also regulates carbohydrate metabolism, participates in the storage of free fatty acids in adipose tissue, and enhances protein synthesis, increasing amino acid uptake by tissues [139].

Some authors have studied whether phytoestrogens can decrease the levels of pro-inflammatory adipokines such as leptin and resistin or increase adiponectin, an anti-inflammatory hormone, as well as regulate the secretion of insulin, glucagon, and ghrelin. Ghrelin, a recently discovered hormone related to cardiovascular health, is involved in feeding behavior, energy homeostasis, and carbohydrate metabolism. It therefore participates in body weight maintenance, which is crucial for vascular health [140].

4.1. Pregnancy

Only one study has evaluated the relationship between phytoestrogens and cardiovascular health during pregnancy. Shi et al. analyzed the association between urinary concentrations of isoflavonoids and cardiometabolic risk markers using data from 299 pregnant women from the NHANES cohort [141]. Those in the fourth quartile of isoflavones had lower levels of insulin and insulin resistance compared to women in the first quartile. None of the individual isoflavonoids (daidzein, equol, and O-desmethylangolensin) in urine were significantly associated with insulin levels.

4.2. Adults

To date, two American cross-sectional studies have examined the relationship between phytoestrogens and cardiovascular-related hormones in healthy adults. In one, only lignan intake seemed to be associated with lower fasting insulin in men [142], whereas the other study reported no significant differences [143]. Ferguson et al. took a different approach, inducing transient endotoxemia in young and healthy volunteers and then analyzing the ability of dietary phytoestrogens to reverse the inflammatory response. They found a significant decrease of insulin sensitivity with the higher intake of isoflavones. The participants were asked to follow a healthy diet but did not receive counseling related to soy food intake. Moreover, similar trends were found in two independent cohorts (MECHE and NHANES) [144].

Six RCTs have evaluated the effect of phytoestrogens on cardiovascular health. The participants in four studies were at high cardiovascular risk [145–148], in one they were men with increased risk of colorectal cancer [149], and in the other they were healthy men [150]. Interventions included isoflavones [149,150], soy nuts [145], daidzein [146], genistein [148], and S-equol [147] administered for periods ranging from 4 weeks to 6 months. Three of the trials found no significant effects on insulin, leptin, or adiponectin [145–147]. However, Amanat et al. report that a daily dose of 250 mg of genistein administered to non-alcoholic fatty liver patients for 8 weeks reduced insulin levels [148]. Maskarinec et al. concluded that men who consumed soy early in life had higher levels of leptin, although no association was observed with soy intake during adulthood [150]. Finally, the results of the trial with subjects at high colorectal cancer risk suggested that isoflavones might reduce the insulin-growth factor but only in equol producers [147].

4.3. Postmenopausal Women

Most studies on phytoestrogen intake and cardiometabolic hormones have evaluated insulin and insulin resistance (HOMA-IR) in postmenopausal women. The largest observational study included 301 women from The Netherlands and used food frequency questionnaires to assess dietary isoflavone and lignan intake. Individuals with a high lignan diet had lower blood pressure but no significant associations with insulin were observed [151]. In another cross-sectional study women in the highest quartile of lignan or enterolactone intake had better anthropometric profiles and insulin sensitivity [152].

Among published clinical trials, a research group from Italy has carried out several studies monitoring cardiovascular risk factors in women receiving 54 mg of genistein. After a 6-month intervention in 60 healthy women, a decrease in insulin and insulin resistance was observed [110]. Similar results were obtained after 12 and 24 months of intervention in a related study in 389 osteopenic postmenopausal women, who received the same dose of genistein plus calcium and vitamin D [153], the values remaining consistent after an extra year of follow-up in a sub-cohort [154]. Examining the role of metabolic status, Villa et al. divided the intervention group into normo- and hyperinsulinemic patients and found that genistein improved insulin sensitivity indexes only in in the latter [71]. Similarly, women with metabolic syndrome who consumed 54 mg of genistein had lower levels of fasting insulin and HOMA-IR, and higher levels of adiponectin than the placebo group [155,156]. More recently, a research group from Iran assessed the effectiveness of 108 mg of genistein on different metabolic factors in 54 women with type-2 diabetes mellitus in a 12-week intervention. As in the other studies, genistein reduced insulin sensitivity [157].

Other RCTs have used soy isoflavones instead of genistein, administering daily doses of 40–160 mg, far higher than the phytoestrogen intake reported in observational studies. For example, in one RCT the mean daily isoflavone intake in the highest tertile was 11.4 mg [151] as opposed to a total mean intake of 0.06 mg in an observational study [152]. Most of the trials with isoflavones have been performed in healthy postmenopausal women for durations ranging from 8 weeks to 24 months. Generally, the studied vascular-related hormones are leptin, adiponectin, and insulin, although in few cases, ghrelin and resistin have also been evaluated. Results from these trials are ambiguous. Whereas most report no significant changes in any of the aforementioned hormones [158–160], others have found beneficial effects on insulin markers in the treatment group compared to the control [118,161–163], or a significant increase in adiponectin peripheral levels [164]. Overall, we can conclude that phytoestrogen therapy did not change hormone levels in obese postmenopausal women [70,165], whereas among diabetic women in a randomized cross-over trial there was a significant decrease in insulin resistance in the soy consumers compared to the placebo group [109].

5. Effect of Phytoestrogen Intake on Hormones Related to Stress Response

No significant changes in cortisol were observed in healthy women or in those at cardiometabolic risk after consuming soy isoflavones for 2–6 months [18,23,53,95,126]. However, differences between equol excretors and non-excretors have been described in premenopausal women, levels being lower in those who produce this metabolite [60].

6. Effect of Phytoestrogen Intake on Hormones Related to Bone Remodeling

Estrogen plays a key role in bone metabolism, contributing to bone mass acquisition in puberty and helping to maintain normal bone density in adulthood [166]. Given that phytoestrogens are structurally similar to estrogens, they can bind to ERs in bone and exert estrogenic actions [167].

Most studies examining the impact of phytoestrogens on bone health measure osteocalcin (OC), a metabolic regulatory hormone secreted by osteoblasts, as it is a sensitive biomarker for bone formation [168]. Parathyroid hormone (PTH), secreted by the parathyroid glands, plays an important role in calcium and phosphate metabolism. As well as stimulating bone turnover, there is increasing evidence that PTH may also promote bone formation [169].

6.1. Children

Early-life exposure to soy protein formula did not produce any change in OC and PTH in a clinical study of 48 children [29]. Even though the available data suggest that phytoestrogen intake does not affect bone-related hormones in early stages of life, more studies are needed to clarify this relationship.

6.2. Premenopausal Women

The reported effects of dietary phytoestrogen on bone health in premenopausal women are inconsistent. Kwak H.S. et al. found an increase in serum OC after the administration of 120 mg/day of soy-isoflavones for three menstrual cycles. They also observed that high genistein-excretors in the soy group had higher concentrations of OC, suggesting that individual variation may affect the metabolism and functions of isoflavones [54]. However, previous studies report unaltered OC levels [170,171], indicating a need for more research on the phytoestrogen effects on bone metabolism in premenopausal women.

6.3. Postmenopausal Women

After menopause, estrogen concentrations decrease dramatically, triggering a greater risk of osteoporosis [172]. Phytoestrogens might improve bone health due to their estrogenic effects, and it has been hypothesized that they could reduce the risk of osteoporosis. Chiechi L.M. et al. and Scheiber M.D. et al. report an increase in OC concentrations in postmenopausal women who consumed a soy-rich diet for 6 and 3 months, respectively. Although uncorroborated by the majority of studies, these results indicate a stimulation of osteoblast activity and suggest that soy may have beneficial effects on bone health [173,174]. It has been suggested that longer treatments may be necessary to produce any change in bone metabolism, but to date neither shorter nor longer studies have reported any alterations in OC related to phytoestrogen intake [74–77,96,97,107,170,175–179].

In contrast, beneficial effects on bone metabolism through mechanisms of action not involving OC have been described in healthy postmenopausal women [77,97,175–179]. Lambert M.N.T. et al. demonstrated that red clover-derived isoflavones combined with probiotics attenuated estrogen-deficient bone mineral density loss and improved bone turnover even in postmenopausal women with osteopenia [177]. Moreover, a recent meta-analysis and systematic review of RCT with perimenopausal and postmenopausal women concluded that isoflavones can be effective in preserving bone mineral density and attenuating accelerated bone resorption [103]. A possible explanation for these contrasting results could be that estrogens are predominantly antiresorptive agents, so the beneficial effects of phytoestrogens may arise from decreased bone resorption by osteoclasts rather than increased bone formation by osteoblasts.

Lastly, administration of isoflavones or genistein alone for 1 to 24 months did not alter PTH in postmenopausal women [78,92,180–183]. Only a cross-sectional study carried out with Chinese women found that postmenopausal women with a high intake of isoflavone had lower serum PTH levels [184].

7. Effect of Phytoestrogen Intake on Insulin-Like Growth Factors

Insulin growth factor 1 (IGF-1) is part of the growth hormone (GH)—IGF-1 axis and is mostly produced in the liver in response to GH stimulation. Among many other functions, IGF-1 binds its receptor on osteoblasts and enhances bone formation, so any changes in this hormone will have an impact on bone health [185]. Consequently, some studies have used IGF-1 and its binding proteins IGFBP-1 and IGFBP-3 as bone turnover biomarkers.

In addition, several epidemiological studies have shown that higher levels of IGF-1 are associated with an increased risk of different types of cancer. IGF-1 exerts its actions by binding to the IGF-1 receptor, which is expressed in most tissues of the body and stimulates cell proliferation (Cohen DH 2012). Apart from higher levels of IGF-1, several cancers also overexpress its receptor IGF-1R, which has a negative impact on their progression. IGF-2 also appears to be associated with gastrointestinal and gynecological tumors [186].

It has been hypothesized that phytoestrogens may interfere with the IGF system through their effects on steroid hormone physiology or by disrupting GH and IGF signaling [187]. However, the limited evidence in humans is inconclusive, as studies have found both positive and negative results.

7.1. Premenopausal Women

To date, only two RCTs have evaluated phytoestrogen effects on IGF-1 and its binding proteins in premenopausal women. In the first study, groups of 14 women consumed soy protein isolates providing 8 mg (control), 65 mg (low dose), or 130 mg (high dose) of isoflavones daily for three menstrual cycles. The low dose significantly increased IGF-1 concentrations compared to the high dose only in the periovulatory phase of the menstrual cycle, although no value was significantly different compared to the control group. A similar result was obtained with IGFBP-3; its concentrations were increased by the low dose diet compared with the high dose in the early follicular phase, but they did not differ from those of the control group [170]. The other study assessed the effects of red clover-derived isoflavone supplementation on IGF-1, IGFBP-1, and IGFBP-3 and its role in breast cancer prevention. This one-month intervention resulted in a non-significant reduction in IGF-1, but this was likely due to differences in IGF-1 levels at baseline between the placebo and the control group. Interestingly, the IGF status was found to be influenced by the stage of the menstrual cycle [188].

Epidemiological data does not support a phytoestrogen effect on IGF levels either. A Japanese cross-sectional study reported that there was no correlation between soy products and isoflavone intake and serum IGF-1 and IGFBP-3 in 261 premenopausal women [189]. Another observational study in women living in Japan and Hawaii also failed to find an association between tofu intake and IGF-1, IGFBP-3, and IGF-1 molar ratio in premenopausal women [190].

7.2. Postmenopausal Women

Most clinical studies on IGFs in postmenopausal women have failed to find a protective effect of phytoestrogens against osteoporosis, breast cancer, or colorectal cancer. One of the most recent found no impact on IGF-1 in women with osteopenia after a 24-month intervention [183], which is consistent with other studies reporting that isoflavone supplementation did not alter the IGF system [170,188,191]. Similar results have been obtained for lignan consumption. After administering flaxseed lignans for 3 months, Lucas E.A. et al. found that IGF-I and IGFBP-3 levels were unaltered [88]. An RCT in which 103 postmenopausal women consumed 400 or 800 mg of EGCG for 2 months found no significant changes in IGF-1 or IGFBP-3, although the latter tended to increase in both groups [91].

In contrast with these results, a study comparing the effects of soy protein and milk-based protein reported that both supplements increased IGF-1 levels. Further stratification showed that soy protein had a more pronounced effect on women who were not on hormone replacement therapy [192]. A cross-sectional study found an association between phytoestrogens and growth factors, specifically an inverse association between tofu intake and IGF-1 levels and the molar ratio in postmenopausal women, whereas no changes were observed in those who had never used hormone replacement therapy [190]. However, a similar observational study performed in participants of the Singapore Chinese Health Study did not find any association between soy intake and the IGF-1, IGFBP-3, and IGF molar ratio [193].

7.3. Men

It is well established that higher circulating IGF-1 levels are associated with an increased risk of PCa [194], and most studies assessing phytoestrogen effects on adult men have consequently focused on PCa patients. In one of two clinical trials with PCa patients, no changes in IGF-1 or IGFBP-3 were observed after a 3–6-month intervention consisting of 200 mg/day of soy isoflavones [37] and in the other Bylund A. et al. (2003) also found that IGF-1 levels remained unaltered after the administration of rye bran bread for 3 weeks [41]. Conversely, a cross-sectional study with 312 men reported a positive association between soy intake and the IGF-1, IGFBP-3, and IGF molar ratio [193].

8. Conclusions

This review has summarized the results of studies on the effects of dietary phytoestrogens on endocrine regulation in humans. Although preclinical studies (in vitro and in animal models) show phytoestrogens to be potentially estrogenic compounds, triggering anti-estrogenic effects in the organism, the results of epidemiological studies are ambiguous.

The impact of phytoestrogens can vary according to the life stage (Figure 3). There is particular concern about how they may affect pregnant women, as this has been poorly studied. Soy isoflavones appear not to have any influence on sex and thyroid hormones, bone remodeling and IGF. However, a study focused on cardiometabolic risk reported a decrease in the level of insulin and insulin resistance in pregnant women consuming higher amounts of isoflavones. Although phytoestrogens transfer from maternal blood to the fetus, no effects have been observed in early life. Nor have endocrine changes been found in infants fed with soy formula, except in a retrospective study carried out in the first year of life of infants with congenital hypothyroidism, which reported an increase of TSH but no conclusive effects on thyroid function. Nevertheless, consumption of phytoestrogens in conditions of insufficient iodine and hypothyroidism may negatively affect thyroid function and favor endocrine imbalance, although such effects have not been observed in euthyroid individuals living in areas with enough supply of iodine. In later stages of childhood, an increase of androgens and decrease of estrogens associated with dietary phytoestrogens have been observed in girls and boys, respectively.

In adulthood, endocrine changes arising from phytoestrogen consumption are unclear, although goitrogenic activity has been observed in men. Effects on sex hormones and IGFs in men are ambiguous, as studies report contradictory results. PCa risk in patients with PCa was unaltered, whereas equol producers with colorectal cancer risk showed a decrease of IGF. Results regarding cardiometabolic risk-related hormones are inconclusive in healthy subjects. Although higher levels of leptin have been reported in early life, no association has been identified in adulthood. However, a reduction in insulin levels was found in patients with non-alcoholic fatty liver.

In premenopausal women, usually studied separately from postmenopausal women, uncertain results have been obtained regarding sex hormones, breast cancer protection, and bone remodeling. Nor has evidence been provided for phytoestrogens affecting IGF levels. Whereas no significant changes in thyroid function were observed, a decrease of free-T3 was found in healthy young females. Among stress response-related hormones, no significant changes in cortisol are described in healthy women or in those at cardiometabolic risk, but a lower production of cortisol is reported in equol-excretors. In postmenopause, the results reported for sex hormones are also ambiguous. However, possible goitrogenic activity derived from phytoestrogen consumption opens up a path for future research. Apart from that, an ameliorative effect has been observed in the cardiometabolic profile of hyperinsulinemic patients, individuals with metabolic syndrome and diabetes. Regarding bone remodeling, the effects of phytoestrogens on OC concentrations are unclear, and their beneficial impact may arise instead from reducing bone resorption by osteoclasts. The results obtained for PHT and IGF are unconvincing, precluding the drawing of any conclusions.

In general, the available evidence for an association between dietary phytoestrogens and endocrine biomarkers is inconclusive. The disparity in results may be due to differences in the type and concentration of the compounds administered and the variety of matrices, which could influence phytoestrogen bioavailability and consequently the effect on hormonal function. Also, while most studies analyze circulating hormones, others report the urinary excretion of metabolites. There is a clear need for further carefully designed studies to elucidate the effects of phytoestrogen consumption on the endocrine system.

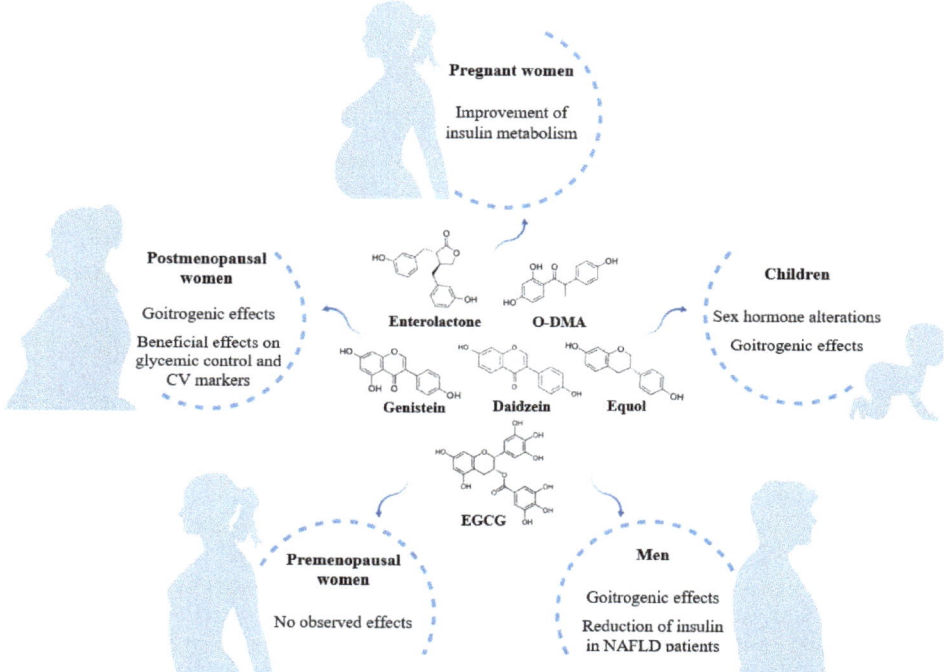

Figure 3. Summary of the effects of dietary phytoestrogens at different life stages. NAFLD: non-alcoholic fatty liver disease.

9. Future Directions

Based on the available literature, we can conclude that intake of phytoestrogens does have some physiological effects in humans related to hormone regulation, but like hormones, the benefits depend on the stage of life. Some factors such as dose and type of compounds, as well as matrices englobing these phytoestroestrogens (food, capsule, etc.) affect their bioavailability and, therefore, the observed results. Most of the research is focused on postmenopausal women and only some have explored the effects during pregnancy and early stages of life. For instance, the effect of phytoestrogen intake on pubertal development has been poorly studied and could lead to interesting results. In order to do that, well-designed intervention trials are key to shed some light on this topic, especially regarding associations that are controversial.

Author Contributions: Conceptualization, A.T.-R. and S.H.-B.; Bibliography searching methodology, S.H.-B.; Writing—original draft preparation, I.D.-L., M.Y.-A., A.S.-H., A.T.-R., and S.H.-B.; Writing—review and editing, A.T.-R. and S.H.-B.; Supervision, A.T.-R. and S.H.-B. All authors have read and agreed to the published version of the manuscript.

Funding: This research received no external funding.

Conflicts of Interest: The authors declare no conflict of interest.

References

1. Viggiani, M.T.; Polimeno, L.; Di Leo, A.; Barone, M. Phytoestrogens: Dietary intake, bioavailability, and protective mechanisms against colorectal neoproliferative lesions. *Nutrients* **2019**, *11*, 1709. [CrossRef] [PubMed]
2. Bennetau-Pelissero, C. Risks and benefits of phytoestrogens: Where are we now. *Curr. Opin. Clin. Nutr. Metab. Care* **2016**, *19*, 477–483. [CrossRef] [PubMed]
3. Zamora-Ros, R.; Knaze, V.; Luján-Barroso, L.; Kuhnle, G.G.C.; Mulligan, A.A.; Touillaud, M.; Slimani, N.; Romieu, I.; Powell, N.; Tumino, R.; et al. Dietary intakes and food sources of phytoestrogens in the European Prospective Investigation into Cancer and Nutrition (EPIC) 24-hour dietary recall cohort. *Eur. J. Clin. Nutr.* **2012**, *66*, 932–941. [CrossRef] [PubMed]
4. Bedell, S.; Nachtigall, M.; Naftolin, F. The pros and cons of plant estrogens for menopause. *J. Steroid Biochem. Mol. Biol.* **2014**, *139*, 225–236. [CrossRef]
5. Rietjens, I.M.C.M.; Louisse, J.; Beekmann, K. The potential health effects of dietary phytoestrogens. *Br. J. Pharmacol.* **2017**, *174*, 1263–1280. [CrossRef]
6. De Pascual-Teresa, S.; Hallund, J.; Talbot, D.; Schroot, J.; Williams, C.M.; Bugel, S.; Cassidy, A. Absorption of isoflavones in humans: Effects of food matrix and processing. *J. Nutr. Biochem.* **2006**, *17*, 257–264. [CrossRef]
7. Patisaul, H.B.; Jefferson, W. The pros and cons of phytoestrogens. *Front. Neuroendocrinol.* **2010**, *31*, 400–419. [CrossRef]
8. Křížová, L.; Dadáková, K.; Kašparovská, J.; Kašparovský, T. Isoflavones. *Molecules* **2019**, *24*, 1076. [CrossRef]
9. Hüser, S.; Guth, S.; Joost, H.G.; Soukup, S.T.; Köhrle, J.; Kreienbrock, L.; Diel, P.; Lachenmeier, D.W.; Eisenbrand, G.; Vollmer, G.; et al. Effects of isoflavones on breast tissue and the thyroid hormone system in humans: A comprehensive safety evaluation. *Arch. Toxicol.* **2018**, *92*, 2703–2748. [CrossRef]
10. Desmawati, D.; Sulastri, D. Phytoestrogens and Their Health Effect. *Maced. J. Med. Sci.* **2019**, *7*, 495–499. [CrossRef]
11. Bilancio, A.; Migliaccio, A. Phosphoinositide 3-Kinase Assay in Breast Cancer Cell Extracts. *Methods Mol. Biol.* **2014**, *1204*, 145–153. [CrossRef] [PubMed]
12. Migliaccio, A.; Castoria, G.; de Falco, A.; Bilancio, A.; Giovannelli, P.; Di Donato, M.; Marino, I.; Yamaguchi, H.; Appella, E.; Auricchio, F. Polyproline and Tat transduction peptides in the study of the rapid actions of steroid receptors. *Steroids* **2012**, *77*, 974–978. [CrossRef] [PubMed]
13. Di Donato, M.; Giovannelli, P.; Cernera, G.; Di Santi, A.; Marino, I.; Bilancio, A.; Galasso, G.; Auricchio, F.; Migliaccio, A.; Castoria, G. Non-genomic androgen action regulates proliferative/migratory signaling in stromal cells. *Front. Endocrinol.* **2015**, *5*, 225 [CrossRef]
14. Nicholls, J.; Lasley, B.L.; Nakajima, S.T.; Setchell, K.D.R.; Schneeman, B.O. Effects of Soy Consumption on Gonadotropin Secretion and Acute Pituitary Responses to Gonadotropin-Releasing Hormone in Women. *J. Nutr.* **2002**, *132*, 708–714. [CrossRef] [PubMed]
15. Jefferson, W.N. Adult Ovarian Function Can Be Affected by High Levels of Soy. *J. Nutr.* **2010**, *140*, 2322S–2325S. [CrossRef] [PubMed]
16. Lord, R.S.; Bongiovanni, B.; Bralley, J.A. Estrogen metabolism and the diet-cancer connection: Rationale for assessing the ratio of urinary hydroxylated estrogen metabolites. *Altern. Med. Rev.* **2002**, *7*, 112–129. [PubMed]
17. Tamaya, T. Phytoestrogens and reproductive biology. *Reprod. Med. Biol.* **2005**, *4*, 225–229. [CrossRef]
18. Duncan, A.M.; Underhill, K.E.; Xu, X.; LaValleur, J.; Phipps, W.R.; Kurzer, M.S. Modest hormonal effects of soy isoflavones in postmenopausal women *J. Clin. Endocrinol. Metab.* **1999**, *84*, 3479–3484. [CrossRef]
19. Verkasalo, P.K.; Appleby, P.N.; Davey, G.K.; Key, T.J. Soy milk intake and plasma sex hormones: A cross-sectional study in pre- and postmenopausal women (EPIC-Oxford). *Nutr. Cancer* **2001**, *40*, 79–86. [CrossRef]

20. Wang, L.-Q. Mammalian phytoestrogens: Enterodiol and enterolactone. *J. Chromatogr. B* **2002**, *777*, 289–309. [CrossRef]
21. Zhao, E.; Mu, Q. Phytoestrogen biological actions on mammalian reproductive system and cancer growth. *Sci. Pharm.* **2011**, *79*, 1–20. [CrossRef] [PubMed]
22. Xu, X.; Duncan, A.M.; Merz, B.E.; Kurzer, M.S. Effects of soy isoflavones on estrogen and phytoestrogen metabolism in premenopausal women. *Cancer Epidemiol. Biomark. Prev.* **1998**, *7*, 1101–1108.
23. Brown, B.D.; Thomas, W.; Hutchins, A.; Martini, M.C.; Slavin, J.L. Types of dietary fat and soy minimally affect hormones and biomarkers associated with breast cancer risk in premenopausal women. *Nutr. Cancer* **2002**, *43*, 22–30. [CrossRef] [PubMed]
24. Nagata, C.; Iwasa, S.; Shiraki, M.; Ueno, T.; Uchiyama, S.; Urata, K.; Sahashi, Y.; Shimizu, H. Associations among maternal soy intake, isoflavone levels in urine and blood samples, and maternal and umbilical hormone concentrations (Japan). *Cancer Causes Control* **2006**, *17*, 1107–1113. [CrossRef] [PubMed]
25. Wada, K.; Nakamura, K.; Masue, T.; Sahashi, Y.; Ando, K.; Nagata, C. Soy intake and urinary sex hormone levels in preschool Japanese children. *Am. J. Epidemiol.* **2011**, *173*, 998–1003. [CrossRef] [PubMed]
26. Todaka, E.; Sakurai, K.; Fukata, H.; Miyagawa, H.; Uzuki, M.; Omori, M.; Osada, H.; Ikezuki, Y.; Tsutsumi, O.; Iguchi, T.; et al. Fetal exposure to phytoestrogens—The difference in phytoestrogen status between mother and fetus. *Environ. Res.* **2005**, *99*, 195–203. [CrossRef]
27. Adlercreutz, H.; Yamada, T.; Wahala, K.; Watanabe, S. Maternal and neonatal phytoestrogens in Japanese women during birth. *Am. J. Obstet. Gynecol.* **1999**, *180*, 737–743. [CrossRef]
28. Franke, A.A.; Lai, J.F.; Halm, B.M. Absorption, distribution, metabolism, and excretion of isoflavonoids after soy intake. *Arch. Biochem. Biophys.* **2014**, *559*, 24–28. [CrossRef]
29. Giampietro, P.G.; Bruno, G.; Furcolo, G.; Casati, A.; Brunetti, E.; Spadoni, G.L.; Galli, E. Soy protein formulas in children: No hormonal effects in long-term feeding. *J. Pediatr. Endocrinol. Metab.* **2004**, *17*, 191–196. [CrossRef]
30. Cao, Y.; Calafat, A.M.; Doerge, D.R.; Umbach, D.M.; Bernbaum, J.C.; Twaddle, N.C.; Ye, X.; Rogan, W.J. Isoflavones in urine, saliva, and blood of infants: Data from a pilot study on the estrogenic activity of soy formula. *J. Expo. Sci. Environ. Epidemiol.* **2009**, *19*, 223–234. [CrossRef]
31. Adgent, M.A.; Umbach, D.M.; Zemel, B.S.; Kelly, A.; Schall, J.I.; Ford, E.G.; James, K.; Darge, K.; Botelho, J.C.; Vesper, H.W.; et al. A Longitudinal Study of Estrogen-Responsive Tissues and Hormone Concentrations in Infants Fed Soy Formula. *J. Clin. Endocrinol. Metab.* **2018**, *103*, 1899–1909. [CrossRef] [PubMed]
32. Maskarinec, G.; Morimoto, Y.; Novotny, R.; Nordt, F.J.; Stanczyk, F.Z.; Franke, A.A. Urinary sex steroid excretion levels during a soy intervention among young girls: A pilot study. *Nutr. Cancer* **2005**, *52*, 22–28. [CrossRef] [PubMed]
33. Nagata, C.; Inaba, S.; Kawakami, N.; Kakizoe, T.; Shimizu, H. Inverse association of soy product intake with serum androgen and estrogen concentrations in Japanese men. *Nutr. Cancer* **2000**, *36*, 14–18. [CrossRef] [PubMed]
34. Tanaka, M.; Fujimoto, K.; Chihara, Y.; Torimoto, K.; Yoneda, T.; Tanaka, N.; Hirayama, A.; Miyanaga, N.; Akaza, H.; Hirao, Y. Isoflavone supplements stimulated the production of serum equol and decreased the serum dihydrotestosterone levels in healthy male volunteers. *Prostate Cancer Prostatic Dis.* **2009**, *12*, 247–252. [CrossRef] [PubMed]
35. Applegate, C.C.; Rowles, J.L.; Ranard, K.M.; Jeon, S.; Erdman, J.W. Soy consumption and the risk of prostate cancer: An updated systematic review and meta-analysis. *Nutrients* **2018**, *10*, 40. [CrossRef] [PubMed]
36. Dalais, F.S.; Meliala, A.; Wattanapenpaiboon, N.; Frydenberg, M.; Suter, D.A.I.; Thomson, W.K.; Wahlqvist, M.L. Effects of a diet rich in phytoestrogens on prostate-specific antigen and sex hormones in men diagnosed with prostate cancer. *Urology* **2004**, *64*, 510–515. [CrossRef] [PubMed]
37. Hussain, M.; Banerjee, M.; Sarkar, F.H.; Djuric, Z.; Pollak, M.N.; Doerge, D.; Fontana, J.; Chinni, S.; Davis, J.; Forman, J.; et al. Soy Isoflavones in the Treatment of Prostate Cancer. *Nutr. Cancer* **2003**, *47*, 111–117. [CrossRef]
38. Pendleton, J.M.; Tan, W.W.; Anai, S.; Chang, M.; Hou, W.; Shiverick, K.T.; Rosser, C.J. Phase II trial of isoflavone in prostate-specific antigen recurrent prostate cancer after previous local therapy. *BMC Cancer* **2008**, *8*, 132. [CrossRef]

39. Hamilton-Reeves, J.M.; Banerjee, S.; Banerjee, S.K.; Holzbeierlein, J.M.; Thrasher, J.B.; Kambhampati, S.; Keighley, J.; Van Veldhuizen, P. Short-Term Soy Isoflavone Intervention in Patients with Localized Prostate Cancer: A Randomized, Double-Blind, Placebo-Controlled Trial. *PLoS ONE* **2013**, *8*, e68331. [CrossRef]
40. Fischer, L.; Mahoney, C.; Jeffcoat, A.R.; Koch, M.A.; Thomas, B.F.; Valentine, J.L.; Stinchcombe, T.; Boan, J.; Crowell, J.A.; Zeisel, S.H. Clinical characteristics and pharmacokinetics of purified soy isoflavones: Multiple-dose administration to men with prostate neoplasia. *Nutr. Cancer* **2004**, *48*, 160–170. [CrossRef]
41. Bylund, A.; Lundin, E.; Zhang, J.X.; Nordin, A.; Kaaks, R.; Stenman, U.H.; Åman, P.; Adlercreutz, H.; Nilsson, T.K.; Hallmans, G.; et al. Randomised controlled short-term intervention pilot study on rye bran bread in prostate cancer. *Eur. J. Cancer Prev.* **2003**, *12*, 407–415. [CrossRef] [PubMed]
42. Bosland, M.C. The role of steroid hormones in prostate carcinogenesis. *J. Natl. Cancer Inst. Monogr.* **2000**, *2000*, 39–66. [CrossRef] [PubMed]
43. Shaneyfelt, T.; Husein, R.; Bubley, G.; Mantzoros, C.S. Hormonal predictors of prostate cancer: A meta-analysis. *J. Clin. Oncol.* **2000**, *18*, 847–853. [CrossRef] [PubMed]
44. Hamilton-Reeves, J.M.; Vazquez, G.; Duval, S.J.; Phipps, W.R.; Kurzer, M.S.; Messina, M.J. Clinical studies show no effects of soy protein or isoflavones on reproductive hormones in men: Results of a meta-analysis. *Fertil. Steril.* **2010**, *94*, 997–1007. [CrossRef]
45. Ho, S.M.; Lee, M.T.; Lam, H.M.; Leung, Y.K. Estrogens and Prostate Cancer: Etiology, Mediators, Prevention, and Management. *Endocrinol. Metab. Clin. N. Am.* **2011**, *40*, 591–614. [CrossRef]
46. Hamilton-Reeves, J.; Rebello, S.; Thomas, W.; Slaton, J.; Kurzer, M. Soy protein isolate increases urinary estrogens and the ratio of 2:16alfa-hydroxyesterone in men at high risk of prostate cancer. *J. Nutr.* **2007**, *137*, 2258–2263. [CrossRef]
47. Lu, L.J.; Anderson, K.E.; Grady, J.J.; Nagamani, M. Effects of soya consumption for one month on steroid hormones in premenopausal women: Implications for breast cancer risk reduction. *Cancer Epidemiol. Biomark. Prev.* **1996**, *5*, 63–70.
48. Lu, L.J.; Cree, M.; Josyula, S.; Nagamani, M.; Grady, J.J.; Anderson, K.E. Increased urinary excretion of 2-hydroxyestrone but not 16α-hydroxyestrone in premenopausal women during a soya diet containing isoflavones. *Cancer Res.* **2000**, *60*, 1299–1305.
49. Lu, L.J.; Anderson, K.E.; Grady, J.J.; Nagamani, M. Effects of an isoflavone-free soy diet on ovarian hormones in premenopausal women. *J. Clin. Endocrinol. Metab.* **2001**, *86*, 3045–3052. [CrossRef]
50. Maskarinec, G.; Beckford, F.; Morimoto, Y.; Franke, A.A.; Stanczyk, F.Z. Association of estrogen measurements in serum and urine of premenopausal women. *Biomark. Med.* **2015**, *9*, 417–424. [CrossRef]
51. Kapiszewska, M.; Miskiewicz, M.; Ellison, P.T.; Thune, I.; Jasienska, G. High tea consumption diminishes salivary 17β-estradiol concentration in Polish women. *Br. J. Nutr.* **2006**, *95*, 989–995. [CrossRef] [PubMed]
52. Cassidy, A.; Bingham, S.; Setchell, K. Biological effects of isoflavones in young women: Importance of the chemical composition of soyabean products *Br. J. Nutr.* **1995**, *74*, 587–601. [CrossRef] [PubMed]
53. Romualdi, D.; Costantini, B.; Campagna, G.; Lanzone, A.; Guido, M. Is there a role for soy isoflavones in the therapeutic approach to polycystic ovary syndrome? Results from a pilot study. *Fertil. Steril.* **2008**, *90*, 1826–1833. [CrossRef] [PubMed]
54. Kwak, H.S.; Park, S.Y.; Kim, M.G.; Yim, C.H.; Yoon, H.K.; Han, K.O. Marked individual variation in isoflavone metabolism after a soy challenge can modulate the skeletal effect of isoflavones in premenopausal women. *J. Korean Med. Sci.* **2009**, *24*, 867–873. [CrossRef] [PubMed]
55. Maskarinec, G.; Williams, A.E.; Inouye, J.S.; Stanczyk, F.Z.; Franke, A.A. A randomized isoflavone intervention among premenopausal women. *Cancer Epidemiol. Biomark. Prev.* **2002**, *11*, 195–201.
56. Martini, M.C.; Dancisak, B.B.; Haggans, C.J.; Thomas, W.; Slavin, J.L. Effects of soy intake on sex hormone metabolism in premenopausal women. *Nutr. Cancer* **1999**, *34*, 133–139. [CrossRef] [PubMed]
57. Tsuji, M.; Tamai, Y.; Wada, K.; Nakamura, K.; Hayashi, M.; Takeda, N.; Yasuda, K.; Nagata, C. Associations of intakes of fat, dietary fiber, soy isoflavones, and alcohol with levels of sex hormones and prolactin in premenopausal Japanese women. *Cancer Causes Control* **2012**, *23*, 683–689. [CrossRef]
58. Maskarinec, G.; Ollberding, N.J.; Conroy, S.M.; Morimoto, Y.; Pagano, I.S.; Franke, A.A.; Gentzschein, E.; Stanczyk, F.Z. Estrogen levels in nipple aspirate fluid and serum during a randomized soy trial. *Cancer Epidemiol. Biomark. Prev.* **2011**, *20*, 1815–1821. [CrossRef]
59. Morimoto, Y.; Conroy, S.M.; Pagano, I.S.; Isaki, M.; Franke, A.A.; Nordt, F.J.; Maskarinec, G. Urinary estrogen metabolites during a randomized soy trial. *Nutr. Cancer* **2012**, *64*, 307–314. [CrossRef]

60. Duncan, A.M.; Merz-Demlow, B.E.; Xu, X.; Phipps, W.R.; Kurzer, M.S. Premenopausal equol excretors show plasma hormone profiles associated with lowered risk of breast cancer. *Cancer Epidemiol. Biomark. Prev.* **2000**, *9*, 581–586.
61. Setchell, K.D.R.; Clerici, C.; Lephart, E.D.; Cole, S.J.; Heenan, C.; Castellani, D.; Wolfe, B.E.; Nechemias-Zimmer, L.; Brown, N.M.; Lund, T.D.; et al. S-equol, a potent ligand for estrogen receptor β, is the exclusive enantiomeric form of the soy isoflavone metabolite produced by human intestinal bacterial flora. *Am. J. Clin. Nutr.* **2005**, *81*, 1072–1079. [CrossRef] [PubMed]
62. Phipps, W.R.; Martini, M.C.; Lampe, J.W.; Slavin, J.L.; Kurzer, M.S. Effect of flax seed ingestion on the menstrual cycle. *J. Clin. Endocrinol. Metab.* **1993**, *77*, 1215–1219. [CrossRef] [PubMed]
63. Haggans, C.J.; Travelli, E.J.; Thomas, W.; Martini, M.C.; Slavin, J.L. The effect of flaxseed and wheat bran consumption on urinary estrogen metabolites in premenopausal women. *Cancer Epidemiol. Biomark. Prev.* **2000**, *9*, 719–725.
64. Cassidy, A.; Bingham, S.; Setchell, K.D. Biological effects of a diet of soy protein rich in isoflavones on the menstrual cycle of premenopausal women. *Am. J. Clin. Nutr.* **1994**, *60*, 333–340. [CrossRef]
65. Maskarinec, G.; Franke, A.A.; Williams, A.E.; Hebshi, S.; Oshiro, C.; Murphy, S.; Stanczyk, F.Z. Effects of a 2-year randomized soy intervention on sex hormone levels in premenopausal women. *Cancer Epidemiol. Biomark. Prev.* **2004**, *13*, 1736–1744. [CrossRef]
66. Nagata, C.; Takatsuka, N.; Inaba, S.; Kawakami, N.; Shimizu, H. Effect of Soymilk Consumption on Serum Estrogen Concentrations in Premenopausal Japanese Women. *J. Natl. Cancer Inst.* **1998**, *90*, 1830–1835. [CrossRef]
67. Watanabe, S.; Terashima, K.; Sato, Y.; Arai, S.; Eboshida, A. Effects of isoflavone supplement on healthy women. *BioFactors* **2000**, *12*, 233–241. [CrossRef]
68. Kumar, N.B.; Cantor, A.; Allen, K.; Riccardi, D.; Cox, C.E. The specific role of isoflavones on estrogen metabolism in premenopausal women. *Cancer* **2002**, *94*, 1166–1174. [CrossRef]
69. Nelson, H.D. Menopause. *Lancet* **2008**, *371*, 760–770. [CrossRef]
70. Llaneza, P.; González, C.; Fernández-Iñarrea, J.; Alonso, A.; Díaz, F.; Pérez-López, F.R. Soy isoflavones improve insulin sensitivity without changing serum leptin among postmenopausal women. *Climacteric* **2012**, *15*, 611–620. [CrossRef]
71. Villa, P.; Costantini, B.; Suriano, R.; Perri, C.; Macrì, F.; Ricciardi, L.; Panunzi, S.; Lanzone, A. The differential effect of the phytoestrogen genistein on cardiovascular risk factors in postmenopausal women: Relationship with the metabolic status. *J. Clin. Endocrinol. Metab.* **2009**, *94*, 552–558. [CrossRef] [PubMed]
72. Villa, P.; Amar, I.D.; Bottoni, C.; Cipolla, C.; Dinoi, G.; Moruzzi, M.C.; Scambia, G.; Lanzone, A. The impact of combined nutraceutical supplementation on quality of life and metabolic changes during the menopausal transition: A pilot randomized trial. *Arch. Gynecol. Obstet.* **2017**, *296*, 791–801. [CrossRef]
73. Rosa Lima, S.M.R.; Bernardo, B.F.A.; Yamada, S.S.; Reis, B.F.; Da Silva, G.M.D.; Longo Galvão, M.A. Effects of Glycine max (L.) Merr. soy isoflavone vaginal gel on epithelium morphology and estrogen receptor expression in postmenopausal women: A 12-week, randomized, double-blind, placebo-controlled trial. *Maturitas* **2014**, *78*, 205–211. [CrossRef]
74. Tousen, Y.; Ezaki, J.; Fujii, Y.; Ueno, T.; Nishimuta, M.; Ishimi, Y. Natural S-equol decreases bone resorption in postmenopausal, non-equol-producing Japanese women: A pilot randomized, placebo-controlled trial. *Menopause* **2011**, *18*, 563–574. [CrossRef] [PubMed]
75. Wu, J.; Oka, J.; Higuchi, M.; Tabata, I.; Toda, T.; Fujioka, M.; Fuku, N.; Teramoto, T.; Okuhira, T.; Ueno, T.; et al. Cooperative effects of isoflavones and exercise on bone and lipid metabolism in postmenopausal Japanese women: A randomized placebo-controlled trial. *Metabolism* **2006**, *55*, 423–433. [CrossRef] [PubMed]
76. Wu, J.; Oka, J.; Tabata, I.; Higuchi, M.; Toda, T.; Fuku, N.; Ezaki, J.; Sugiyama, F.; Uchiyama, S.; Yamada, K.; et al. Effects of isoflavone and exercise on BMD and fat mass in postmenopausal Japanese women: A 1-year randomized placebo-controlled trial. *J. Bone Miner. Res.* **2006**, *21*, 780–789. [CrossRef] [PubMed]
77. Zhang, G.; Qin, L.; Shi, Y. Epimedium-derived phytoestrogen flavonoids exert beneficial effect on preventing bone loss in late postmenopausal women: A 24-month randomized, double-blind and placebo-controlled trial. *J. Bone Miner. Res.* **2007**, *22*, 1072–1079. [CrossRef]
78. Spence, L.A.; Lipscomb, E.R.; Cadogan, J.; Martin, B.; Wastney, M.E.; Peacock, M.; Weaver, C.M. The effect of soy protein and soy isoflavones on calcium metabolism in postmenopausal women: A randomized crossover study. *Am. J. Clin. Nutr.* **2005**, *81*, 916–922. [CrossRef]

79. Reed, S.D.; Newton, K.M.; LaCroix, A.Z.; Grothaus, L.C.; Grieco, V.S.; Ehrlich, K. Vaginal, endometrial, and reproductive Hormone Findings: Randomized, placebo-controlled trial of black cohosh, multibotanical Herbs, and dietary soy for vasomotor symptoms: The Herbal Alternatives for Menopause (HALT) Study. *Menopause* **2008**, *15*, 51–58. [CrossRef]
80. Evans, M.; Elliott, J.G.; Sharma, P.; Berman, R.; Guthrie, N. The effect of synthetic genistein on menopause symptom management in healthy postmenopausal women: A multi-center, randomized, placebo-controlled study. *Maturitas* **2011**, *68*, 189–196. [CrossRef]
81. Wu, W.-H.; Kang, Y.-P.; Wang, N.-H.; Jou, H.-J.; Wang, T.-A. Sesame Ingestion Affects Sex Hormones, Antioxidant Status, and Blood Lipids in Postmenopausal Women. *J. Nutr.* **2006**, *136*, 1270–1275. [CrossRef]
82. Foth, D.; Nawroth, F. Effect of soy supplementation on endogenous hormones in postmenopausal women. *Gynecol. Obstet. Investig.* **2003**, *55*, 135–138. [CrossRef]
83. Baird, D.D.; Umbach, D.M.; Lansdell, L.; Hughes, L.; Setchell, K.D.; Weinberg, R.; Haney, F.; Wilcox, J.; Mclachian, J.A. Dietary Intervention Study to Assess Estrogenicity of Dietary Soy Among Postmenopausal Women. *J. Clin. Endocrinol. Metab.* **1995**, *80*, 1685–1690.
84. Murray, M.J.; Meyer, W.R.; Lessey, B.A.; Oi, R.H.; DeWire, R.E.; Fritz, M.A. Soy protein isolate with isoflavones does not prevent estradiol-induced endometrial hyperplasia in postmenopausal women: A pilot trial. *Menopause* **2003**, *10*, 456–464. [CrossRef]
85. Wu, A.H.; Stanczyk, F.Z.; Martinez, C.; Tseng, C.C.; Hendrich, S.; Murphy, P.; Chaikittisilpa, S.; Stram, D.O.; Pike, M.C. A controlled 2-mo dietary fat reduction and soy food supplementation study in postmenopausal women. *Am. J. Clin. Nutr.* **2005**, *81*, 1133–1141. [CrossRef]
86. Lee, C.C.; Bloem, C.J.; Kasa-Vubu, J.Z.; Liang, L.-J. Effect of oral phytoestrogen on androgenicity and insulin sensitivity in postmenopausal women. *Diabetes Obes. Metab.* **2012**, *14*, 315–319. [CrossRef]
87. Goldin, B.R.; Brauner, E.; Adlercreutz, H.; Ausman, L.M.; Lichtenstein, A.H. Hormonal response to diets high in soy or animal protein without and with isoflavones in moderately hypercholesterolemic subjects. *Nutr. Cancer* **2005**, *51*, 1–6. [CrossRef]
88. Lucas, E.A.; Wild, R.D.; Hammond, L.J.; Khalil, D.A.; Juma, S.; Daggy, B.P.; Stoecker, B.J.; Arjmandi, B.H. Flaxseed improves lipid profile without altering biomarkers of bone metabolism in postmenopausal women. *J. Clin. Endocrinol. Metab.* **2002**, *87*, 1527–1532. [CrossRef]
89. Rashid, A.; Khurshid, R.; Latif, A.; Ahmad, N.; Aftab, L. Role of phytoestrogen in suppressing bone turnover in a group of postmenopausal women. *J. Ayub Med. Coll. Abbottabad* **2010**, *22*, 201–204.
90. Rios, D.R.A.; Rodrigues, E.T.; Cardoso, A.P.Z.; Montes, M.B.A.; Franceschini, S.A.; Toloi, M.R.T. Lack of effects of isoflavones on the lipid profile of Brazilian postmenopausal women. *Nutrition* **2008**, *24*, 1153–1158. [CrossRef]
91. Wu, A.H.; Spicer, D.; Stanczyk, F.Z.; Tseng, C.C.; Yang, C.S.; Pike, M.C. Effect of 2-month controlled green tea intervention on lipoprotein cholesterol, glucose, and hormone levels in healthy postmenopausal women. *Cancer Prev. Res.* **2012**, *5*, 393–402. [CrossRef]
92. Morabito, N.; Crisafulli, A.; Vergara, C.; Gaudio, A.; Lasco, A.; Frisina, N.; D'Anna, R.; Corrado, F.; Pizzoleo, M.A.; Cincotta, M.; et al. Effects of genistein and hormone-replacement therapy on bone loss in early postmenopausal women: A randomized double-blind placebo-controlled study. *J. Bone Miner. Res.* **2002**, *17*, 1904–1912. [CrossRef]
93. Levis, S.; Strickman-Stein, N.; Ganjei-Azar, P.; Xu, P.; Doerge, D.R.; Krischer, J. Soy isoflavones in the prevention of menopausal bone loss and menopausal symptoms: A randomized, double-blind trial. *Arch. Intern. Med.* **2011**, *171*, 1363–1369. [CrossRef]
94. Pino, A.M.; Valladares, L.E.; Palma, M.A.; Mancilla, A.M.; Yáñez, M.; Albala, C. Dietary isoflavones affect sex hormone-binding globulin levels in postmenopausal women. *J. Clin. Endocrinol. Metab.* **2000**, *85*, 2797–2800. [CrossRef]
95. Persky, V.W.; Turyk, M.E.; Wang, L.; Freels, S.; Chatterton, R., Jr.; Barnes, S.; Erdman, J., Jr.; Sepkovic, D.W.; Bradlow, H.L.; Potter, S. Effect of Soy Protein on Endogenous Hormones in Postmenopausal Women. *Am. J. Clin. Nutr.* **2002**, *75*, 145–153. [CrossRef]
96. Oh, H.Y.; Kim, S.S.; Chung, H.Y.; Yoon, S. Isoflavone supplements exert hormonal and antioxidant effects in postmenopausal Korean women with diabetic retinopathy. *J. Med. Food* **2005**, *8*, 1–7. [CrossRef]
97. Uesugi, S.; Watanabe, S.; Ishiwata, N.; Uehara, M.; Ouchi, K. Effects of isoflavone supplements on bone metabolic markers and climacteric symptoms in Japanese women. *BioFactors* **2004**, *22*, 221–228. [CrossRef]

98. Sapbamrer, R.; Visavarungroj, N.; Suttajit, M. Effects of dietary traditional fermented soybean on reproductive hormones, lipids, and glucose among postmenopausal women in northern thailand. *Asia Pac. J. Clin. Nutr.* **2013**, *22*, 222–228. [CrossRef]
99. Hutchins, A.M.; Martini, M.C.; Olson, B.A.; Thomas, W.; Joanne, L.; Slavin, J.L. Flaxseed Consumption Influences Endogenous Hormone Concentrations in Postmenopausal Women. *Nutr. Cancer* **2009**, *5581*, 37–41. [CrossRef]
100. Sturgeon, S.R.; Heersink, J.L.; Volpe, S.L.; Bertone-Johnson, E.R.; Puleo, E.; Stanczyk, F.Z.; Sabelawski, S.; Wähälä, K.; Kurzer, M.S.; Bigelow, C. Effect of dietary flaxseed on serum levels of estrogens and androgens in postmenopausal women. *Nutr. Cancer* **2008**, *60*, 612–618. [CrossRef]
101. Törmälä, R.; Appt, S.; Clarkson, T.B.; Mueck, A.O.; Seeger, H.; Mikkola, T.S.; Ylikorkala, O. Impact of soy supplementation on sex steroids and vascular inflammation markers in postmenopausal women using tibolone: Role of equol production capability. *Climacteric* **2008**, *11*, 409–415. [CrossRef]
102. Low, Y.L.; Taylor, J.I.; Grace, P.B.; Dowsett, M.; Scollen, S.; Dunning, A.M.; Mulligan, A.A.; Welch, A.A.; Luben, R.N.; Khaw, K.T.; et al. Phytoestrogen exposure correlation with plasma estradiol in postmenopausal women in European Prospective Investigation of Cancer and Nutrition-Norfolk may involve diet-gene interactions. *Cancer Epidemiol. Biomark. Prev.* **2005**, *14*, 213–220.
103. Lambert, M.N.T.; Hu, L.M.; Jeppesen, P.B. A systematic review and meta-analysis of the effects of isoflavone formulations against estrogen-deficient bone resorption in peri- and postmenopausal women. *Am. J. Clin. Nutr.* **2017**, *106*, 801–811. [CrossRef]
104. Haggans, C.J.; Hutchins, A.M.; Olson, B.A.; Thomas, W.; Martini, M.C.; Slavin, J.L. Effect of flaxseed consumption on urinary estrogen metabolites in postmenopausal women. *Nutr. Cancer* **1999**, *33*, 188–195. [CrossRef]
105. Brooks, J.D.; Ward, W.E.; Lewis, J.E.; Hilditch, J.; Nickell, L.; Wong, E.; Thompson, L.U. Supplementation with flaxseed alters estrogen metabolism in postmenopausal women to a greater extent than does supplementation with an equal amount of soy 1-3. *Am. J. Clin. Nutr.* **2004**, *79*, 318–325. [CrossRef]
106. Sturgeon, S.R.; Volpe, S.L.; Puleo, E.; Bertone-Johnson, E.R.; Heersink, J.; Sabelawski, S.; Wahala, K.; Bigelow, C.; Kurzer, M.S. Effect of flaxseed consumption on urinary levels of estrogen metabolites in postmenopausal women. *Nutr. Cancer* **2010**, *62*, 175–180. [CrossRef]
107. Scambia, G.; Mango, D.; Signorile, P.G.; Angeli, R.A.; Palena, C.; Gallo, D.; Bombardelli, E.; Morazzoni, P.; Riva, A.; Mancuso, S. Clinical effects of a standardized soy extract in postmenopausal women: A pilot study. *Menopause* **2000**, *7*, 105–111. [CrossRef]
108. Sosvorová, L.; Mikšátková, P.; Bičíková, M.; Kaňová, N.; Lapčík, O. The presence of monoiodinated derivates of daidzein and genistein in human urine and its effect on thyroid gland function. *Food Chem. Toxicol.* **2012**, *50*, 2774–2779. [CrossRef]
109. Jayagopal, V.; Albertazzi, P.; Kilpatrick, E.S.; Howarth, E.M.; Jennings, P.E.; Hepburn, D.A.; Atkin, S.L. Beneficial effects of soy phytoestrogen intake in postmenopausal women with type 2 diabetes. *Diabetes Care* **2002**, *25*, 1709–1714. [CrossRef]
110. Crisafulli, A.; Altavilla, D.; Marini, H.; Bitto, A.; Cucinotta, D.; Frisina, N.; Corrado, F.; D'Anna, R.; Squadrito, G.; Adamo, E.B.; et al. Effects of the phytoestrogen genistein on cardiovascular risk factors in postmenopausal women. *Menopause* **2005**, *12*, 186–192. [CrossRef]
111. Basaria, S.; Wisniewski, A.; Dupree, K.; Bruno, T.; Song, M.; Yao, F.; Ojumu, A.; John, M.; Dobs, A.S. Effect of High-Dose Isoflavones on Cognition, Quality of life, Androgens, and Lipoprotein in Post-Menopausal Women. *J. Endocrinol. Investig.* **2009**, *32*, 150–155. [CrossRef]
112. Baber, R.J.; Templeman, C.; Morton, T.; Kelly, G.E.; West, L. Randomized placebo-controlled trial of an isoflavone supplement and menopausal symptoms in women. *Climacteric* **1999**, *2*, 85–92. [CrossRef]
113. Kapoor, R.; Ronnenberg, A.; Puleo, E.; Chatterton, R.T.; Dorgan, J.F.; Seeram, N.P.; Sturgeon, S.R. Effects of Pomegranate Juice on Hormonal Biomarkers of Breast Cancer Risk. *Nutr. Cancer* **2015**, *67*, 1113–1119. [CrossRef]
114. Monroe, K.R.; Murphy, S.P.; Henderson, B.E.; Kolonel, L.N.; Stanczyk, F.Z.; Adlercreutz, H.; Pike, M.C. Dietary fiber intake and endogenous serum hormone levels in naturally postmenopausal Mexican American women: The multiethnic cohort study. *Nutr. Cancer* **2007**, *58*, 127–135. [CrossRef]
115. Low, Y.L.; Dunning, A.M.; Dowsett, M.; Folkerd, E.; Doody, D.; Taylor, J.; Bhaniani, A.; Luben, R.; Khaw, K.T.; Wareham, N.J.; et al. Phytoestrogen exposure is associated with circulating sex hormone levels in postmenopausal women and interact with ESR1 and NR1I2 gene variants. *Cancer Epidemiol. Biomark. Prev.* **2007**, *16*, 1009–1016. [CrossRef]

116. Wu, A.H.; Stanczyk, F.Z.; Seow, A.; Lee, H.P.; Yu, M.C. Soy intake and other lifestyle determinants of serum estrogen levels among postmenopausal Chinese women in Singapore. *Cancer Epidemiol. Biomark. Prev.* **2002**, *11*, 844–851.
117. Messina, M.; Redmond, G. Effects of soy protein and soybean isoflavones on thyroid function in healthy adults and hypothyroid patients: A review of the relevant literature. *Thyroid* **2006**, *16*, 249–258. [CrossRef]
118. Sathyapalan, T.; Manuchehri, A.M.; Thatcher, N.J.; Rigby, A.S.; Chapman, T.; Kilpatrick, E.S.; Atkin, S.L. The effect of soy phytoestrogen supplementation on thyroid status and cardiovascular risk markers in patients with subclinical hypothyroidism: A randomized, double-blind, crossover study. *J. Clin. Endocrinol. Metab.* **2011**, *96*, 1442–1449. [CrossRef]
119. Li, J.; Teng, X.; Wang, W.; Chen, Y.; Yu, X.; Wang, S.; Li, J.; Zhu, L.; Li, C.; Fan, C.; et al. Effects of dietary soy intake on maternal thyroid functions and serum anti-thyroperoxidase antibody level during early pregnancy. *J. Med. Food* **2011**, *14*, 543–550. [CrossRef]
120. Milerová, J.; Čeřovská, J.; Zamrazil, V.; Bílek, R.; Lapčík, O.; Hampl, R. Actual levels of soy phytoestrogens in children correlate with thyroid laboratory parameters. *Clin. Chem. Lab. Med.* **2006**, *44*, 171–174. [CrossRef]
121. Conrad, S.C.; Chiu, H.; Silverman, B.L. Soy formula complicates management of congenital hypothyroidism. *Arch. Dis. Child.* **2004**, *89*, 37–40. [CrossRef]
122. Zung, A.; Shachar, S.; Zadik, Z.; Kerem, Z. Soy-derived isoflavones treatment in children with hypercholesterolemia: A pilot study. *J. Pediatr. Endocrinol. Metab.* **2010**, *23*, 133–141. [CrossRef]
123. Hampl, R.; Ostatnikova, D.; Celec, P.; Putz, Z. Lapčík, O.; Matucha, P. Short-term Effect of Soy Consumption on Thyroid Hormone Levels and Correlation with Phytoestrogen Level in Healthy Subjects. *Endocr. Regul.* **2008**, *42*, 53–61.
124. Sathyapalan, T.; Rigby, A.S.; Bhasin, S.; Thatcher, N.J.; Kilpatrick, E.S.; Atkin, S.L. Effect of soy in men with type 2 diabetes mellitus and subclinical hypogonadism: A randomized controlled study. *J. Clin. Endocrinol. Metab.* **2017**, *102*, 425–433. [CrossRef]
125. Zhou, Y.; Alekel, D.L.; Dixon, P.M.; Messina, M.; Reddy, M.B. The effect of soy food intake on mineral status in premenopausal women. *J. Women's Health* **2011**, *20*, 771–780. [CrossRef]
126. Duncan, A.M.; Merz, B.E.; Xu, X.; Nagel, T.C.; Phipps, W.R.; Kurzer, M.S. Soy Isoflavones Exert Modest Hormonal Effects in Premenopausal Women. *J. Clin. Endocrinol. Metab.* **1999**, *84*, 192–197. [CrossRef]
127. Mittal, N.; Hota, D.; Dutta, P.; Bhansali, A.; Suri, V.; Aggarwal, N.; Marwah, R.K.; Chakrabarti, A. Evaluation of effect of isoflavone on thyroid economy & autoimmunity in oophorectomised women: A randomised, double-blind, placebo-controlled trial. *Indian J. Med. Res.* **2011**, *133*, 633–640.
128. Khaodhiar, L.; Ricciotti, H.A.; Li, L.; Pan, W.; Schickel, M.; Zhou, J.; Blackburn, G.L. Daidzein-rich isoflavone aglycones are potentially effective in reducing hot flashes in menopausal women. *Menopause* **2008**, *15*, 125–132. [CrossRef]
129. Ryan-Borchers, T.; Chew, B.; Park, J.S.; McGuire, M.; Fournier, L.; Beerman, K. Effects of Dietary and Supplemental Forms of Isoflavones on Thyroid Function in Healthy Postmenopausal Women. *Top. Clin. Nutr.* **2007**, *23*, 13–22. [CrossRef]
130. Pop, E.A.; Fischer, L.M.; Coan, A.D.; Gitzinger, M.; Nakamura, J.; Zeisel, S.H. Effects of a high daily dose of soy isoflavones on DNA damage, apoptosis, and estrogenic outcomes in healthy postmenopausal women: A phase I clinical trial. *Menopause* **2008**, *15*, 684–692. [CrossRef]
131. Bitto, A.; Polito, F.; Atteritano, M.; Altavilla, D.; Mazzaferro, S.; Marini, H.; Adamo, E.B.; D'Anna, R.; Granese, R.; Corrado, F.; et al. Genistein aglycone does not affect thyroid function: Results from a three-year, randomized, double-blind, placebo-controlled trial. *J. Clin. Endocrinol. Metab.* **2010**, *95*, 3067–3072. [CrossRef]
132. Alekel, D.L.; Genschel, U.; Koehler, K.J.; Hofmann, H.; Van Loan, M.D.; Beer, B.S.; Hanson, L.N.; Peterson, C.T.; Kurzer, M.S. Soy Isoflavones for Reducing Bone Loss Study: Effects of a 3-year trial on hormones, adverse events, and endometrial thickness in postmenopausal women. *Menopause* **2015**, *22*, 185–197. [CrossRef]
133. Steinberg, F.M.; Murray, M.J.; Lewis, R.D.; Cramer, M.A.; Amato, P.; Young, R.L.; Barnes, S.; Konzelmann, K.L.; Fischer, J.G.; Ellis, K.J.; et al. Clinical outcomes of a 2-y soy isoflavone supplementation in menopausal women. *Am. J. Clin. Nutr.* **2011**, *93*, 356–367. [CrossRef]
134. Liu, Y.; Vu, V.; Sweeney, G. Examining the Potential of Developing and Implementing Use of Adiponectin-Targeted Therapeutics for Metabolic and Cardiovascular Diseases. *Front. Endocrinol. Lausanne* **2019**, *10*, 842. [CrossRef]

135. Ouchi, N.; Parker, J.L.; Lugus, J.J.; Walsh, K. Adipokines in inflammation and metabolic disease. *Nat. Rev. Immunol.* **2011**, *11*, 85–97. [CrossRef]
136. Kwon, H.; Pessin, J.E. Adipokines mediate inflammation and insulin resistance. *Front. Endocrinol. Lausanne* **2013**, *4*, 71. [CrossRef]
137. Su, X.; Peng, D. Adipokines as novel biomarkers of cardio-metabolic disorders. *Clin. Chim. Acta* **2020**, *507*, 31–38. [CrossRef]
138. Müller, T.D.; Finan, B.; Bloom, S.R.; D'Alessio, D.; Drucker, D.J.; Flatt, P.R.; Fritsche, A.; Gribble, F.; Grill, H.J.; Habener, J.F.; et al. Glucagon-like peptide 1 (GLP-1). *Mol. Metab.* **2019**, *30*, 72–130. [CrossRef]
139. Kojta, I.; Chacińska, M.; Błachnio-Zabielska, A. Obesity, Bioactive Lipids, and Adipose Tissue Inflammation in Insulin Resistance. *Nutrients* **2020**, *12*, 1305. [CrossRef]
140. Tokudome, T.; Otani, K.; Miyazato, M.; Kangawa, K. Ghrelin and the heart. *Peptides* **2019**, *111*, 42–46. [CrossRef]
141. Shi, L.; Ryan, H.H.; Jones, E.; Moore Simas, T.A.; Lichtenstein, A.H.; Sun, Q.; Hayman, L.L. Urinary Isoflavone Concentrations Are Inversely Associated with Cardiometabolic Risk Markers in Pregnant U.S. Women. *J. Nutr.* **2014**, *144*, 344–351. [CrossRef]
142. Van der Schouw, Y.T.; Sampson, L.; Willett, W.C.; Rimm, E.B. The Usual Intake of Lignans but Not That of Isoflavones May Be Related to Cardiovascular Risk Factors in U.S. Men. *J. Nutr.* **2005**, *135*, 260–266. [CrossRef]
143. Rohrmann, S.; Shvetsov, Y.B.; Morimoto, Y.; Wilkens, L.R.; Monroe, K.R.; Le Marchand, L.; Franke, A.A.; Kolonel, L.N.; Maskarinec, G. Self-reported dietary flavonoid intake and serum markers of inflammation: The multiethnic cohort. *Cancer Causes Control* **2018**, *29*, 601–607. [CrossRef]
144. Ferguson, J.F.; Ryan, M.F.; Gibney, E.R.; Brennan, L.; Roche, H.M.; Reilly, M.P. Dietary isoflavone intake is associated with evoked responses to inflammatory cardiometabolic stimuli and improved glucose homeostasis in healthy volunteers. *Nutr. Metab. Cardiovasc. Dis.* **2014**, *24*, 996–1003. [CrossRef]
145. Reverri, E.J.; Lasalle, C.D.; Franke, A.A.; Steinberg, F.M. Soy provides modest benefits on endothelial function without affecting inflammatory biomarkers in adults at cardiometabolic risk. *Mol. Nutr. Food Res.* **2015**, *59*, 323–333. [CrossRef]
146. Qin, Y.; Shu, F.; Zeng, Y.; Meng, X.; Wang, B.; Diao, L.; Wang, L.; Wan, J.; Zhu, J.; Wang, J.; et al. Daidzein Supplementation Decreases Serum Triglyceride and Uric Acid Concentrations in Hypercholesterolemic Adults with the Effect on Triglycerides Being Greater in Those with the GA Compared with the GG Genotype of ESR-β RsaI. *J. Nutr.* **2014**, *144*, 49–54. [CrossRef]
147. Usui, T.; Tochiya, M.; Sasaki, Y.; Muranaka, K.; Yamakage, H.; Himeno, A.; Shimatsu, A.; Inaguma, A.; Ueno, T.; Uchiyama, S.; et al. Effects of natural S-equol supplements on overweight or obesity and metabolic syndrome in the Japanese, based on sex and equol status. *Clin. Endocrinol. Oxf.* **2013**, *78*, 365–372. [CrossRef]
148. Amanat, S.; Eftekhari, M.H.; Fararouei, M.; Bagheri Lankarani, K.; Massoumi, S.J. Genistein supplementation improves insulin resistance and inflammatory state in non-alcoholic fatty liver patients: A randomized, controlled trial. *Clin. Nutr.* **2018**, *37*, 1210–1215. [CrossRef]
149. Vrieling, A.; Rookus, M.A.; Kampman, E.; Bonfrer, J.M.G.; Korse, C.M.; Van Doorn, J.; Lampe, J.W.; Cats, A.; Witteman, B.J.M.; van Leeuwen, F.E.; et al. Isolated Isoflavones Do Not Affect the Circulating Insulin-Like Growth Factor System in Men at Increased Colorectal Cancer Risk. *J. Nutr.* **2007**, *137*, 379–383. [CrossRef]
150. Maskarinec, G.; Oum, R.; Chaptman, A.K.; Ognjanovic, S. Inflammatory markers in a randomised soya intervention among men. *Br. J. Nutr.* **2009**, *101*, 1740–1744. [CrossRef]
151. Kreijkamp-Kaspers, S.; Kok, L.; Bots, M.L.; Grobbee, D.E.; Van Der Schouw, Y.T. Dietary phytoestrogens and vascular function in postmenopausal women: A cross-sectional study. *J. Hypertens.* **2004**, *22*, 1381–1388. [CrossRef]
152. Morisset, A.S.; Lemieux, S.; Veilleux, A.; Bergeron, J.; John Weisnagel, S.; Tchernof, A. Impact of a lignan-rich diet on adiposity and insulin sensitivity in post-menopausal women. *Br. J. Nutr.* **2009**, *102*, 195–200. [CrossRef]
153. Atteritano, M.; Marini, H.; Minutoli, L.; Polito, F.; Bitto, A.; Altavilla, D.; Mazzaferro, S.; D'Anna, R.; Cannata, M.L.; Gaudio, A.; et al. Effects of the phytoestrogen genistein on some predictors of cardiovascular risk in osteopenic, postmenopausal women: A two-year randomized, double-blind, placebo-controlled study. *J. Clin. Endocrinol. Metab.* **2007**, *92*, 3068–3075. [CrossRef]

154. Marini, H.; Bitto, A.; Altavilla, D.; Burnett, B.P.; Polito, F.; Di Stefano, V.; Minutoli, L.; Atteritano, M.; Levy, R.M.; Frisina, N.; et al. Efficacy of genistein aglycone on some cardiovascular risk factors and homocysteine levels: A follow-up study. *Nutr. Metab. Cardiovasc. Dis.* **2010**, *20*, 332–340. [CrossRef]
155. Irace, C.; Marini, H.; Bitto, A.; Altavilla, D.; Polito, F.; Adamo, E.B.; Arcoraci, V.; Minutoli, L.; Di Benedetto, A.; Di Vieste, G.; et al. Genistein and endothelial function in postmenopausal women with metabolic syndrome. *Eur. J. Clin. Investig.* **2013**, *43*, 1025–1031. [CrossRef]
156. Squadrito, F.; Marini, H.; Bitto, A.; Altavilla, D.; Polito, F.; Adamo, E.B.; D'Anna, R.; Arcoraci, V.; Burnett, B.P.; Minutoli, L.; et al. Genistein in the metabolic syndrome: Results of a randomized clinical trial. *J. Clin. Endocrinol. Metab.* **2013**, *98*, 3366–3374. [CrossRef]
157. Braxas, H.; Rafraf, M.; Karimi Hasanabad, S.; Asghari Jafarabadi, M. Effectiveness of Genistein Supplementation on Metabolic Factors and Antioxidant Status in Postmenopausal Women with Type 2 Diabetes Mellitus. *Can. J. Diabetes* **2019**, *43*, 490–497. [CrossRef]
158. Hall, W.L.; Vafeiadou, K.; Hallund, J.; Bugel, S.; Reimann, M.; Koebnick, C.; Zunft, H.J.F.; Ferrari, M.; Branca, F.; Dadd, T.; et al. Soy-isoflavone-enriched foods and markers of lipid and glucose metabolism in postmenopausal women: Interactions with genotype and equol production. *Am. J. Clin. Nutr.* **2006**, *83*, 592–600. [CrossRef]
159. Nadadur, M.; Stanczyk, F.Z.; Tseng, C.C.; Kim, L.; Wu, A.H. The Effect of Reduced Dietary Fat and Soy Supplementation on Circulating Adipocytokines in Postmenopausal Women: A Randomized Controlled 2-Month Trial. *Nutr. Cancer* **2016**, *68*, 554–559. [CrossRef]
160. Matvienko, O.A.; Alekel, D.L.; Genschel, U.; Ritland, L.; Van Loan, M.D.; Koehler, K.J. Appetitive hormones, but not isoflavone tablets, influence overall and central adiposity in healthy postmenopausal women. *Menopause* **2010**, *17*, 594–601. [CrossRef]
161. Llaneza, P.; González, C.; Fernandez-Iñarrea, J.; Alonso, A.; Diaz, F.; Arrott, I.; Ferrer-Barriendos, J. Soy isoflavones, diet and physical exercise modify serum cytokines in healthy obese postmenopausal women. *Phytomedicine* **2011**, *18*, 245–250. [CrossRef]
162. Sathyapalan, T.; Aye, M.; Rigby, A.S.; Thatcher, N.J.; Dargham, S.R.; Kilpatrick, E.S.; Atkin, S.L. Soy isoflavones improve cardiovascular disease risk markers in women during the early menopause. *Nutr. Metab. Cardiovasc. Dis.* **2018**, *28*, 691–697. [CrossRef]
163. Cheng, S.Y.; Shaw, N.S.; Tsai, K.S.; Chen, C.Y. The hypoglycemic effects of soy isoflavones on postmenopausal women. *J. Women's Health* **2004**, *13*, 1080–1086. [CrossRef]
164. Charles, C.; Yuskavage, J.; Carlson, O.; John, M.; Tagalicud, A.S.; Maggio, M.; Muller, D.C.; Egan, J.; Basaria, S. Effects of high-dose isoflavones on metabolic and inflammatory markers in healthy postmenopausal women. *Menopause* **2009**, *16*, 395–400. [CrossRef]
165. Christie, D.R.; Grant, J.; Darnell, B.E.; Chapman, V.R.; Gastaldelli, A.; Sites, C.K. Metabolic effects of soy supplementation in postmenopausal Caucasian and African American women: A randomized, placebo-controlled trial. *Am. J. Obstet. Gynecol.* **2010**, *203*, 153.e1–153.e9. [CrossRef]
166. Almeida, M.; Laurent, M.R.; Dubois, V.; Claessens, F.; O'Brien, C.A.; Bouillon, R.; Vanderschueren, D.; Manolagas, S.C. Estrogens and androgens in skeletal physiology and pathophysiology. *Physiol. Rev.* **2017**, *97*, 135–187. [CrossRef]
167. Chiang, S.S.; Pan, T.M. Beneficial effects of phytoestrogens and their metabolites produced by intestinal microflora on bone health. *Appl. Microbiol. Biotechnol.* **2013**, *97*, 1489–1500. [CrossRef]
168. Seibel, M.J. Biochemical markers of bone remodeling. *Endocrinol. Metab. Clin. N. Am.* **2003**, *32*, 83–113. [CrossRef]
169. Goltzman, D. Physiology of Parathyroid Hormone. *Endocrinol. Metab. Clin. N. Am.* **2018**, *47*, 743–758. [CrossRef]
170. Wangen, K.E.; Duncan, A.M.; Merz-Demlow, B.E.; Xu, X.; Marcus, R.; Phipps, W.R.; Kurzer, M.S. Effects of soy isoflavones on markers of bone turnover in premenopausal and postmenopausal women. *J. Clin. Endocrinol. Metab.* **2000**, *85*, 3043–3048. [CrossRef]
171. Zittermann, A.; Geppert, J.; Baier, S.; Zehn, N.; Gouni-Berthold, I.; Berthold, H.K.; Reinsberg, J.; Stehle, P. Short-term effects of high soy supplementation on sex hormones, bone markers, and lipid parameters in young female adults. *Eur. J. Nutr.* **2004**, *43*, 100–108. [CrossRef] [PubMed]
172. Drake, M.T.; Clarke, B.L.; Lewiecki, E.M. The Pathophysiology and Treatment of Osteoporosis. *Clin. Ther.* **2015**, *37*, 1837–1850. [CrossRef] [PubMed]

173. Chiechi, L.M.; Secreto, G.; D'Amore, M.; Fanelli, M.; Venturelli, E.; Cantatore, F.; Valerio, T.; Laselva, G.; Loizzi, P. Efficacy of a soy rich diet in preventing postmenopausal osteoporosis: The Menfis randomized trial. *Maturitas* **2002**, *42*, 295–300. [CrossRef]
174. Scheiber, M.D.; Liu, J.H.; Subbiah, M.T.R.; Rebar, R.W.; Setchell, K.D.R. Dietary Inclusion of Whole Soy Foods Results in Significant Reductions in Clinical Risk Factors for Osteoporosis and Cardiovascular Disease in Normal Postmenopausal Women. *Menopause* **2001**, *8*, 384–392. [CrossRef]
175. Ye, Y.B.; Tang, X.Y.; Verbruggen, M.A.; Su, Y.X. Soy isoflavones attenuate bone loss in early postmenopausal Chinese women: A single-blind randomized, placebo-controlled trial. *Eur. J. Nutr.* **2006**, *45*, 327–334. [CrossRef]
176. Roudsari, A.H.; Tahbaz, F.; Hossein-Nezhad, A.; Arjmandi, B.; Larijani, B.; Kimiagar, S.M. Assessment of soy phytoestrogens' effects on bone turnover indicators in menopausal women with osteopenia in Iran: A before and after clinical trial. *Nutr. J.* **2005**, *4*, 3–7. [CrossRef]
177. Lambert, M.N.T.; Thybo, C.B.; Lykkeboe, S.; Rasmussen, L.M.; Frette, X.; Christensen, L.P.; Jeppesen, P.B. Combined bioavailable isoflavones and probiotics improve bone status and estrogen metabolism in postmenopausal osteopenic women: A randomized controlled trial. *Am. J. Clin. Nutr.* **2017**, *106*, 909–920. [CrossRef]
178. Uesugi, T.; Fukui, Y.; Yamori, Y. Beneficial Effects of Soybean Isoflavone Supplementation on Bone Metabolism and Serum Lipids in Postmenopausal Japanese Women: A Four-Week Study. *J. Am. Coll. Nutr.* **2002**, *21*, 97–102. [CrossRef]
179. Gambacciani, M.; Ciaponi, M.; Cappagli, B.; Piaggesi, L.; Genazzani, A.R. Effects of combined low dose of the isoflavone derivative ipriflavone and estrogen replacement on bone mineral density and metabolism in postmenopausal women. *Maturitas* **1997**, *28*, 75–81. [CrossRef]
180. Weaver, C.M.; Martin, B.R.; Jackson, G.S.; McCabe, G.P.; Nolan, J.R.; McCabe, L.D.; Barnes, S.; Reinwald, S.; Boris, M.E.; Peacock, M. Antiresorptive effects of phytoestrogen supplements compared with estradiol or risedronate in postmenopausal women using 41Ca methodology. *J. Clin. Endocrinol. Metab.* **2009**, *94*, 3798–3805. [CrossRef]
181. Pérez-Alonso, M.; Briongos, L.S.; Ruiz-Mambrilla, M.; Velasco, E.A.; Linares, L.; Cuellar, L.; Olmos, J.M.; De Luis, D.; Dueñas-Laita, A.; Pérez-Castrillón, J.L. The Effect of Genistein Supplementation on Vitamin D Levels and Bone Turnover Markers during the Summer in Healthy Postmenopausal Women: Role of Genotypes of Isoflavone Metabolism. *Lifestyle Genom.* **2017**, *10*, 139–145. [CrossRef] [PubMed]
182. Vupadhyayula, P.M.; Gallagher, J.C.; Templin, T.; Logsdon, S.M.; Smith, L.M. Effects of soy protein isolate on bone mineral density and physical performance indices in postmenopausal women—A 2-year randomized, double-blind, placebo-controlled trial. *Menopause* **2009**, *16*, 320–328. [CrossRef] [PubMed]
183. Marini, H.; Minutoli, L.; Polito, F.; Bitto, A.; Altavilla, D.; Atteritano, M.; Gaudio, A.; Mazzaferro, S.; Frisina, A.; Frisina, N.; et al. Effects of the phytoestrogen genistein on bone metabolism in osteopenic postmenopausal women: A randomized trial. *Ann. Intern. Med.* **2007**, *146*, 839–847. [CrossRef] [PubMed]
184. Mei, J.; Yeung, S.S.C.; Kung, A.W.C. High dietary phytoestrogen intake is associated with higher bone mineral density in postmenopausal but not premenopausal women. *J. Clin. Endocrinol. Metab.* **2001**, *86*, 5217–5221. [CrossRef]
185. Bahamonde, M.; Misra, M. Potential applications for rhIGF-I: Bone disease and IGFI. *Growth Horm. IGF Res.* **2020**, *52*, 101317. [CrossRef]
186. Gallagher, E.J.; LeRoith, D. Minireview: IGF, insulin, and cancer. *Endocrinology* **2011**, *152*, 2546–2551. [CrossRef]
187. Scarth, J.P. Modulation of the growth hormone-insulin-like growth factor (GH-IGF) axis by pharmaceutical, nutraceutical and environmental xenobiotics: An emerging role for xenobiotic-metabolizing enzymes and the transcription factors regulating their expression. A rev. *Xenobiotica* **2006**, *36*, 119–218. [CrossRef]
188. Campbell, M.J.; Woodside, J.V.; Honour, J.W.; Morton, M.S.; Leathem, A.J.C. Effect of red clover-derived isoflavone supplementation on insulin-like growth factor, lipid and antioxidant status in healthy female volunteers: A pilot study. *Eur. J. Clin. Nutr.* **2004**, *58*, 173–179. [CrossRef]
189. Nagata, C.; Shimizu, H.; Takami, R.; Hayashi, M.; Takeda, N.; Yasuda, K. Dietary soy and fats in relation to serum insulin-like growth factor-1 and insulin-like growth factor-binding protein-3 levels in premenopausal Japanese women. *Nutr. Cancer* **2003**, *45*, 185–189. [CrossRef]

190. Takata, Y.; Maskarinec, G.; Rinaldi, S.; Kaaks, R.; Nagata, C. Serum insulin-like growth factor-I levels among women in Hawaii and Japan with different levels of tofu intake. *Nutr. Cancer* **2006**, *56*, 136–142. [CrossRef]
191. Vrieling, A.; Rookus, M.A.; Kampman, E.; Bonfrer, J.M.G.; Bosma, A.; Cats, A.; Van Doorn, J.; Korse, C.M.; Witteman, B.J.M.; Van Leeuwen, F.E.; et al. No effect of red clover-derived isoflavone intervention on the insulin-like growth factor system in women at increased risk of colorectal cancer. *Cancer Epidemiol. Biomark. Prev.* **2008**, *17*, 2585–2593. [CrossRef] [PubMed]
192. Arjmandi, B.H.; Khalil, D.A.; Smith, B.J.; Lucas, E.A.; Juma, S.; Payton, M.E.; Wild, R.A. Soy protein has a greater effect on bone in postmenopausal women not on hormone replacement therapy, as evidenced by reducing bone resorption and urinary calcium excretion. *J. Clin. Endocrinol. Metab.* **2003**, *88*, 1048–1054. [CrossRef] [PubMed]
193. Probst-Hensch, N.M.; Wang, H.; Goh, V.H.H.; Seow, A.; Lee, H.P.; Yu, M.C. Determinants of circulating insulin-like growth factor I and insulin-like growth factor binding protein 3 concentrations in a cohort of Singapore men and women. *Cancer Epidemiol. Biomark. Prev.* **2003**, *12*, 739–746. [CrossRef]
194. Rowlands, M.A.; Gunnell, D.; Harris, R.; Vatten, L.J.; Holly, J.M.P.; Martin, R.M. Circulating insulin-like growth factor peptides and prostate cancer risk: A systematic review and meta-analysis. *Int. J. Cancer* **2009**, *124*, 2416–2429. [CrossRef] [PubMed]

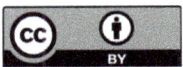

© 2020 by the authors. Licensee MDPI, Basel, Switzerland. This article is an open access article distributed under the terms and conditions of the Creative Commons Attribution (CC BY) license (http://creativecommons.org/licenses/by/4.0/).

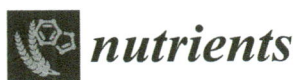

Review

Metabolic Impact of Flavonoids Consumption in Obesity: From Central to Peripheral

Viviana Sandoval [1,†], Hèctor Sanz-Lamora [1,2,†], Giselle Arias [1], Pedro F. Marrero [1,3,4], Diego Haro [1,3,4,*] and Joana Relat [1,2,4,*]

1. Department of Nutrition, Food Sciences and Gastronomy, School of Pharmacy and Food Sciences, Food Torribera Campus, University of Barcelona, E-08921 Santa Coloma de Gramenet, Spain; vivianapazsandovals@gmail.com (V.S.); h.sanz.lamora@gmail.com (H.S.-L.); giselle.arias@upr.edu (G.A.); pedromarrero@ub.edu (P.F.M.)
2. Institute of Nutrition and Food Safety of the University of Barcelona (INSA-UB), E-08921 Santa Coloma de Gramenet, Spain
3. Institute of Biomedicine of the University of Barcelona (IBUB), E-08028 Barcelona, Spain
4. CIBER Physiopathology of Obesity and Nutrition (CIBER-OBN), Instituto de Salud Carlos III, E-28029 Madrid, Spain
* Correspondence: dharo@ub.edu (D.H.); jrela@ub.edu (J.R.); Tel.: +93-0403-3690 (D.H.); +34-9340-20862 (J.R.)
† Both authors contributed equally to this work.

Received: 21 July 2020; Accepted: 5 August 2020; Published: 10 August 2020

Abstract: The prevention and treatment of obesity is primary based on the follow-up of a healthy lifestyle, which includes a healthy diet with an important presence of bioactive compounds such as polyphenols. For many years, the health benefits of polyphenols have been attributed to their anti-oxidant capacity as free radical scavengers. More recently it has been described that polyphenols activate other cell-signaling pathways that are not related to ROS production but rather involved in metabolic regulation. In this review, we have summarized the current knowledge in this field by focusing on the metabolic effects of flavonoids. Flavonoids are widely distributed in the plant kingdom where they are used for growing and defensing. They are structurally characterized by two benzene rings and a heterocyclic pyrone ring and based on the oxidation and saturation status of the heterocyclic ring flavonoids are grouped in seven different subclasses. The present work is focused on describing the molecular mechanisms underlying the metabolic impact of flavonoids in obesity and obesity-related diseases. We described the effects of each group of flavonoids in liver, white and brown adipose tissue and central nervous system and the metabolic and signaling pathways involved on them.

Keywords: non-alcoholic fatty liver disease; obesity; flavonoids; lipid metabolism; metabolic regulation; adipose tissue; brain

1. Introduction

Overnutrition and unhealthy diets together with physical inactivity cause an impairment in the metabolic homeostasis that lead to the development of pathologies such as obesity, type 2 diabetes, cardiovascular diseases (CVD) and more recently this kind of lifestyle has also been linked to neuroinflammation and neurodegenerative diseases [1–5].

The metabolic syndrome (MetS) is the medical term used to define the concomitance in an individual of some of the following alterations: hyperglycemia and/or insulin resistance, arterial hypertension, dyslipidemia and central or abdominal obesity [6]. It is currently one of the main public health problems worldwide and its incidence increases significantly each year, affecting almost 25% of the adult population today and has been directly associated to a greater risk of suffering from CVD or type 2 diabetes among others [3].

Obesity is one of the most important trigger for many of the other alterations include in the MetS. Obesity is essentially caused by an imbalance between energy intake and energy expenditure that initially causes an expansion of the white adipose tissue (WAT) to store the overfeed as triglycerides (TG). Some evidences indicate that at some point, WAT fails to adequately keep the surplus of nutrients and together with an insufficient differentiation of new adipocytes lead to an off-WAT accumulation of lipids in peripheral relevant organs. This ectopic accumulation of lipids causes lipotoxicity that may be, at least in part, responsible of the metabolic obesity-related metabolic dysfunctions [7]. It seems obvious that defects in WAT functionality together with peripheral lipotoxicity are the key points in the onset of metabolic syndrome (MetS) [8]. Looking for a way to restore lipid homeostasis and reduce lipotoxicity but also to diminish adipose tissue inflammation and macrophage infiltration many research groups are focused on identifying specific dietary patterns or foods capable to counteract these effects to finally revert obesity and its comorbidities.

Furthermore, it has been described that long-term hyperglycemia and diabetes complications induce impairments in the hippocampal synaptic plasticity as well as cognitive deficits [9] and increase the risk for Alzheimer disease [10,11] and depressive illness [12]. On the other side, diet-induced hypothalamic inflammation and mitochondrial dysfunction result in the onset and development of obesity and related metabolic diseases. It has been shown that, in rats, high fat diet (HFD) induces metabolic inflammation in the central nervous system (CNS), particularity in the hypothalamus [13].

The prevention of MetS and obesity is primary based on the follow-up of a healthy lifestyle, which includes, among other recommendations, a healthy diet. In this context, the Mediterranean Diet (DietMEd) has shown beneficial effects on the prevention and treatment of MetS and obesity by reducing chronic low-grade inflammation, improving endothelial function and reducing cardiovascular risk [14–16]. The study of Prevention with Mediterranean Diet (Predimed) has shown that high adherence to this nutritional profile is effective in the primary and secondary prevention of CVD, diabetes and obesity [17–24]. DietMed is characterized by a high consumption of foods rich in bioactive compounds such as polyphenols to whose have been attributed a large part of the health effects of this diet [18,23,25–28].

In this review, we have summarized the current knowledge on the metabolic effects of a specific group of polyphenols, the flavonoids, and the molecular mechanisms underlying these effects.

Concretely, the main goal of the present work is to describe the molecular mechanisms underlying the anti-obesity effects of flavonoids in three target organs/tissues: liver, adipose tissues (WAT and brown adipose tissue (BAT)) and central nervous system (CNS).

We choose a high variety of obesity models, sources and doses of flavonoids to identify the metabolic and signaling pathways involved in the effects of each subclass of flavonoids (anthocyanins, flavanols, flavanones, flavonols, isoflavones, flavones and chalcones) in these tissues/organs. Only studies in humans and experimental approaches whit animal models from the last years have been included, thus avoiding cell culture experimental approaches except when relevant.

2. Polyphenols and Metabolism

Polyphenols are the most abundant phytochemicals in nature. They are widely distributed in fruits, vegetables, and highly present in foods like legumes, cocoa, some cereals as well as in some beverages, such as tea, coffee and wine [29]. Polyphenols are not essential nutrients for humans but research in nutrition, including epidemiological studies, randomized controlled trials, in vivo and in vitro assays with animal models and cell lines, has shown that long-term and acute intakes can have beneficial effects on weight management and chronic diseases such as CVD, obesity, type 2 diabetes, the onset and development of some cancers and cognitive function [13,30–37].

The effects of polyphenols are directly related to their bioavailability. It is assumed that just the 5%-10% of the total dietary polyphenol intake is absorbed directly through the stomach and/or small intestine, the rest reaches the colon where they are transformed by the microbiota [38–40]. After being absorbed, polyphenols undergo phase I and II metabolism (sulfation, glucuronidation, methylation, and glycine conjugation) in the liver [29]. Polyphenol metabolites derived from liver metabolism may interact, among others, with adipose tissue, pancreas, muscle, and liver, where they exert their bioactivity.

Polyphenols have been divided in two main families: flavonoids and non-flavonoids, that are subdivided into several subclasses. For many years, the health benefits of polyphenols have been attributed to their anti-oxidant capacity as free radical scavengers. More recently it has been described that polyphenols activate other cell-signaling pathways that are not related to ROS production but rather involved in metabolic regulation [23,41].

Flavonoids

Flavonoids are widely distributed in the plant kingdom when are used for vegetables for growing and defensing. They are structurally characterized by two benzene rings and a heterocyclic pyrone ring and based on the oxidation and saturation status of the heterocyclic ring flavonoids are grouped in seven different subfamilies (Table 1).

Table 1. Flavonoids subclasses: compounds, representative food sources and chemical structures.

Compounds	Representative Food Source	Subclass	Chemical Structure
Cyanidin Delphinidin Malvidin Peonidin		Anthocyanins	
(+)-Catechin (−)-Epicatechin (−)-Epigallocatechin (−)-Epigallocatechin gallate Procyanidin dimer B2		Flavanols	
Hesperetin Hesperidin Naringenin Naringin Eriodyctiol		Flavanones	
Kaempferol Myricetin Quercetin Isoquercetin		Flavonols	
Daidzein Genistein		Isoflavones	

Table 1. *Cont.*

Compounds	Representative Food Source	Subclass	Chemical Structure
pigenin Chrysin Luteolin Baicalin Vitexin Nobiletin		Flavones	
Butein Licochalcone Isoliquiritigenin Xanthohumol		Chalcones	

Flavonoids are abundant in food and beverages highly consumed by human population including fruits, vegetables, tea, cocoa or wine [42] and in global are the bioactive compounds more largely associated with a reduced risk of all-cause mortality, type 2 diabetes [43–46], CVD [36,47], obesity and its comorbidities such as non-alcoholic fatty liver disease (NAFLD) [48–50] and more recently they have been described as potential therapeutic agents against cognitive pathologies such as Alzheimer's disease (AD) [42,51,52] or cerebrovascular alterations [47].

The molecular mechanisms underlying the beneficial effects of flavonoids have been widely studied and, in many cases, involved the activation of the AMP-activated protein kinase (AMPK). AMPK is a key enzyme for the control of lipid metabolism and adipogenesis. AMPK phosphorylation and activation promote catabolic processes such as FAO, glucose uptake, or glycolysis as well as inhibits anabolic pathways such as fatty acid synthesis or gluconeogenesis [53].

3. Anthocyanins

Anthocyanins are natural pigments and are responsible for the red-blue color of several flowers, fruits (mainly berries and grapes), roots, seeds (beans) but also of some leaves and cereal grains where they are found in low concentrations. Cyanidin, delphinidin, malvidin and their derivates are the most commonly studied anthocyanins [29,42,54–56].

Anthocyanins have shown antioxidant and anti-inflammatory properties but also positive effects in obesity and its comorbidities [57–60]. Several studies have demonstrated that the intake of anthocyanins by itself or of anthocyanins-rich foods such as berries is able to prevent CVD [61], to reduce body fat accumulation, to improve glucose tolerance/insulin sensitivity, to diminish the levels of fasting glucose, to control body weight in humans and rodents [57,59,62–72] and to increase energy expenditure and fatty acid oxidation (FAO) in mice and humans [59,73–76]. Globally, anthocyanins and anthocyanins-rich foods are able to improve metabolic homeostasis. More recently, anthocyanins have also revealed promising effects on cognitive function [51,77–79].

Part of the anthocyanins metabolic effects occur by regulating adipogenesis, increasing FAO, lipolysis, thermogenesis and mitochondrial biogenesis, regulating satiety and reducing lipogenesis in different tissues and organs and enhancing energy expenditure and body weight progression [74–76,80–83]. Dietary supplementation with anthocyanins improves the lipid profile by favorably controlling the circulating levels of TG, total cholesterol, LDL-cholesterol and HDL-cholesterol [84].

3.1. Anthocyanins Improve the Metabolic Hemostasis in Obesity: The Liver Response

Non-alcoholic fatty liver disease (NAFLD) is characterized by an excessive accumulation of lipids in the livers. Its onset is closely related to obesity where an imbalance between fatty acids input and output causes initially a hepatic steatosis that can progress to NAFLD, non-alcoholic steatohepatitis

(NASH), fibrosis, cirrhosis and in some cases hepatocarcinoma. Anthocyanins and anthocyanins-rich foods extracts or juices have demonstrated in several studies their ability to reduce the hepatic content of TG and lipids [85,86] and their capacity to modulate hepatic metabolism to protect against NAFLD [62,87–89]. Although in most of the published approaches performed with rodent models of obesity or NAFLD, anthocyanins or anthocyanin-rich fruits or extracts significatively reduced the hepatic lipid content and ameliorated the hepatic steatosis profile of these animals [88,90–92] some ineffective approaches have also been described [93–95].

The beneficial effects of anthocyanins in the liver have been linked to the activation of the AMPK, the upregulation of glycolytic and FAO genes and the downregulation of the gluconeogenic and lipogenic genes among others [70–72,96,97].

Mulberry anthocyanin extract administration to type 2 diabetic mice increased the activity of AMPK/peroxisome proliferator-activated receptor gamma coactivator 1 alfa (PGC1α)/p38 mitogen-activated protein kinase (MAPK) and reduced the activity of the acetyl-CoA carboxylase enzyme (ACC), a rate-limiting enzyme of fatty acid synthesis, and of the mammalian target of rapamycin (mTOR) that is involved in protein synthesis regulation and insulin signaling [96]. Similar effects were described in HFD-fed hamsters, where Mulberry water extracts exerted anti-obesity effects by inhibiting lipogenesis (downregulation of fatty acid synthase (FASN) and 3-hydroxy-3-methylglutaryl-coenzyme A (HMG-CoA) reductase) and upregulating PPARα and CPT1A [81]. On its side, honeyberry (*Lonicera caerulea*) extract (HBE) also decreased lipid accumulation in the liver of HFD-obese mice. HBE downregulated the hepatic expression of lipogenic genes such as *sterol regulatory element-binding protein-1 (Srebp-1c), CCAAT/enhancer-binding protein alpha (C/ebpα), Pparγ*, and *Fasn* as well as upregulated the mRNA and protein levels of CPT1a and PPARα, thus enhancing FAO. As mulberry anthocyanin extract, HBE treatment also increased the phosphorylation of AMPK and ACC thus activating and inhibiting these enzymes respectively [98]. On the other hand, in NAFLD-induced rats, blackberry extracts improved insulin sensitivity and dyslipidemia, ameliorated triglyceride and lipid peroxide accumulation and suppressed the mRNA expression of genes involved in fatty-acid synthesis (*Fasn* and *Srebp-1c*) [88]. Finally, purple sweet potato reduced the protein levels of FASN and of the cluster of differentiation 36 (CD36), inactivated the C/EBPβ, restored AMPK activity and increased the protein levels of CPT1a in livers of HFD-fed mice, thus indicating decreased lipogenesis and fatty acid uptake and enhanced FAO [62].

Regarding glucose metabolism, protein-bound anthocyanin compounds of purple sweet potato ameliorate hyperglycemia in obese and diabetic mice by regulating hepatic glucose metabolism. Anthocyanin compounds of purple sweet potato induced the hepatic protein levels of p-AMPK, glucose transporter type 2 (GLUT2), insulin receptor α (IRα), glucokinase (GK), as well as the expression of *phosphofructokinase (Pfk)* and *pyruvate kinase (Pk)*, while gluconeogenic genes, *glucose-6-phosphatase (G6Pase)* and *phosphoenolpyruvate carboxykinase (Pepck)* were downregulated [99]. Further, Saskatoon berry normalized liver expression of *Gk* and *glycogen phosphorylase* and increased *G6Ppase* in diet-induced MetS rats, thus suggesting that Saskatoon berry regulated glycolysis, gluconeogenesis and glycogenesis to improve MetS [100].

Although most of the experimental approaches have been done using anthocyanins-rich extracts, pure compounds have been also analyzed. Cyanidin-3-glucoside (C3G) administration to C57BL/6J obese mice fed a HFD and db/db mice diminished the triglyceride hepatic content and steatosis [73,101], through the blockade of the c-Jun N-terminal kinase activation (JNK) and the promotion of the phosphorylation and nuclear exclusion of the transcription factor Forkhead box protein O1 (FoxO1) [101].

All these data confirm the impact of anthocyanins and even in a more significative way of the anthocyanin-rich foods on metabolism. These effects can be added to their anti-inflammatory, antiapoptotic, pro-autophagic and antioxidant properties in steatotic livers [59,62,102–104].

3.2. Anthocyanins in Adipose Tissue: The Activation of BAT and the Browning of WAT

The impairment of adipose tissue function is strongly associated with the development of obesity and insulin resistance (IR). The activation of BAT and the browning in WAT are considered potential strategies to counteract the metabolic alterations linked to the obese phenotype. Both actions are mechanisms to increase the energy expenditure (EE) through the induction of lipolysis, FAO and thermogenesis and consequently efficient ways to reduce the ectopic lipid accumulation and the lipotoxicity [105–108].

Part of the beneficial effects of anthocyanins on diet-induced obesity are due to their impact on adipose depots. Anthocyanidins regulate lipolysis, FAO, lipogenesis and adipose tissue development [76,109–111]. They affected the adipokines secretion [112], modified the adipocytes-gene expression [33,113,114]. Moreover, anthocyanins are able to improve WAT functionality, to induce browning in WAT [33,57,82,115] or to increase the BAT mass or its activity [57,109,115], thus regulating energy expenditure [59,73]. Moreover, in WAT, anthocyanins ameliorate the obesity-associated inflammation [57,59,116].

In WAT, an anthocyanin-rich bilberry extract ameliorated hyperglycemia and insulin sensitivity through the activation of AMPK that resulted in an increase of the glucose transporter 4 (GLUT4) [72]. On its side, C3G-enriched *Aronia melanocarpa* extract reduced food intake and WAT weight in HFD-fed mice but also suppressed adipogenesis. These animals showed a downregulating in the expression levels of *C/ebpα*, *Srebp1c*, *Acc*, *ATP-citrate lyase*, *Pgc1α*, *Fasn*, and *adipocyte protein 2 (Ap2)* as well as in the circulating levels of leptin [111]. In the same way, in HFD-induced obese mice model, the dietary supplementation with maqui (*Aristotelia chilensis*) improved the body weight gain and glucose metabolism at least in part by modifying the expression of the *carbohydrate responsive element binding protein β (Chrebpβ)*, *the fibroblast growth factor 21 (Fgf21)* and *adiponectin* as well as of the lipogenic and FAO genes [82]. Globally, the maqui supplementation induced the browning of the subcutaneous WAT (scWAT) [82].

The induction of browning is a common phenotype in obese rodent models treated with anthocyanins or anthocyanins-rich foods. The thermogenic and mitochondrial markers were also increased in the inguinal WAT (iWAT) of high fat-high fructose (HF/HFD)-fed mice treated with C3G, thus indicating the browning of this adipose tissue depot and suggesting an increased heat production and energy expenditure (EE) [117]. In db/db mice, C3G and vanillic acid exerted similar effects: increased EE, limited weight gain and upregulated expression of *Ucp1* and other thermogenic and mitochondrial markers, thus indicating the induction of brown-like adipocytes development in the scWAT [73] or iWAT [115]. Freeze dried raspberry decreased WAT hypertrophy induced by HFD and promoted the browning of WAT as it is showed by a higher expression of beige markers such as *Ucp1*, *PR-Domain zinc finger protein 16 (Prdm16)*, *Cytochrome C*, *Cell death inducing DFFA like effector A (Cidea)*, and *Fatty acid elongase 3(Elovl3)*, elevated levels of PGC-1α and Fibronectin type III domain-containing protein 5 (FNDC5)/irisin, and an activation of the AMPK/Sirtuin 1 (SIRT1) pathway [33]. AMPK and Sirt1 are important sensors of the energy status that together with PGC-1α regulate energy homeostasis and stimulate FNDC5/irisin expression, thus inducing beige adipogenesis [118]. The regulation of adipogenesis through the AMPK/SIRT1 pathway has also been described in HFD fed mice treated with maize extract rich in ferulic acid and anthocyanins [119].

In WAT, anthocyanins and anthocyanin-rich foods also improve the inflammatory profile. The administration of a black soybean testa extracts (BBT) to diet-induced obese mice decreased fat accumulation, and the expression of *Acc* and *C/ebpα* and increased the levels of lipolysis proteins such as lipoprotein lipase (LPL), hormone-sensitive lipase (HSL) in mesenteric fat but also showed anti-inflammatory effects [109]. Similar effects were observed in humans where the administration of BBT to overweight or obese individuals decreased the abdominal fat measured as waist and hip circumference and improved the lipid profile [110]. The anti-inflammatory effects have been also achieved with sweet cherry anthocyanins and blueberry (*Vaccinium ashei*) anthocyanins. These anthocyanins reduced the body weight gain, the size of adipocytes and the leptin secretion in HFD-fed mice but also expression of *Il-6* and *Tnfa* genes, thus indicating an amelioration of the deleterious effects of a HFD [114,120].

Besides their effects on WAT, anthocyanins and anthocyanins-rich food also impact on BAT where they promote its activity. In high fructose/HFD-fed animals, besides inducing the browning of WAT, C3G attenuated the development of obesity by promoting the tremorgenic capacity of BAT. C3G upregulated the expression of thermogenic markers such as *Ucp1*, induced the mitochondrial biogenesis and function and finally increased the EE [117]. In db/db mice, C3G and vanillic improved cold tolerance and enhanced BAT activity and induced mitochondrial biogenesis In BAT, anthocyanin and anthocyanin-rich foods upregulated the expression of thermogenic markers (*Ucp1, Prdm16, Cidea* ...), lipid metabolism (*Cpt1a, Hsl, adipose triglyceride lipase (Atgl)*), mitochondrial markers (*mitochondrial transcription factor A (Tfam), Nuclear Respiratory Factor 1 and 2 (Nrf1 and Nrf2)* ...) and transcriptional regulators or coactivators of these processes (*Pparα, Pgc1β, Pgc1α* ...) [73,115].

3.3. In the Central Nervous System (CNS) Anthocyanins Have Been Related to Neuroprotective Effects as Well as in Feeding Behavior

The neuroprotective activity of anthocyanins has been widely evidenced in several epidemiological studies and their potential for the prevention of many neurodegenerative diseases such as Parkinson's disease (PD) and Alzheimer's disease (AD) has been suggested [77,78]. The neuroprotective effects of anthocyanins and C3G correlate with the regulation of molecules upstream of nitric oxide (NO) production, neuroinflammatory response and oxidative stress [79,121–123].

It has been demonstrated that C3G and malvidin 3-O-glucoside (M3G) inhibited the hyperphosphorylation of Tau protein in Alzheimer's disease [124] and berries supplementation have shown neurocognitive benefits in older adults at risk for dementia with mild cognitive impairment [125]. Recent studies highlighted an anti-depressive effect of a maqui-berry extract in a mouse model of a post-stroke depression. In this case the maqui effects were associated to its antioxidant capacity [126]. Otherwise, anthocyanins extracted from dried fruits of *Lycium ruthenicum Murr* have demonstrated a protective role in cerebral ischemia/reperfusion injury in rats [127] by inhibiting cell apoptosis and reducing edema and inflammation.

Besides their role in neuroprotection, anthocyanins modulate the feeding behavior. In rats, anthocyanins from black soybean increase the expression of the gamma-aminobutyric acid B1 receptor (GABAB1R) and decrease the expression of neuropeptide Y (NPY) in the hypothalamus, thus modulating the food intake behavior/body weight control. The upregulation of GABABR1 is followed by a decrease of the activated protein kinase A (PKA) and the phosphorylated cAMP-response element binding protein (CREB), both located downstream of GABAR1 [83]. In a similar way, the administration of an anthocyanin-rich black soybean testa (Glycine max (L.) Merr.) to diet-induced obese mice decreased food intake [109].

4. Flavanols

Flavanols are present in cocoa, tea, red wine, beer and several fruits such as grapes, apricots, apples where they are responsible for their astringency [128]. Flavanols exist as monomers named catechins or as polymers named proanthocyanins. The monomeric forms include: catechin (−)-epicatechin (EC), (−)-epigallocatechin gallate (EGCG), (−)-epigallocatechin (EGC), and (−)-epicatechin gallate (ECG). The proanthocyanins, also known as tannins, are more complex structures (dimers, oligomers, and polymers of catechins) and can be transformed to anthocyanins [29]. Like other flavonoids, flavanols are absorbed between the small intestine and the colon depending on their physicochemical properties and structure [129].

Flavanols possess a health claim related to their role in maintaining the elasticity of blood vessels that was approved in 2014 by the European Food Safety Authority (EFSA) [130].

In humans and animal models, flavanols or flavanols-rich foods (mainly, cocoa or tea derivates) have demonstrated the ability to reduce body weight, decrease waist circumference and fat percentages, improve glucose metabolism in individuals with type 2 diabetes, obesity or MetS and increase energy expenditure [75,131–139]. One of the most described molecular mechanism underlying theses effects are the activation of the AMPK enzyme [140].

Due to the high amount of publications including flavanols and metabolism we just included a representative group of the most recently published and the ones that deepen more on the molecular mechanisms underlying the beneficial effects of flavanols.

4.1. Flavanols Improve Hepatic Steatosis and Glucose/Lipid Metabolism in Obesity Models

In humans and several rodent models of obesity, flavanols have been able to improve blood lipid profile and protect liver from excessive fat deposition and hepatic steatosis [136,141–146]. These effects have been related mostly with an activation of the AMPK and the protein kinase B (PKB/Akt) pathways that finally lead to the suppression of lipogenesis by modulating the expression of *Srebp1c*, *cAMP-response element-binding protein regulated transcription coactivator 2 (Crtc2)*, and *stearyl coenzyme A dehydrogenase-1 (Scdh1)* or the activity of ACC, the inhibition of gluconeogenesis by affecting the levels of *PepcK* and *G6pase* and the increment of FAO by increasing the *Cpt1a* levels. Moreover, flavanols are able to improve cholesterol homeostasis through the regulation of several enzymes from the cholesterol synthesis and bile acids metabolism apart from the modulation of the mRNA expression of apolipoprotein B100 and ATP-binding cassette transporter A1. Most of the approaches included have been done using tea extracts or cocoa flavanols but other extracts with a more diverse composition of flavonoids have been also described in this section [137,143,147–151].

Theabrownin from Pu-erh tea in combination with swinging improved serum lipid profile and prevent development of obesity and insulin resistance in rats fed a high-fat-sugar-salt diet and subjected to a 30-min daily swinging. A transcriptomic analysis in the liver indicated that theabrownin together with exercise activated circadian rhythm, PKA, AMPK, and insulin signaling pathway, increased the levels of cAMP and accelerated the consumption of sugar and fat [142]. Similar results were obtained with HFD-fed mice supplemented with Yunkang green tea and subjected to treadmill exercise. These animals showed a reduction in the body weight gain and liver weight, a lower level of blood glucose, serum total cholesterol (TC), TG, insulin and ALT and an improvement in the fatty liver and hepatic pro-inflammatory profile compared to HFD group. Supplemented and exercised-animals showed a downregulation of the lipid synthesis genes (*Srebp1c, Fasn, Acc*), and an improvement of the hepatic insulin signaling [143].

Furthermore, in obese Zucker rats fed with a HFD and treated with green tea polyphenols a significant reduction on fasting insulin, glucose and lipids and an improvement of the NAFLD were observed. Livers of treated rats had lower levels of alanine aminotransferase (ALT) and aspartate aminotransferase (AST), of inflammatory markers and of TG content and exhibited less lipid droplets. These improvements have been related to an activation of the AMPK pathway and the inhibition of the hepatic lipogenesis (higher levels of the inactive p-ACC and lower levels of SREBP1c) [152]. These effects on lipid metabolism were also observed after the administration of Benifuuki (a tea that contains methylated catechins such as epigallocatechin-3-O-(3-O-methyl) gallate (EGCG3''Me) to high fat/high sucrose diet-fed mice. Benifuuki treatment lowered the levels of TG and NEFA in serum and liver and reduced the expression of hepatic lipogenic genes (*Srebp-1c, Acc1, Fasn* and *Stearoyl-CoA desaturase 1(Scd1)*) [153]. In parallel the use of *Euterpe oleracea* Mart.-derived polyphenols, known by the popular name of açai and rich in catechin and polymeric proanthocyanins, when administered to HFD-fed mice [154] or a pistachio-diet supplementation to diet-induce obese mice exhibited similar impact on lipid metabolism and gene expression modulation [150].

Finally, Oliogonol, a flavanol-rich lychee fruit extract, significantly reduced hepatic lipid content (less lipid droplets and ballooning by downregulating the *Pparγ* and, *Srebp1c* mRNA levels [155] probably via the inhibition of the mTOR activity promoted by the activation of the AMPK enzyme [156]. Moreover, oligonol improved hepatic insulin sensitivity by reducing the phosphorylation of glycogen synthase kinase 3a (GSK3a) and the phosphatase and tension homologue (PTEN) in HFD-induced obese mice [155] as well as inhibiting the mTOR/S6K cascade. The activation of the mTOR/S6K phosphorylates and desensitizes the insulin receptor substrate 1 (IRS1) [157]. In a similar way, GC-(4→8)-GCG, a proanthocyanidin dimer from *Camellia ptilophylla* improved hepatic steatosis and hyperlipidemia in HFD-induced obese mice [158].

Besides on hepatic lipogenesis, tea extracts also impact in FAO. The administration of tea water extracts from green tea, yellow tea, white tea, black tea, raw pu-erh tea and oolong tea decreased TG and total cholesterol levels in serum and liver as well as the hepatic lipid content. Supplemented animals displayed less lipid droplets, the activation of the AMPK and the upregulation of the *Cpt1a* together with the inhibition of the FASN enzyme. These treatments also reduced the inflammation profile linked to HFD [149]. Similar results were obtained with grape seed procyanidin B2 (GSPB2) and a polyphenol extract from *Solanum nigrum* that contains among other different catechins. In db/db mice, GSPB2 decreased body weight and improved the lipid profile in serum (TG, total cholesterol and free fatty acids (FFA)) but also reduced hepatic lipid droplets and TG accumulation. The proposed mechanism implied the AMPK activation, the ACC phosphorylation and *Cpt1a* overexpression, thus inhibiting FA synthesis and increasing FAO [159]. In a similar way, the *Solanum nigrum* polyphenol extract inhibited lipogenesis and enhanced FAO (upregulation of *Cpt1a* and *Pparα*) through the AMPK cascade [151].

In different animal models of obesity and insulin resistance, EGCG has shown the capacity to improve glucose homeostasis, to inhibit gluconeogenesis, FA and cholesterol synthesis and to increase FAO [147,148]. In HFD and STZ-induced type 2 diabetes, EGCG downregulated *Pepck* and *G6Pase* and inhibited SREBP1c, FASN and ACC1. The mechanism underlying these effects is not yet well understood but it has been suggested that EGCG would activate the PXR/CAR-mediated phase II metabolism that through a direct or indirect mechanism would suppress gluconeogenesis and lipogenesis [147]. Moreover, in HFD Wistar rats, EGCG diminished the liver weight, the hepatic hyperlipidemia, animals showed less lipid droplets, reduced serum levels of ALT and AST, TG, total cholesterol and better profile of LDL/HDL but also an ameliorated oxidative stress. In this case, EGCG activated SIRT1, FoXO1 and regulate SREBP2 activity to suppress hepatic cholesterol synthesis. These data point out the downregulation of SREBP2 expression under the SIRT1/FOXO1 signaling pathway as a mechanism to reduce the cholesterol content [148]. Furthermore, EGCG also decreased bile acid reabsorption, which decreased the intestinal absorption of lipids [160]. In the same way, EC administered to a high-fat high cholesterol diet rats reduced serum levels of total cholesterol, LDL and TG while increased HDL [161]. Moreover, EC intake also reduced serum levels of ALT and AST enzymes, the lipid peroxidation and the pro-inflammatory cytokines levels, thus indicating an improvement in the liver functionality. The proposed mechanism of EC included the downregulation of the nuclear receptor liver-X-receptor (LXR), the FASN enzyme and the SIRT1 protein but also the blockade of the Insig-1-SREBP-SCAP pathway that drives the SREBP2 maturation [161].

4.2. Flavanols in Adipose Tissue: Less Adiposity and More Energy Expenditure: The Browning Effect

In humans, some studies described the capacity of green tea to reduce body weight and abdominal fat accumulation [162,163], influence on the body fat mass index, waist circumference, total fat mass and energy expenditure through the induction of browning or BAT activity [164–166] but also to regulate ghrelin secretion and adiponectin levels, to control appetite and decrease nutrient absorption [135,167].

In rodents, the administration of grape seed-derived proanthocyanins to Wistar rats reduced the body weight by limiting food intake and activating EE in scWAT [168] and it has been widely described that in rodent models of obesity, flavanols are able to affect the lipid metabolism of WAT and BAT. Global effects of flavanols in adipose tissues lead to a decrease in adiposity, specially of the WAT depots and in adipocyte size by reducing adipogenesis, the release of adipokines such as leptin and resistin, the modulation of lipid metabolism and the induction of browning [153,155,158,169–174]. In BAT, flavanols caused the activation of thermogenesis and FAO [172–176].

As has been mentioned before, in WAT, flavanols modified lipid metabolism. EGCG reduced the expression of genes related with *de novo* lipogenesis (*Acc1*, *Fasn*, *Scd1*, *C/ebpβ*, *Pparγ* and *Srebp1c*), increased the expression of genes involved in lipolysis (*Hsl*) and lipid oxidization (*Ppara, Acetyl-CoA oxidase (Acox)2*, and medium-chain acyl-CoA dehydrogenase (*Mcad*)) in epididymal (eWAT) and scWAT and highly upregulated the expression of delta-9 desaturase, the enzyme responsible to convert saturated fatty acids to monounsaturated [177]. The activation of the AMPK in HFD-EGGC-treated mice indicated that at least in part the changes in lipid metabolism observed were due to the AMPK phosphorylation [177]. In scWAT, although EGCG increased lipolysis (*Hsl*) and FAO (*Cpt1a*) [168,178], some lipogenic genes (*Acc1, Fasn, Scd1, Pparγ*, and *Srebp1*) has been detected upregulated at the mRNA level but no at protein level [178]. These data suggested that EGCG might have different effects in scWAT and eWAT. Finally, pistachio-diet supplementation to diet-induce obese mice also ameliorated the HFD-induced expression of *Srebp1c, Pparγ*, and *Fatp* [150].

Besides its effects in the liver, the GC-(4→8)-GCG inhibited the expansion of all WAT depots in HFD fed mice. Adipocytes from eWAT were smaller and some of the main adipocyte-associated transcription markers were downregulated (*Srebp1c, C/ebpa* and *Pparγ*), thus indicating a better WAT functionality [158]. The GC-(4→8)-GCG-supplemented mice showed an upregulation of the adiponectin and a downregulation of the leptin mRNA levels as well as an improved inflammatory profile with less macrophage infiltration [158].

Regarding the browning effect of flavanols it has been published that EC increased mitochondrial biogenesis, fatty acid metabolism and upregulated the expression of BAT-specific markers (*Prdm16, Dio2, Ucp1* and *Ucp2*) in WAT in a way that depends on phosphorylation and deacetylation cascades [170]. The authors demonstrated that EC supplementation upregulated the mitochondrial related proteins p-SIRT1, SIRT1, SIRT3, PGC1α, PPARγ, TFAM, NRF1, NRF2, complex II, IV and V and mitofilin [170]. In a similar way, a polyphenolic extract from green tea leaves (GTE) ameliorated the body weight gain caused by a HFD with no changes in calorie intake but reducing the adiposity and the adipocyte size in WAT and BAT. GTE supplementation induced BAT markers in scWAT (higher mRNA levels of *Pgc1α, Cbp/p300-interacting transactivator 1 (Cited1)* and *Prdm16* and of UCP1 protein) and reduced HFD-induced whitening in BAT (lower expression of adipogenic markers *C/ebpa* and *Ap2* and upregulation of *Pgc1α* and *vascular endothelial growth factor-A(165)* (*Vegfa165*)) [171]. These animals also showed an improvement in the inflammatory profile in scWAT and BAT. Finally, a Grape pomace extract (GPE) showed the capacity to induce browning (upregulation of *Pgc1α, Pparγ, Prdm16* and *Ucp1*) in the eWAT of HFD-fed rats [179,180].

Besides tea extracts also cacao components are able to induce browning and BAT activation. Concretely, theobromine alleviated diet-induced obesity in mice by inducing a brown-like phenotype in the iWAT and activated lipolysis and thermogenesis in BAT. In HFD fed mice theobromine inhibited phosphodiesterase-4 (PDE4D) activity in adipose tissue, thus increasing β3-adrenergic receptor (AR) signaling pathway and EE [172]. The inhibition of PDE increases the cellular levels of cAMP levels thus activating the β-AR cascade and finally PKA and UCP1 activity [181].

The capacity of flavanols on activating BAT has been described even with a single dose of a flavanol mixture that included catechins and B type procyanidins or by administering individual components by itself [182]. In these animals, *Ucp1* mRNA expression in BAT and levels of catecholamines in plasma were significantly increased via SNS stimulation but with varying efficacy depending on the stereochemical structure of flavanols [182]. It should be noted that prolonged ingestion of a catechin-rich beverage increased the BAT density with a decrease in extramyocellular lipids in humans [183]. EGCG-supplemented diet-induced obese mice exhibited higher body temperature and more mitochondrial DNA (mtDNA) content in BAT together with an upregulation of the genes related to fatty acid metabolism, thermogenesis and mitochondrial biogenesis (*Ucp1, Ucp2, Prdm16, Cpt1β, Pgc-1α, Nrf1*, and *Tfam*) [184,185] and a downregulation of *Acc*. These effects have been related to an increased activity of the AMPK in BAT [184].

Thermogenesis can also be induced by a polyphenol-rich green tea extract (PGTE) through a mechanism that depends on adiponectin signaling. The treatment with this extract reversed part of the obesity phenotype in WT mice but no in adiponectin KO mice (AdipoKO). PGTE treatment increased EE, BAT thermogenesis, and promoted browning phenotype in the scWAT of WT mice but these effects were blunted in AdipoKO mice [176].

Some data regarding BAT activation by catechins in humans have also described. Different approaches have been done to demonstrate the effects of green tea extract and caffeine over thermogenesis and body weight [186,187]. Short- and long-term effects have been studied with different results and effectiveness but suggesting that catechins and caffeine may act synergistically to control body weight and induce thermogenesis [175,188]. It has been proposed that the thermogenic response to green tea extracts or its components would be mediated, in BAT, by the direct stimulation of the β-adrenergic receptor (β-AR) cascade through the inhibition of the enzyme catechol-O-methyl transferase (COMT), which degrades catecholamines. On its side, caffeine inhibited PDE, thus inducing a sustained activation of the PKA and its downstream cascade [175].

4.3. Flavanols Consumption Induces Energy Expenditure in Peripheral Organs through the Sympathetic Nervous System Activation

Part of the anti-obesity effects of flavanols have been also related to their influence on sympathetic nervous system (SNS) activity. The SNS activation by green tea catechins (GTC) has been associated to their capacity to inhibit COMT. The inhibition of COMT leads to a prolonged activation of the sympathetically-response and of the β-adrenergic cascade that produces cAMP and the activation of the PKA. Caffeine, in turn, is able to inhibit the PDE activity which drives to a sustained activation of the PKA and its downstream response [175]. Then, both effects act synergistically to increase EE, lipolysis and FAO as has been described in the above sections. Some other mechanisms to describe the anti-obesity effects of flavanols include the modulation of food intake. It has been demonstrated that grape-seed proanthocyanins extract (GSPE) reduced food intake in rats fed a cafeteria diet. These animals showed an activation of the STAT3 protein which upregulated the *pro-opiomelanocortin (Pomc)* expression, thus improving the leptin resistance [189].

Moreover, GSPE supplementation reduced the neuroinflammation and increased the expression of SIRT1 [189]. Flavanols has been described as active molecules against diet-induced neuroinflammation. The induction of neuroinflammation and cognitive impairment in rats by feeding them with a high salt and cholesterol diet (HSCD) could be in part reversed by the treatment with different doses of an enriched-tannins fraction of the Indian fruit *Emblica officinalis*. Treatment with this tannin-enriched gooseberry reversed the HSCD-induced behavioral and memory disturbances, neuronal cell death and reduced the levels of cognitive impairment markers. [190]. In the same way, it has been published that, in mice, EGCG attenuated the neuronal damage and insulin resistance caused by a high fat/high fructose diet (HF/HFD). In this case, EGCG upregulated the IRS-1/AKT and the extracellular-signal-regulated kinase (ERK)/CREB/Brain-derived neurotrophic factor (BDNF) signaling pathways. In longer nutritional interventions with the HF/HFD, EGCG was capable to inhibit the MAPK and NF-κB pathways, as well as the expression of inflammatory mediators, such as TNF-α to reverse the neuroinflammation [191]. Similar results were obtained with EGCG-HFD dietary supplementation. The authors demonstrated that EGCG ameliorated the HFD-induced obesity in part by attenuating hypothalamic inflammation through the inhibition of NF-kB and Signal transducer and activator of transcription 3 (STAT3) phosphorylation, as well as the expression and release of inflammatory cytokines, such as TNF-a, IL-6, and IL-1b [185].

Finally, EGCG alleviated part of the cognitive deficits in a mixed model of familial Alzheimer's disease (AD) and type 2 diabetes mellitus (T2DM). The AD mice model APP/PS1 fed with a HFD showed an improvement in peripheral parameters such as insulin sensitivity but also in central memory deficits when treated with EGCG. Synaptic markers and CREB phosphorylation were increased because of an amelioration in the unfolded protein response (UPR) activity via a downregulation of the activation factor 4 (ATF4) levels. Moreover, EGCG decreased brain amyloid β (Aβ) production and plaque burden by increasing the levels of α-secretase (ADAM10) and reduced the neuroinflammation in these animals [192]. Finally, green tea extracts can modulate the redox status of the CNS in obese and lean rats [193].

5. Flavanones

Flavanones are a subfamily of flavonoids widely distributed in *citrus* fruits such as grape, tomatoes, and oranges and are the responsible of the bitter taste of their peel and of their juice. As other flavonoids, flavanones show strong health benefits due to its antioxidant activity but also exhibit antiviral, antimicrobial, antiatherogenic, anti-inflammatory antidiabetic and anti-obesity properties [45,48,75,194,195]. Flavanones are mainly found as aglycones or as glycosylated derivatives [196]. The most studied flavanones are hesperidin, naringenin but also eriodyctiol, isosakuranetin and taxifolin.

Hesperidin and its aglycone, hesperetin are found in citrus fruits, such as limes and lemons, tomatoes and cherries and have demonstrated antidiabetic, neuroprotective, antiallergic, anti-inflammatory anticarcinogenic besides their well-established antioxidant capacity [45,197] Naringenin and its aglycone naringin are found to be more abundant in citrus fruits such as grapefruit orange, lemon but also in tomatoes. Naringenin and derivates have been associated with beneficial effects in cardiovascular diseases, osteoporosis, cancer and have showed anti-inflammatory, antiatherogenic, lipid-lowering, neuroprotective, nephroprotective, hepatoprotective and antidiabetic properties [198,199].

5.1. Flavanones-Dietary Supplementation Ameliorates the NAFLD in Humans

Frequently, liver diseases are initiated by oxidative stress, inflammation and lipid accumulation that lead to an excessive production of extracellular matrix followed by a progression to fibrosis, cirrhosis and hepatocellular carcinoma [200]. In the last years, several studies have demonstrated the capacity of different flavanones to ameliorate liver diseases.

To analyze the positives effects of flavanones in liver different approaches have been used. Some authors worked with hepatic chemical-induced damage being the most used the streptozotocin injection to mice or rats [199,201]. Other authors induced liver damage with diet [199] or worked with genetically obese models. Although flavanones demonstrated positive effects in the different approaches, in this review we focused on the experimental approaches where the liver disease has been induced by diet or where genetically obese-models has been used. Experiments with naringenin, hesperidin and eriodyctiol has been done to evaluate the impact of this flavanones' consumption in NAFLD or liver steatosis.

Naringenin has showed the capacity to restore the activities of liver hexokinase, PK, G6Pase and Fructose 1,6-bisphosphatase from rats fed a high fructose diet to levels similar to healthy non-diabetic animals [202]. In this animal model, naringenin also enhanced liver protein tyrosine kinase (PTK), while reduced protein tyrosine phosphatase (PTP) activity [202]. In addition, administration of naringenin to HF/HSD-fed rats increased the protein levels of PPARα, CPT1a and UCP2 [203]. In a similar way, naringenin increased FAO and the AMPK activity in HFD fed mice where ameliorated the metabolic alterations caused by diet [204]. Similar results were obtained in high-fat/high-cholesterol (HFHC) fed Ldlr -/- mice. In lean Ldlr -/- mice, naringenin induced weight loss and reduce calorie intake, enhanced EE and increased hepatic FAO by upregulating *Pgc1α, Cpt1a and Hsl*, thus indicating that naringenin is also effective in non-obese models [195]. In HFD fed Ldlr -/-, naringenin increased FAO and reduced lipogenesis. Hepatic *Srebp1c* and *Acox1* mRNA levels were downregulated, while *Fgf21, Pgc1α, and Cpt1a* were upregulated by naringenin [205]. Later on, it was published that naringenin prevented obesity, hepatic steatosis, and glucose intolerance in an FGF21-independent way [206]. More recently, it has been described that in obese-mice naringin decreased hepatic liver content (TG and total cholesterol) and activated the AMPK enzyme resulting in reduced expression and protein levels of liver SREBP1C, SREBP2, but increased LDLR. Moreover, these mice showed reduced plasma levels of proprotein convertase subtilisin/kexin type 9 (PCSK9), leptin, insulin, and LDL-C compared to obese non-treated mice [207].

Besides naringenin, naringin and hesperidin effects in liver have also been evaluated. Hesperidin and naringin supplementation in db/db and ob/ob mice regulated hepatic gluconeogenesis and glycolysis, as well as lipid metabolism [208]. Hesperidin stimulated PPARγ, increased the hepatic GK activity and glycogen concentration and reduced the hepatic levels of *Glut2* as well as increased the expression of *Glut4* in WAT [46,208,209]. Moreover, hesperidin prevented hepatic steatosis in western diet-fed rats by preventing the upregulation of lipogenesis-related genes *Srebf1*, and *Scd1* caused by Western diet and the downregulation of *Pparα* and *Cpt1a* expression and CPT1a protein levels [210]. Most of these effects were blunted when hesperidin is combined with capsaicin [210].

In diet-induced obese mice treated with neohesperidin the expression and secretion of FGF21 and the activity of the AMPK/SIRT1/PGC-1α axis were improved [211]. Treatment with neohesperidin improved the steatotic state (less and smaller lipid droplets), reversed the downregulation of hepatic *Pparα* levels while increased the levels of the hepatic *Fgf21* expression and its plasma levels. Finally, neohesperidin treatment phosphorylated AMPK, resulting in a rise of the HFD-downregulated proteins SIRT1 and PGC1α [211]. On its side, eriodyctiol has also demonstrated effects on diet-induced obesity. Diet-induced obese mice supplemented with eriodyctiol showed a reduction of hepatic TG, fatty acids and the size and number of lipid droplets accompanied with an increased fecal excretion of cholesterol and fatty acids [212]. It is worth to mention that eriodyctiol decreased the enzymatic activity of malic enzyme (ME), FASN, phosphatide phosphohydrolase (PAP) and downregulated the expression of *Srepb1c, Acc and Fasn* [212]. These data indicate that eriodyctiol improved the hepatic steatosis caused by a HFD by decreasing hepatic lipogenesis and increasing the hepatic FAO. On the other hand, alpinetin, an O-methylated flavanone, improved HFD-induced NAFLD via ameliorating oxidative stress, inflammatory response and lipid metabolism. Alpinetin decreased *Scd1, Fasn, Srebp1c, Lxrα, Elovl2* and *Irs1* expressions, and increased PPARα levels [213].

In humans a randomized placebo-controlled, double-blind clinical trial with NAFLD patients shown the effect of hesperidin supplementation [214]. Patients who follow healthy lifestyle habits and supplemented their diet with hesperidin have a significant reduction of ALT, glutamyl-transferase, total cholesterol, hepatic steatosis, C reactive protein and TNFα, proving the scope of hesperidin [214]. One of the possible mechanisms underlying the effects of flavanones on metabolism goes through the FGF21 and AMPK/Sirt1/PGC1α signaling axis.

5.2. Flavanones Induce Browning in Adipose Tissue

As other flavonoids, flavanones can also modulate lipid metabolism in adipose tissue as well as induce browning in WAT, and activate in BAT [166] as well as reduce the characteristic obese-macrophage infiltration in adipose tissue [215].

In HFD fed mice, hesperetin supplementation on its side showed metabolic health effects in adipose tissue, concretely is able to reduce mesenteric adipose weight and decrease leptin levels [216]. In this case, lipid metabolism was not changed nor in liver nor in WAT. On the other hand, a characteristic of obesity is the recruitment of immune cells by adipose tissue that leads to metabolic disorders such as insulin resistance. In a short-term HFD mice model, naringenin can suppress neutrophil and macrophage infiltration into adipose tissue [215]. Concretely it can inhibit the expression of several chemokines like MCP-1 and MCP-3 [217]. Eriodyctiol (ED) supplementation on its side lowered the adiposity in diet-induced obese mice by regulating gene expression. ED-supplemented mice showed reduced weight of all the WAT depots but also a downregulated expression of adipocyte genes involved in lipid uptake (*Cd36*, and *Lpl*) and lipogenesis (*Srebp1, Acc, and Scd1*), an upregulation of the *Ucp1*, with no changes in FAO genes such as *Adrb3, Cpt2, Pgc1α, Pgc1β*, and *Cox8b* genes [212].

Another beneficial effect of flavanones in adipose tissue is related to EE and thermogenesis. It has been demonstrated that in human white adipocytes and in scWAT a treatment with naringenin increased the expression of genes associated with thermogenesis and FAO, including *Atgl* and *Ucp1* as well as *Pgc1α* and *Pgc1β* that can mediate the PPARδ-dependent transcriptional responses involved in mitochondrial biogenesis and uncoupling phenotype. Moreover, naringenin administration increased the expression of insulin sensitivity-related proteins such as *Glut4, adiponectin,* and *Chrebp* [218]. These data indicate that naringenin may promote the conversion of human WAT to a brown/beige adipose tissue. Similarly, in HFD-obese mouse model, the induction of brown-like adipocyte formation on WAT was described by supplementing the diet with a flavanones-rich extract from *Citrus reticulata* [219]. The main phytochemical components of a water extraction of *Citrus reticulata* in were synephrine, narirutin, hesperidin, nobiletin, and tangeretin. Among flavanones, citrus also contain synephrine that is an alkaloid which binds to $β_3AR$ in adipose tissue promoting lipolysis and thermogenesis [220]. Dietary supplementation with this citrus extract reduced body weight gain, epididymal fat weight, fasting blood glucose, serum levels of TG and total cholesterol, and lipid accumulation in liver and WAT as well as activated FAO and induced the browning phenotype [219]. These animals showed increased levels of *Ucp1* in the iWAT and an upregulation of *Prdm16, transmembrane protein 26 (Tmem26), cluster of differentiation 137 (CD137),* and *Cidea* [219].

In the same way it has been published that hesperidin induced browning in retroperitoneal WAT (rWAT) but not in iWAT of Western diet-fed rats. Hesperidin decreased the size of adipocytes and induced the formation of multilocular and positive-UCP1 and CIDEA brown-like adipocytes. Besides the induction browning, hesperidin also enhanced the expression of *Ucp1* in BAT [221]. In contrast, it has been recently published a study where not hesperidin but its monoglycosyl has the capacity to induce brown-like adipocyte formation in HFD-fed mice [222]. In this case, α-monoglucosyl hesperidin increased EE and reduced body fat accumulation by stimulating the browning phenotype in the iWAT. iWAT adipocytes of supplemented mice exhibited a multilocular phenotype and were UCP1-positive cells. The iWAT of these animals also showed increased levels of COXIV. No effects were observed in BAT nor in other WAT depots [222].

In a human randomized double-blind placebo-controlled trial with moderate high BMI subjects, it's shown that glycosylated hesperidin decreased significantly abdominal and subcutaneous fat area when is supplemented with caffeine [223].

5.3. Flavanones Are Neuroprotective against Several CNS Injuries

There is low information about the effects of flavanones on CNS to combat obesity. It has been demonstrated that quercetin, naringenin and berberine can modulate glucose homeostasis in the brain of STZ-induced diabetic rats through the regulation of glucose transporters and other key components of insulin signaling pathway [224].

Most of the studies that show the neuroprotective role of flavanones have been performed using animal with CNS-induced injuries. In a rat model of global cerebral ischemia reperfusion (I/R), pinocembrin (a honey flavanone) exerted antioxidant, anti-inflammatory and anti-apoptotic effects. [225] as well as inhibited autophagy on the hippocampus [226]. Moreover, naringenin and eriodyctiol exert effects in ischemic stroke, promoting cortical cell proliferation, inhibiting apoptosis and reducing oxidative stress in rodent models [227,228]. In a similar way, the induction of neurotoxicity by lipopolysaccharide (LPS) administration in mice can be ameliorated by the coadministration of hesperetin or naringenin that reduced the expression of inflammatory cytokines, attenuated the generation of reactive oxygen species/lipid peroxidation and enhanced the antioxidant capacity in CNS [229,230]. Furthermore, hesperetin enhanced synaptic integrity, cognition and memory processes by increasing the levels p-CREB, postsynaptic density protein-95 (PSD-95) and syntaxin proteins [229] and naringenin decreased the acetylcholinesterase (AChe) activity [230]. Other mental stresses such as social defeat stress, depression and autistic-like behaviors can also be counteract with flavanones in rodent models [231–233]. Hesperidin and naringenin have demonstrated positive effects by increasing the resilience through a reduction in the levels of interleukins and corticosterone thus suppressing the chronic inflammation caused by kynurenine pathway related to depression [234] and inhibiting the AChe activity, the oxidative stress as well as neuroinflammation [235].

6. Flavonols

Flavonols are widely distributed in plants and are present as minor compound in many polyphenol-rich foods. Their synthesis is stimulated by light and they accumulate in the skin of fruits and vegetables being absent in the flesh. The main dietetic flavonols are quercetin, kaempferol, isorhamnetin, fisetin, and myricetin [48,236,237].

Quercetin is found in capers, lovage (*Levisticum officinale*) apples, seeds of tomatoes, berries, red onions, grapes, cherries, broccoli, pepper, coriander, citrus fruits, fennel, flowers, leaves pepper and teas (*Camellia sinensis*) and it is the skeleton of other flavonoids, such as hesperidin, naringenin, and rutin. Rutin, rutoside or sophorin are the glycosylated form of quercetin and can be extracted from buckwheat, oranges, grapes, lemons, limes, peaches, and berries [238]. Kaempferol is abundant in apples, grapes, onions, tomatoes, teas, potatoes, beans, broccoli, spinaches, and some edible berries. Isorhamnetin is commonly found in medicinal plants such as ginko (*Ginkgo biloba*), sea-buckthorn (*Hippophae rhamnoides*) and *Oenanthe javanica*. Myricetin is found in teas, wines, berries, fruits and vegetables. Fisetin is abundant in apples, grapes, persimmon, cucumber, onions and strawberries. Finally, morin is present in *Prunus dulcis*, *Chlorophora tinctoria* L., and fruits such as guava and figs [45].

As other groups of flavonoids, flavonols have shown healthy effects. They exhibit anticarcinogenic, anti-inflammatory, and antioxidant activities but also anti-obesity and antidiabetic properties in animal models and in humans where flavonols consumption has been associated to a lower risk of type 2 diabetes [43,236–243]. Some flavonols inhibited carbohydrate absorption thus lowering postprandial blood glucose mainly through the inhibition of the α-glucosidase activity but also by inhibiting glucose transporters (GLUT2, SGLT1) or other enzymes such as maltase or saccharase [236]. Finally, a combination of quercetin and resveratrol have shown the capacity to reduce obesity in HFD-fed rats by modulating gut microbiota [244].

Due to the high number of publications and previous reviews [45,48,238], in the present work only the most recent data have been included.

6.1. Flavonols Exert Beneficial Effects on Lipid Steatosis by Regulating Lipid Metabolism, Inflammation and Oxidative Stress

Quercetin enhanced hepatic insulin sensitivity and reduced liver fat content and ameliorated hepatic steatosis [245]. Quercetin diminished the mRNA and protein levels of CD36 and MSR1, upregulated the levels of LC3II and downregulated p62 and mTOR thus suggesting an autophagy lysosomal degradation as the potential hepatoprotective mechanism of quercetin [245]. From another point of view the effects and mechanisms of quercetin against NAFLD were analyzed through a metabolomic approach [246]. Treatment with quercetin decreased AST and ALT levels in serum and reduced lipid droplets and hepatocyte swelling in rats fed a high fat/high sucrose diet. A metabolomic analysis indicated that quercetin modified fatty acid- inflammation- and oxidative stress-related metabolites among others. In this case, the effects of quercetin were more evident in 30-day NAFLD induction than in 50 days, thus indicating that dietary quercetin may be beneficial in early stages of NAFLD development [246]. Besides the effects of quercetin alone there are several studies where quercetin is used in combination with other compounds. The beneficial effects of quercetin in NAFLD development increased synergistically when quercetin is administered within benifuuki, a tea that contains EGCG. Both compounds administered to rats fed high fat/high cholesterol diet were more effective to downregulate *Fasn* and *Scd1* showing higher effects on their lipid-lowering effects alone [247]. In a similar way, the combination of quercetin with resveratrol ameliorated fatty liver in rats by improving the antioxidant capacity of the liver [248]. Finally, a combination of borage seed oil (as a source of linoleic (18:2n-6; LA) and gamma-linolenic (18:3n-6; GLA) acids and quercetin improved liver steatosis in obese rats [249].

On its side, isoquercetin (IQ), a glucoside derivative of quercetin has demonstrated beneficial effects in NAFLD by improving hepatic lipid accumulation via an AMPK dependent way in HFD-induced NAFLD rats [250]. Concretely, IQ treatment enhanced the phosphorylation of AMPK and ACC and reversed the downregulation of liver kinase β1 (LKβ1) and Calcium/calmodulin-dependent protein kinase kinase-1 (CaMKK1) caused by HFD. The activation of AMPK modulated the expression of lipogenic and lipolytic genes, such as *Fasn, Srebp1c, Pparγ and Cpt1a*. Moreover, IQ supplementation upregulated PPARα and downregulated nuclear factor-kB (NF-kB) protein levels [250].

As quercetin, kaempferol is also able to reduce lipid accumulation in liver of obese rodent models. In dyslipidemia-induced mice, kaempferol inhibited PKB (Akt) and SREBP-1 activities and blocked the Akt/mTOR pathway, thus inducing hepatic autophagy and decreasing hepatic lipid content [251]. Similarly, in ApoE deficient mice fed with a HFD, kaempferol attenuated metabolic syndrome via interacting with LXR receptors and inhibiting posttranslational activation of SREBP-1. Both effects contributed to the reduction of plasma and serum TG [252].

Other flavonols with positive effect in the liver are fisetin, dihydromyricetin or rutin. Obese rats fed with a high fat/high sucrose diet and supplemented with fisetin showed a decreased in body weight and hepatic lipid content as well as an improvement in the lipid profile (low levels of TG, total cholesterol, LDL) and liver functionality (reduced levels of ALT and AST). The hepatic nuclear receptor 4α (HNF4α) has been pointed out as the key factor in the hepatic effects of fisetin. Fisetin upregulated *Hnf4a* gene expression, increased nuclear lipin-1 levels. Moreover, fisetin promoted FAO, diminished FASN activity, enhanced hepatic antioxidant capacity and decreased the hepatic poly (ADP-ribose) polymerase 1 (PARP1) activity, a DNA repair enzyme, and thioredoxin-interacting protein (TXNIP) that is important for maintaining the redox status [253]. Through the regulation of SIRT3 signaling, dihydromyricetin have showed the ability to ameliorate NAFLD in HFD-fed mice. Dihydromyricetin increased *Sirt3* expression via activation of the AMPK/PGC1α/estrogen-related receptor α (ERRα) cascade thus improving mitochondrial capacity and restored redox homeostasis [254]. In a similar way, rutin lowered TG content and the abundance of lipid droplets in NAFLD-induced HFD fed mice. Rutin treatment restored the expression of *Pparα* and *Cpt1a* and *Cpt2*, while downregulated *Srebp-1c*, *diglyceride acyltransferase 1 and 2 (Dgat-1 and 2* and *Acc*. These effects enhanced FAO and diminished lipid synthesis. In addition, rutin repressed the autophagy in the liver [255]. On its side, the rutin derivate, troxerutin (TRX), has also demonstrated effectiveness against metabolic disorders in a rat model of hereditary hypertriglyceridemia (HHTg) non-obese model of MetS [256]. The treatment with TRX lowered the levels of hepatic cholesterol and reduced the expression of cholesterol and lipid synthesis genes (*Hydroxymethylglutaryl-CoA reductase* (*Hmgcr*), *Srebp2* and *Scd1*) as well as decreased lipoperoxidation and increased the activity of antioxidant enzymes [256]. Moreover, these animals exhibited higher levels of adiponectin in serum [256].

Besides the effects of flavonols by itself, favonols-rich extracts have also been tested in fatty liver-associated diseases. A *Sicyos angulatus* extract that contains kaempferol as the main flavonol administered to a HFD-induced obese mice lowered plasma levels of ALT and AST and the hepatic lipid content. The *Sicyos angulatus* extract impacted on lipid metabolism by repressing the expression of genes related to fatty acid and TG synthesis (*Acc1, Fasn Scd1* and *Dgat*) and of the key transcription factors that regulate lipogenesis (*Srebp-1c* and *Pparγ*) [257]. Another source of kaempferol, quercetin and derivates is Sanglan Tea (SLT), a Chinese medicine-based formulation consumed for the effective management of obesity-associated complications. It has been demonstrated that dietary SLT supplementation prevented body weight gain and fatty liver and ameliorated insulin resistance in HFD-induced obese mice. SLT improved the serum lipid profile (lower levels of TG, Total cholesterol and LDL) and reduced the ALT and AST circulating levels. The liver of these animals displayed less lipid droplets and a downregulation of the lipogenic genes *(Lxrα, Fasn, Acacb, Srebf-1,* and *Scd1*) and the adipogenesis-related genes (*Pparγ, C/ebpα* and *Ap2*) that are induced under HFD [258].

In a similar way, the flower of *Prunus persica* commonly known as peach blossom has demonstrated that capacity to reduce body weight, abdominal fat mass, serum glucose, ALT, AST, and liver and spleen weights compared to a HFD fed mice. This flower is rich in flavonoids and phenolic phytochemicals with chlorogenic acid, kaempferol, quercetin and its derivatives as its major compounds. The supplementation with this flower suppressed hepatic expression of lipogenic genes (*Scd1, Scd2,*

Fasn) and increased the mRNA levels of FAO genes (*Cpt1a*), thus modifying he lipid metabolism in HFD-fed mice [259]. Furthermore, a mulberry leaf powder also showed effects on liver gene expression in a mice model of hepatic steatosis induced by a western diet. Liver weight, plasma TG and liver enzymes ALT and AST were reduced in treated-animals. A global hepatic gene expression analysis revealed that supplemented mice displayed a downregulation in inflammation-related genes and an upregulation in liver regeneration-related genes [260]. Finally, a 70% ethanol extract from leaves of *Moringa oleifera (MO)* that contains different flavonols and flavones such as quercetin and kaempferol and their derivates. reduced glucose and insulin but also the total cholesterol, TG and LDL serum and increased the HDL in high-fat diet obese rats as well as downregulated hepatic expression of *Fasn* and *Hmgcr* [261].

Through a network pharmacological approach Nie et al. [262] highlighted that Chaihu shugan powder (CSP) may exert its beneficial effects against NAFLD through the interaction of its main compounds with nuclear receptors. Through a molecular docking approach, they screened PPARγ, FXR, PPARα, RARα and PPARδ and quercetin, kaempferol, naringenin, isorhamnetin and nobiletin interactions. To confirm the results of docking, an in vivo approach was done using NAFLD-induced rats. The NAFLD-induced rats treated with CSP exhibited ameliorated effects in body weight, hepatic histopathology and serum and liver lipids. Moreover, the mRNA levels of *Pparγ*, *FXR*, *Pparα* and *Rarα* were modified suggesting nuclear receptors regulation as a potential molecular mechanism underlying the effects of CSP [262].

Adiponectin signaling and AMPK activation have been also pointed out as possible mechanisms underlying the effects of flavonols in the liver. An extract of black soybean leaves (EBL), which mainly contains quercetin glycosides and isorhamnetin glycosides was administered to HFD-fed mice. EBL supplementation reduced body weight, fasting glucose, TG, total cholesterol and non-esterified fatty acid levels as well as hepatic steatosis. EBL supplementation increased the levels of adiponectin and the expression of adiponectin-receptors in the liver (AdipoR1 and AdipoR2) thus restoring adiponectin signaling pathway [263]. Downstream of the adiponectin signaling there is the activation of AMPK and FAO, the suppression of fatty acid synthesis and the improvement of insulin signaling [264]. Moreover, the mRNA levels of *Pgc1*, *Pparα*, *Pparδ*, *Pparγ*, *Acc*, *Fasn*, *Cpt1a*, *Glut2*, *FoxO1* and *Irs1* were partially or totally normalized in HFD-EBL-supplemented animals [263].

Finally, it has been described that part of the mechanisms involving the hepatic beneficial effects of flavonols may be mediated by gut microbiota. An experimental approach of gut microbiota transplantation revealed a gut–liver axis where the *Akkermansia* genus have a key role on the quercetin protecting effects against obesity-associated NAFLD development. [247]. In a similar way, kaempferol blunted part of the effects of HFD in gut microbiota diversity. HFD fed mice displayed a reduced microbial diversity that it is mostly reversed by kaempferol [265]. Furthermore, IQ combined with inulin attenuated weight gain, improved glucose tolerance and insulin sensitivity and reduced lipid accumulation in the liver, adipocyte hypertrophy in WAT and diminished the circulating levels of leptin in HFD-fed mice probably through the modulation of gut microbiota [266].

6.2. Flavonols Impact on WAT Where They Modulate Lipid Metabolism and Induce Browning

Several studies with animal models showed that flavonols can protect mice or rats from HFD obesity by reducing body weight gain and lipid accumulation in WAT via reducing inflammation, modifying lipid metabolism, increasing EE, inducing browning of WAT and activating BAT [174,242,267–269].

Quercetin and quercetin-rich red onior (ROE) ameliorated diet-induced WAT expansion and inflammation in HFD-fed mice [270]. Quercetin and ROE ameliorated adipocyte size and number compared to HFD fed mice in WAT depots and induced a multilocular phenotype typical of BAT [270]. Moreover, quercetin and ROE diminished the HFD-increased levels of leptin. Besides its impact on adipose tissue phenotype, quercetin and ROE supplementation also attenuated the inflammatory profile induced by HFD in WAT [270]. Similarly, a quercetin-rich supplement administered to diet-induced obese rats decreased body fat and adipocyte size of the perirenal WAT as well as increased adiponectin circulating levels [271]. Quercetin-rich supplement attenuated the upregulation of genes related to lipid synthesis such as *Acc, Fasn, HMG-CoA reductase, Lpl, Ap2,* and *Fatty acid transporter protein 1 (Fatp1)* caused by HFD; and upregulated the HFD-downregulated genes such as *Atgl, Hsl, Ampk, Acox, Pparα,* and *Cpt1a* [271]. In diet-induced obese mice quercetin administration decreased plasma TG levels without affecting food intake, body composition, or EE [272]. Quercetin enhanced the uptake of [^{3}H]-oleate derived from labeled lipoprotein-like particles in the scWAT [272]. On the other side Perdicaro et al. demonstrated that quercetin attenuated adipose tissue hypertrophy, reduced the adipocyte size but activated the adipogenesis in HFD-fed rats. Quercetin supplemented rats showed increased levels of angiogenic (*Vascular endothelial growth factor 1* and *2 (Vegf1, Vegf2)*) and adipogenic (*Pparg* and *C/ebpa*) markers but also mitigated inflammation, and reticulum stress [273].

Together with their capacity to modulate lipid metabolism, flavonols are also able to induce browning in WAT depots. Quercetin treatment increased the expression of *Ucp1, Pgc1α* and *Elovl3* in WAT [272,274]. In a similar way, the administration of onion peel extract (rich in quercetin) to HFD-fed mice upregulated markers of BAT (*Prdm16, Pgc1α, Ucp1, Fgf21, Cidea*) in perirenal and scWAT [275]. It has been described that the induction of browning was mediated at least in part through the activation of the AMPK and the SIRT1 or via sympathetic stimulation. The quercetin-supplemented HFD-fed mice displayed higher levels of plasma norepinephrine and of PKA protein levels in scWAT [274]. Besides the activation of PKA signaling, it has been described that quercetin also increased SIRT1 protein levels and pAMPK in visceral WAT [276]. Although most of the studies showed positive effects of quercetin, this flavonol did not induce significant effects on the adipose tissue weights of rats fed an obesogenic diet except when combined with resveratrol (RSV). The treatment with quercetin and RSV but not with just quercetin or RSV promoted multilocular UCP1-positive adipocytes that also displayed increased levels of browning markers (*Cidea, bone morphogenic protein 4 (Bmp4), Homeobox C9 (Hoxc9), Solute Carrier Family 27 Member 1 (Slc27a1), Tmem26* and *proton/amino acid symporter (Pat2)*) and genes related to catabolic pathways (*Atgl* and *ATP synthase subunit delta (Atp5d)*) in perirenal WAT. Regarding BAT, the supplementation with RSV and quercetin upregulated *Cidea* and *Ucp1* expression, thus indicating more thermogenic capacity in this tissue [277].

It is worth to mention that quercetin effectiveness is specie dependent. Studies in rats usually showed more effects than in mice whilst in humans the results are still unclear. In rodent models the levels of quercetin reached after its administration are higher than in humans [269]. Similar to quercetin, isoquercetin (IQ), a quercetin glycoside with greater bioavailability than quercetin, also exerts positive effects in WAT. In normal diet-fed mice IQ supplementation decreased WAT weight and increased pAMPK levels in WAT as well as in liver and muscle. Moreover, IQ reduced the expression of *Pparγ, C/ebpα, C/ebpβ* and *Srebp1* whilst increased the expression of *Ucp2, Pgc1α, Prdm16, Sirt1* and *Cpt1a* in WAT, suggesting less adipogenesis, enhanced FAO and browning [278].

On its side, rutin administration to db/db mice and diet-induced mice reduced body weight gain and improved adiposity (smaller lipid droplets) mainly by increasing EE [279]. These animals exhibited higher core temperature when submitted to a cold environment indicating enhanced BAT activity. Rutin-treated animals overexpressed BAT markers (*Ucp1, Cidea, Prdm16*), FAO-related genes (*Cpt1a, Mcad, Pparα and Pgc1α*), mitochondrial biogenic transcription factors (*tfam, Nrf1, Nrf2*) and more copies of mitochondrial DNA in BAT [279]. Besides BAT, rutin also affected scWAT, where induces browning (upregulation of BAT-specific genes, including *Ucp1, Pgc1α, Pgc1β, Cpt1a, Pparα, Tfam, Nrf1* and *Nrf2*...) [279]. The molecular mechanism underlying these effects may go through the Sirt1 activation. It has been demonstrated that rutin was able to directly bind to Sirt1 protein and activate the SIRT/PGC1α/NRF2/Tfam signaling pathway [279]. On the other hand, rutin combined with exercise (treadmill running) in diet-induced obese mice increased the mRNA levels of *adiponectin*, the protein levels of PPARγ, the binding immunoglobulin protein (BIP), and the phosphorylated form of c-Jun terminal quinase (JNK) and reduced disulfide-bond A oxidoreductase-like protein (DsbA-L). These profile indicated an improvement on the ER stress and on adipose tissue functionality [280].

When instead of flavonols, plant extracts were used similar effects were observed. A 70% ethanol extract of *Moringa oleifera* (MO) that mainly contains quercetin, kaempferol and their derivates induced the expression of *Glut4*, *adiponectin*, *omentin* and upregulated *Pparα* and *melanocortin-4 receptor (MC4R)* on the WAT of diet-induced obese rats. [261]. *Cuscuta pedicellata* and some of its isolated compounds, including kaempferol, quercetin and some derivates were suggested to have an anti-obesity effect in HFD-fed rats. Supplemented animals showed a reduction in HOMA-IR and oxidative stress as well as exhibited an upregulation of *Ucp1* and *Cpt1a* expression in BAT [281]. Finally, through a high-throughput metabolomic approach it has been described that the consumption of a hawthorn ethanol extract that contains chlorogenic acid, hyperoside, isoquercetin, rutin, vitexin, quercetin, and apigenin affected several metabolic pathways including: fatty acid biosynthesis, galactose metabolism, biosynthesis of unsaturated fatty acids, arginine and proline metabolism, alanine, aspartate and glutamate metabolism, glycerolipid metabolism and steroid biosynthesis [282].

6.3. Flavonols: Neuroprotection in Neurodegenerative Diseases

Flavonols have shown neuroprotective effects in neurodegenerative diseases. Quercetin, rutin and some other flavonols have exhibited positive effects against pathologies such as Alzheimer's Disease (AD), Parkinson's disease, Huntington's Disease, multiple sclerosis, brain ischemic injury, epilepsy neurotoxins but also for aging cognitive alterations [238,283–288]. Furthermore, flavonols have also demonstrated beneficial effects in the CNS alterations caused by HFD.

It is well-known that HFD induces oxidative stress in brain that may lead to neurodegenerative diseases. In HFD-fed mice, quercetin ameliorated the cognitive and memory impairment and enhanced the expression of *phosphatidylinositol-4,5-bisphosphate 3-kinase (PI3K)*, *PKB/Akt*, *Creb*, and *brain-derived neurotrophic factor (Bdnf)* [289]. In a similar way, in HFD-fed mice, *Acer okamotoanum* and its main bioactive compound isoquercitin improved cognitive function by inhibiting the ROS production, the lipid peroxidation and nitric oxide formation, thus reducing oxidative stress [290]. Furthermore, it has been described that obesity induces hypothalamic inflammation and activates microglia. In diet-induced obese mice, quercetin supplementation reduced the levels of inflammatory cytokines and microglia activation markers in the hypothalamus [291]. Quercetin has also showed positive effects in streptozotocin (STZ)-induced AD rats where improved memory impairment and the anxiogenic-like behavior induced by STZ. In these rats, quercetin prevented the acetylcholinesterase (AChE) overactivity and the increased malondialdehyde levels caused by STZ [292]. Finally, quercetin showed capacity to modulate several kinases signaling cascades involved in synaptic plasticity such as the PI3K/Akt, protein kinase C (PKC) and mitogen-activated protein kinase (MAPK) [293].

7. Isoflavones

Isoflavones, also known as phytoestrogens, are flavonoids with a limited distribution in plant kingdom. They are found in leguminous plants such as soybean, kudzu, red clover, fava beans, alfalfa, chickpeas or peanuts but also soy-based foods (tofu, soymilk, miso …) and some pants such the *Puerariae* genus [42,294]. Genistein and daidzein are the most representative dietary isoflavones.

Although there are several human clinical studies studying soy isoflavone consumption and diabetes the data obtained are not conclusive. Some evidence suggests that long-term intake of isoflavones may improve insulin resistance in type 2 diabetic patients and have anti-obesity effects [295–299]. In animal studies, isoflavones have showed antidiabetic and anti-obesity activities [45,236,297,300]. The beneficial effects of isoflavones include the improvement of insulin sensitivity, lipid profile and adiposity [45,49,301–303].

7.1. Isoflavones Reduced H Steatosis by Modulating Lipid Metabolism

Like many of the other flavonoids, isoflavones also exert an hepatoprotective action [49]. A recent publication using data of the National Health and Nutrition Examination Survey from 1999 to 2010 in the USA describes an inverse correlation between urinary genistein levels and serum ALT levels in males but not in females [304]. On the other hand, in NAFLD-rodent models, genistein supplementation decreased fat accumulation, inflammation, hepatic steatosis and liver fibrosis in animal models and in humans [302]. These effects on hepatic steatosis have been described both in short- and long-term interventions [305].

One of the mechanisms proposed is the blockade of aldose reductase (AR)/polyol pathway. It has been described that some isoflavones are AR inhibitors. The inhibition of the AR/polyol pathway reduces fructose production and hepatic fat accumulation in high glucose diets as well as improved PPARα activity and enhanced FAO, thus attenuating liver steatosis in HFD-obese models [306]. Moreover, the blockade of AR/polyol pathway reduced the CYP2E1-mediated oxidative stress [306]. Other mechanism suggested for isoflavones is the downregulation of PPARγ and fat-specific protein 27 (FSP27) together with a reduction of fatty acid synthesis and increased lipolysis [307]. This mechanism was described in female rats fed with a 20% casein-diet and supplemented with soy isoflavones [307].

Effects via the activation of AMPK has been also described for genistein [308,309]. Hepatic activation of AMPK drives to an inhibition of cholesterol and fatty acid synthesis and an enhancement of FAO [310]. In high fat/high sucrose-fed rats, genistein improved lipid metabolism and ameliorated hepatic lipid accumulation. P-AMPK and p-ACC were increased while SREBP1 protein levels were decreased. Moreover, genistein downregulated the expression of *Fasn, glycerol-3-phosphate acyltransferase (Gpat)* as well as upregulated *Ppara, Cpt1a* and *Acox* [309]. A similar effect on NAFLD has been described with Puerarin, a major bioactive isoflavone compound isolated from the roots of the *Pueraria lobata*. Puerarin attenuated NAFLD development in high fat/high sucrose-fed mice via the activation of the Poly(ADP-ribose) polymerase 1 (PARP-1)/PI3K/Akt signaling pathway and lately the improvement of the mitochondrial function [311]. In HFD-obese mice, puerarin reduced TG, total cholesterol and leptin serum levels as well as decreased the hepatic lipid content. Puerarin inactivated FASN and activated AMPK, CPT and HSL as well as increased the protein levels of PPARγ. These data indicated that puerarin regulated lipid metabolism by reducing lipid synthesis and enhancing lipid consumption [312].

Positive effects on NAFLD has been also observed by combining soluble soybean polysaccharides and genistein. This combination increased the bioavailability of genistein and administered to HFD-fed mice prevented weight gain, oxidative stress inflammation and dyslipidemia. These effects on lipid profile have been related to an activation of AMPK and PPARα/PPARγ pathways and changes in the mRNA levels of *Fasn, Acc, Srebp1c* and *adipose differentiation-related protein (Adrp)* [313].

Besides genistein some of its derivatives are also active. Sophoricoside, a genistein derivate isolated from the *Sophora japonica* L, has been tested in high fructose-fed mice. Administration of sophoricoside diminished body and liver weight as well as reduced hepatic cholesterol and TG and serum levels of ALT, AST and LDL whilst increased the levels of circulating HDL. Moreover, the livers of treated-mice displayed a better inflammatory profile and an increased antioxidant capacity [314]. Calycosin, an o-methylated isoflavone showed positive effects against NAFLD-induced in HFD-fed mice. Calycosin improved insulin sensitivity, decreased the levels of ALT and AST and increased the levels of adiponectin. In the liver, calycosin blocked gluconeogenesis and lipogenesis by suppressing PEPCK G6Pase, SREBP1c and FASN, as well as induced the expression of *Gsk3β, Glut4*, increased the phosphorylation of Irs1 and Irs2 and activated farnesoid X receptor (FXR) [315].

Similar to isolated compounds, soy isoflavones (that includes genistein, daidzein and glycitein) or a soy protein preparation also reverted hepatic steatosis when administered to obese female Zucker or HFD-obese rats. Soy isoflavones reduced hepatic lipid accumulation, improved serum levels of ALT and downregulated *Srebp1c* and *Fasn* levels as well as increased the protein levels of PPARα indicating less lipogenesis and more FAO [316]. In a similar way, the intake of soy protein with isoflavones decreased the liver steatosis, reduced the levels of AST and ALT and increased the levels of leptin in female Zucker obese rats [305].

Apart from the effects of isoflavones on lipid metabolism they also exhibit anti-inflammatory properties. Genistein protected against NAFLD by targeting the arachidonic acid cascade that is responsible for the chronic inflammation [317]. Genistein supplementation to HFD-fed mice blocked the synthesis of ciclooxigeanse-1 activity and thromboxane A2 [317]. Other mechanism to explain the anti-inflammatory effect of genistein is the promotion of miR-451 [318]. In humans a randomized controlled trial described that genistein supplementation improved the inflammatory state in NAFLD patients [319].

7.2. Isoflavones Ameliorate the Weight Gain in Diet-Induced Obesity Models and Improve Lipid Metabolism in Adipose Tissue

It has been widely described that isoflavones are able to control food satiety and appetite, to ameliorate the body weight gain and fat accumulation in rodent models of obesity, to modulate fatty acid metabolism and to induce browning and BAT activation which make its use in nutritional interventions as a promising approach for weight management therapies [269]. Isoflavones reach and affect adipose tissue as it was demonstrated through a whole-transcriptome microarray analysis of the perigonadal WAT from mice fed either control diet or a soybean extract diet containing a genistein/daidzein mix. This study described the impact of soy isoflavones on adipose tissue describing 437 downregulated genes and 546 upregulated [320].

In HFD-fed rats, soy isoflavones attenuated diet-induced obesity mainly by reducing the visceral WAT depot (lower hypertrophy and less lipid accumulation). Soy isoflavones supplementation downregulated fat synthesis (reduced SREBP1 protein levels) and upregulated lipolysis (increased ATGL protein levels) in visceral WAT via the activation of AMPK and the inhibition of SREBP1 [321]. In a similar way, 6,8-diprenylgenistein (DPG), a major isoflavone of *Cudrania tricuspidata* fruits decreased the body weight of HFD-induced obese mice at least in part by the suppression of de novo lipogenesis via the AMPK activation [322]. This isoflavone reduced the expression of lipogenic genes by regulating Pparγ and C/EBPα transcriptional activity as well as leptin and adiponectin levels. DPG also regulated ACC and HMGCR [322].

Isoflavones are also present in fermented soy products. The heathy properties of these products have been also evaluated. Fermented soybean meal (SBM) administered to HFD-fed rats showed positive effects on the obese profile of these animals. The body weight gain, as well as weights of abdominal and epididymal fat were reduced. Also, the lipid profile was improved. Supplemented rats exhibited lower levels of TG, total cholesterol and LDL and higher levels of HDL compared to HFD-non supplemented rats. Moreover, in WAT, there were a decrease on the hepatic lipogenesis (downregulation of *Fasn* and *Acc*) and an increase on lipolysis (upregulation of *Lpl*) [323].

Besides their effects on lipid metabolism, isoflavones also induce browning and BAT activation [166]. Genistein administration to HFD-fed mice reduced body weight gain and scWAT mass and induced the expression of *Ucp1* and *Cidea* in WAT, indicating a browning phenotype [324]. Genistein may induce the browning phenotype by a direct upregulation of *Ucp1* expression or through an indirect pathway that would imply irisin signaling. Irisin is a myokine that induces the expression of *Ucp1* and *Tmem26* in preadipocytes [325]. This indirect mechanism describes an induction of the PGC-1α/FNDC5 pathway in skeletal muscle that lead to an increase of irisin production and secretion [325].

Formononetin and puerarin also modulate adipogenesis and thermogenesis. Formononetin attenuated visceral fat accumulation and increased EE in HFD-fed mice [326,327]. In vitro, this isoflavone downregulated *Pparγ*, *C/ebpα* and *Srebp1* probably via AMPK/β-catenin signal transduction pathway that drove its antiadipogenic effect [326]. Moreover, formononetin induced *Ucp1* expression in primary culture of mouse adipocytes [327]. In a similar way, *Puerariae lobata* root extracts (PLR) activated browning in iWAT and regulated BAT activity [328]. PLR treatment caused weight loss and improved glucose metabolism in diet-induced obese mice as well as increased EE. In BAT, PLR upregulated *Ucp1* expression (but no other thermogenic markers) and in iWAT induced the expression of BAT markers (*Ucp1*, *Pparγ1*, *Pparγ2* and *Pparα*), thus indicating a brown-like phenotype [328].

Several studies focused on describing the mechanisms underlying the isoflavones' effects have been performed in ovariectomized mice or rats. These models mimic menopausal stage in humans and are useful to analyze the potential role of isoflavones to counteract the increase of the adipose tissue that takes place during this period of life. In these rodent models, isoflavones exert positive effects on body weight gain and food intake as well as in fat pats enlargement [297]. In HFD-fed ovariectomized rats the administration of genistein decreased the body weight gain, improved insulin sensitivity and reduced plasma TG and cholesterol [329]. In liver, genistein blocked the lipogenic pathway by inhibiting p-ACC, SREBP-1, FASN and CD36 proteins. In retroperitoneal WAT, genistein diminished adiposity and adipocyte hypertrophy, inflammatory phenotype and induced browning. In iWAT, genistein-supplemented rats exhibited higher levels of UCP1, PRDM16, PGC-1α and CIDEA proteins and *Ppargc1a* and *Ucp-1* mRNAs [329]. Furthermore, isoflavones supplementation can modulate the metabolic effects of estradiol treatments in ovariectomized rats [330]. Finally, calycosin has demonstrated positive effects perivascular adipose tissue of obese mice. Through the adiponectin/AMPK/ endothelial nitric oxide synthase (eNOS) pathway, calycosin is able to restore at least in part the perivascular adipose tissue functionality [331].

7.3. Isoflavones Have Become Engaging Flavonoids in Neuronal Diseases due to Their Estrogenic-Like Structure and Its High Antioxidant Capacity

Obesity is a risk factor for neurodegenerative diseases essentially because it causes the neuroinflammation and oxidative stress. Isoflavones can ameliorate part of these effects as well as affect food intake and feeding behavior.

It has been described that daidzein administered to HFD-fed rats reduced food intake and attenuated body weight gain as well as improved glucose tolerance, adiponectin and leptin levels and increased the 17b-estradiol. In rat hippocampus, daidzein enhanced cell proliferation and reduced apoptosis and gliosis, thus exerting a neuroprotective effect against the brain injuries caused by diet [332]. On the other side, doenjang, a Korean traditional fermented soybean pastry alleviated hippocampal neuronal loss and enhanced cell proliferation in HFD-fed mice as well as reduced oxidative stress markers (less oxidative metabolites and lower levels of oxidative stress- and neuroinflammation-related genes). Dietary doenjang reduced Aβ and tau phosphorylation [333]. Furthermore, genistein has shown the capacity to improve metabolism and induce browning via hypothalamus gene expression regulation. Through a transcriptome analysis it was identified that the hypothalamic expression of *urocortin 3 (Ucn3)*, *decidual protein induced by progesterone (Depp)*, and *stanniocalcin1 (Stc1)* correlated with the browning markers in WAT and with insulin sensitivity [324].

Regarding neurodegenerative diseases isoflavones have shown protective properties. An extract of soybean isoflavone reduced the elevated oxidative stress parameters and reversed the overproduction of Aβ in rats with colchicine-induced neuronal damage [334]. In the same way, daidzein alone or mixed with genistein and glycitin isoflavones could reverse the cognitive impairments produced by scopolamine injection by activating the cholinergic system and the BDNF/ERK/CREB signaling pathway in mice [335,336], thus reinforcing the idea that soy isoflavones may be a good candidate for the treatment of neurodegenerative diseases. Besides the BDNF/ERK/CREB signaling pathway, it has been postulated that the Nrf2 signaling pathway can also be underlying the neuroprotective effects of isoflavones [337].

8. Flavones

Flavones is one of the largest groups of flavonoids with a high degree of chemical diversity. Some of the richest sources of flavones are parsley, celery, peppermint, and sage, which predominantly contain apigenin and luteolin as well as maize and citrus fruits. In general, flavones are found as glucosides in citrus fruits, vegetables, herbs and grains and although they represent a small fraction of the total flavonoid intake, they have shown health effects and anti-obesity properties [338,339]. As it is going to described latter, most of the studies that investigate the beneficial effects of flavones use them as aglycone and a scarce number of approaches deepen on the effects of flavones when consumed within the whole food and a feasible doses or in combination with other bioactive compounds.

8.1. Flavones Improved Liver Steatosis and Hepatic Inflammation

Flavones such as apigenin, luteolin, baicalin, vitexin, nobiletin among others prevented NAFLD and hepatic steatosis mainly by modulating lipid metabolism (increasing FAO and decreasing lipogenesis) and reducing oxidative stress and inflammation [340–345].

As many other flavonoids, some flavones also exert their hepatic effects by activating the AMPK enzyme. Vitexin, an apigenin flavone glucoside, for instance, when administered to HFD-fed mice reduced body and liver weight, triglyceride and cholesterol content in serum and liver and circulating levels of ALT and AST. Moreover, vitexin regulated lipid metabolism suppressing de novo lipogenesis by downregulating the expression of *Pparγ*, *C/ebpα*, *Srebp1c*, *Fasn*, and *Acc* and enhancing FAO and lipolysis by increasing the expression of *Pparα*, *Cpt1a* and *Atgl*) in an AMPK-dependent way that has been suggested may be activated by the binding of vitexin to the Leptin receptor [345].

In a similar way, luteolin, the principal yellow dye compound from *Reseda luteola*, or luteolin-enriched artichoke leaf extract alleviated hepatic alterations caused by a HFD by exerting anti-inflammatory activities and modulating lipid metabolism. Luteolin treatment of HFD-fed mice reduced hepatic lipotoxicity by improving the inflammatory profile, decreasing the extracellular matrix, enhancing the antioxidant capacity of the liver and increasing the FFA flux between liver and WAT [346]. A crosstalk between adipose tissue and liver has been suggested to explain the effects of luteolin on hepatic steatosis [347]. Moreover, luteolin and luteolin-enriched artichoke leaf extract administered to HFD-fed mice prevented hepatic steatosis (less and smaller lipid droplets, lower levels of *Cidea*) and insulin resistance by suppressing lipogenesis and gluconeogenesis (suppression of PEPCK and G6Pase activities) and increasing FAO (more CPT1a activity and higher expression of *Pparα*, *Pgc1α* and *Pgc1β*) [342]. The repression of hepatocyte nuclear factor 4a and of LXR/SREBP1c signaling pathway has been described as putative molecular mechanisms for luteolin improvement of liver steatosis and NAFLD [348,349].

Regarding the capacity of flavones to modulate FAO, it has been described through a quantitative proteomic study that baicalin may act as an allosteric activator of CPT1a enzyme thus increasing the FA entrance to the mitochondria to undergo the β-oxidation in the liver [343]. Moreover, baicalin attenuated liver alterations by regulating the AMPK/ACC pathway in diet-induced obese mice [350]. Finally, baicalin is also a potent anti-inflammatory and antioxidant compound in a way that as other flavones also implied the nuclear erythroid 2-related factor 2 (Nrf2) activity in a cholestatic mice model [351].

It has been described that some flavones exert their hepatoprotective effects via the activation of the Nrf2 transcription factor. Nrf2 is a positive regulator of the expression of genes involved in the protection against oxidative stress as well as a negative regulator of genes that promote hepatic steatosis [352,353]. In this context, apigenin and scutellarin exerted their hepatoprotective activity via the activation of Nrf2. Scutellarin is a natural compound of *Erigeron breviscapus* (vant.) that in a HFD-fed mice attenuated obesity. It repressed lipogenesis and promoted FAO and cholesterol output besides its anti-inflammatory activity [340]. Moreover it has been described that scutellarin increased mRNA and/or protein levels of PPARγ, PGC1α, Nrf2, haem oxygenase-1 (HO-1), glutathione S-transferase (GST), NAD(P)H quinone dehydrogenase 1 (NQO1) and PI3K and AKT, whilst reduced nuclear factor kappa B (NF-κB), Kelch-like ECH-associated protein 1 (Keap1) [354,355]. By contrast, apigenin administration to HFD-fed mice inhibited the expression of PPARγ target genes via the translocation to the nucleus and activation of the Nrf2 transcription factor that seems to block PPARγ activity. Apigenin treatment downregulated the expression of genes related to lipid droplet formation (*Cidea*, *Plin2*, fat storage inducing transmembrane protein 1 and 2 and) as well as genes involved in FA uptake

(*Fabp1* and *Lpl*), FAO (*Cpt1a, Pdk4, Acox1, Acaa2*) and lipogenesis (*Fasn, Scd11, Acaca*) [341]. On the other side, apigenin may act as a PPARγ modulator in a mouse model of obesity where it activated the p65/PPARγ complex translocation into the nucleus, thereby decreasing the NF-κB activation and favoring the M2 macrophage polarization [356] or blocking NLRP3 inflammasome assembly and the ROS production [357]. The capacity of flavones to modulate PPARγ activity and induce macrophage polarization to M2 phenotype has also been described for Chrysin in a HFD-fed mice model [358].

Finally, wogonin have shown beneficial effects on the liver steatosis development in a mice NAFLD model [359]. Concretely wogonin administration to HFD fed mice ameliorated the NAFLD progression via enhancing the PPARα/Adiponectin receptor R2 (AdipoR2) pathway. Wogonin induced the hepatic activity of PPARα and upregulated the levels of the AdipoR2. Moreover, wogonin also reduced the inflammatory profile and alleviated the hepatic oxidative stress [359].

Besides their effects alone, the combination of flavones with other bioactive compounds or polyphenols-rich extracts have also shown positive effects against hepatic steatosis [360].

8.2. Flavones Improved the Adipose Tissue Inflammation and Reduced the Macrophages Infiltration as Well as Enhanced the Thermogenic Capacity

Although flavones have been widely studied for their antioxidant and anti-inflammatory properties [338] their capacity to impact on adipose tissue metabolism and functionality cannot be underestimated.

Besides its reduction of the inflammatory phenotype in adipose tissue, apigenin administration to diet-induced obese mice ameliorated the body weight increment, reduced the visceral adiposity by inhibiting the adipogenesis via a STAT3/CD36 signaling pathway [361], decreased leptin and increased adiponectin [362] and induced energy expenditure mainly by promoting lipolysis and FAO as well as browning of WAT [363]. In scWAT, apigenin-treated mice exhibited a downregulation of adipogenic genes (*Pparγ, Lpl* and *aP2*) and of genes involved in lipogenesis (*Fasn* and *Scd1*) and a promotion of lipolysis by increasing the mRNA levels of *Atgl, Hsl, Forkhead box protein O1 (FoxO1)* and *Sirt1*. In BAT there is an increment of the p-AMPK and p-ACC levels, thus indicating that FAO is enhanced in this fat depot after apigenin administration. Finally, apigenin activated the thermogenesis in BAT (upregulation of *Ucp1* and *Pgc1α*) and induced the browning phenotype in scWAT (upregulation of *Ucp1, Pgc1α, Tmem26, Cited1*) [363]. Similar results were obtained with vitexin. Vitexin administration reduced the adipocyte size of HFD-fed mice and increased the p-AMPK levels in eWAT followed by a downregulation of C/EBPa and FASN protein levels [364].

In the case of nobiletin and luteolin, their administration to HFD-fed mice improved the fibrotic and inflammatory profile in adipose tissue and reduced the macrophage infiltration and polarization [344,346,365,366]; but in contrast with other flavones they increased the mRNA expression of FAO- (*Pparα, Cox8b,* and *Cpt1a*) and lipogenic (*Pparγ, Srebp1c, Fasn* and *Scd1*) -related genes simultaneously [342,344] as well as CPT1 and FASN activity [344] in WAT. The simultaneously activation of both metabolic pathways in adipose tissues has been demonstrated as a way to maintain thermogenesis in BAT [367,368] and as a marker of browning in WAT [82]. In the case of luteolin, its administration either in HFD-fed or low-fat-fed mice activated browning and thermogenesis in mice via the AMPK/PGC1α cascade. Under the AMPK/PGC1α signal, luteolin increased energy expenditure in HFD-fed mice and upregulated the mRNA levels of *Pgc1α, PPARα, Cidea* and *Sirt1* in BAT as well as *Ucp1 Pgc1α, Tmem26, Cidea, PPARα, Sirt1, Elovl3* and *Cited1* in scWAT [369]. Moreover, the increased of PPARγ protein levels in WAT has been linked to an alleviation of the hepatic lipotoxicity in HFD-fed mice [347]. Similar effects were observed with baicalein that administered to HFD-fed mice decreased pP38MAPK, pERK and PPARγ levels and increased pAKT, PGC1α and UCP1 as well as the presence of GLUT4 in cell membranes of the eWAT. Globally, baicalein reversed the glucose intolerance and insulin resistance produced by HFD [370].

Besides the effects of each compound by itself some flavones-rich extracts or foods or combinations of different bioactive compounds have been evaluated regarding their potential therapeutic role against obesity and its metabolic and inflammatory features [371,372].

8.3. Flavones and Obesity in the CNS- No Clear Evidences

There are few studies describing the potential role of flavones in obesity-related central alterations. Just luteolin has been demonstrated a protective effect against HFD-induced cognitive effects in obese mice. Luteolin administration alleviated neuroinflammation, oxidative stress and neuronal insulin resistance as well as improved the Morris water maze (MWM) and step-through task and increased the levels of BDNF [373]. Other effects of flavones described recently are anxiolytic-like activity [374], neuroprotection against gamma-radiation [375] treatment of glioblastoma [376], amelioration of the hypoxia-reoxygenation injury [377] or inhibition of the neuroinflammation caused by LPS [378].

9. Chalcones

Chalcones is a group of polyphenolic compounds with a broad structural diversity. Chalcones are precursors of other flavonoids and responsible for the golden yellow pigments found in flowers, fruits, vegetables, spices, teas and different plant tissues. Although their metabolism in the gastrointestinal tract and their rate of absorption are not still completely known, chalcones have shown a wide variety of biological activities. Several studies have demonstrated that, either from natural sources or synthetic, chalcones can impact on glucose and lipid metabolism and their health benefits have been studied in relation to type 2 diabetes [379]. Chalcones have shown hypoglycemic capacity, the ability to modulate food intake and activate AMPK, as well as antioxidant, anti-inflammatory, anticancer, anti-obesity, hepatoprotective and neuroprotective properties [380–392] Although there are no many studies in humans the effects of chalcones in the obese phenotype in animal models are similar to the ones described for other flavonoids, thus suggesting a potential therapeutic role of these group of bioactive compounds.

9.1. The Hepatoprotective Role of Chalcones

Chalcones have hepatoprotective properties in NAFLD, alcoholic fatty liver, drug- and toxicant-induced liver injury, and liver cancer [381]. It has been described that chalcones are able to inhibit the synthesis of triglycerides and the lipogenesis, to increase FAO, and to modulate adiponectin production and signaling.

Licochalcone F, a novel synthetic retrochalcone, has shown anti-inflammatory properties when administered to diet-induced obese mice. Licochalcone F inhibited TNFa-induced NF-kB activation and the mRNA expression of several pro-inflammatory markers. In the liver licochalcone F alleviated hepatic steatosis, by decreasing lipid droplets and glycogen deposition [380]. On its side, Licochalcone A, a chalcone isolated from *Glycyrrhiza uralensis*, administered to HFD-fed mice, reduced body weight, decreased serum triglycerides, LDL free fatty acids and fasting blood glucose, ameliorated hepatic steatosis, reduced lipid droplet accumulation [393]. In the liver, licochalcone A downregulated the protein levels of SREBP1c, PPARγ, and FASN as well as increased the phosphorylation of HSL, ATGL and ACC enzymes [393]. Moreover, licochalcone A increase the protein levels of CPT1A and stimulated SIRT1 and AMPK activity [393]. Taken together, licochalcone A ameliorated obesity and NAFLD in mice at least in part by reducing the fatty acid synthesis and increasing lipolysis and FAO via the activation of the SIRT1/AMPK pathway.

In a mouse model of HFD-induced obesity, *trans*-chalcone reduced the ALT levels and increased the HDL [394]. Similarly, in a mouse model of non-alcoholic steatohepatitis KK-Ay mice, xanthohumol, the chalcone from beer hops (*Humulus lupulus* L.), diminished hepatic inflammation and prevented from the expression of profibrogenic genes in the liver [395] as well as lowered hepatic fatty acid synthesis through the downregulation of *Srebp1c* expression and promoted FAO by upregulating the mRNA expression of *Pparα* in KK-Ay mice [396]. Moreover, in HFD-fed mice, xanthohumol prevented body weight gain; decreased glycemia, triglyceride and cholesterol, and improved insulin sensitivity. Xanthohumol activated the hepatic and skeletal muscle AMPK, downregulated the expression of *Srebp1c* and *Fasn* and inhibited the activity of ACC, thus reducing the lipogenic pathway [386,397].

According to these data, aspalathin a C-glucosyl dihydrochalcone present in rooibos tea from *Aspalathus linearis*, also activated AMPK and reduced the expression of hepatic enzymes and transcriptional regulators that are associated with either gluconeogenesis and/or lipogenesis (*Acc*, *Fasn*, *Scd*) in diabetic *ob/ob* mice [388,398]. Furthermore, Aspalathin-enriched green rooibos extract (GRE) improved hepatic insulin resistance via the regulation of the PI3K/AKT and AMPK Pathways [399]. In obese insulin resistant rats GRE upregulated the expression of *Glut2*, *insulin receptor (Insr)*, *Irs1* and *Irs2*, as well as *Cpt1a* [399]. Finally, Isoliquiritigenin at a low dose ameliorated insulin resistance and NAFLD in diet-induced obese mice. Isoliquiritigenin administration to HFD-fed mice decreased body fat mass and plasma cholesterol as well as alleviated hepatic steatosis (smaller lipid droplets) with no changes in TG and FFA serum levels [400]. It has been described that isoliquiritigenin suppressed the expression of lipogenic genes (*Fasn* and *Scd1*) and increased FAO activity. Moreover, isoliquiritigenin improved the insulin signaling in the liver and muscle [400].

Besides chalcones, chalcones-enriched products like Safflower yellow or ashitaba have demonstrated hepatoprotective properties. In mice fed with HFD, Safflower yellow improved lipid profile and alleviated fatty liver in a mechanism that has been associated to a reduction of the biosynthesis of intracellular cholesterol. Safflower yellow significantly reduced the levels of total cholesterol, triglycerides, LDL-cholesterol and the LDL/HDL ratio [401]. On its side, ashitaba (*Angelica keiskei*) extract showed hepatoprotective activity in fructose-induced dyslipidemia due to increased expression of FAO genes in the liver. Treatment with this extract upregulated the expression of the *Acox1*, *Mcad*, *ATP-binding membrane cassette transporter A1 (ABCA1)* and *apolipoprotein A1 (Apo-A1)* [402]. In a similar way, this extract exerted hepatoprotective effects in HFD-fed mice. Ashitaba extract reduced plasma levels of cholesterol, glucose, and insulin, lowered triglyceride and cholesterol content in the liver, inhibited hepatic lipogenesis by downregulating *Srebp1* and *Fasn* and activated FAO by upregulating the expression of *Cpt1A* and *Ppara* [403]. The proposed mechanism underlying this hepatic metabolic effects is an activation of the AMPK enzyme in the liver [403].

In some of the studies the hepatoprotective role of chalcones has been linked to the adiponectin production. Concretely, trans-chalcone administration to high cholesterol diet-induced liver fibrosis increased the serum levels of adiponectin and the hepatic antioxidant enzymes, thus alleviating liver damage [404]. Similarly, xanthohumol and ashitaba extract or licochalcone A also increased the adiponectin expression and secretion [393,403,405].

9.2. Chalcones in the Adipose Tissue, Upregulation of Adiponectin, Induction of Browning and Enhancement of Energy Expenditure

As has been mentioned above, chalcones induce adiponectin expression and secretion but also improve adipocytes function and reduce fat depots. Different molecular mechanisms underlying these effects has been described.

The treatment of obese mice with licochalcone F to reduced adipocyte size and ameliorated macrophage infiltration in WAT depots as well as enhanced Akt signaling and reduced p38 MAPK pathway [380]. On its side, the administration of Licochalcone A, isoliquiritigenin or a *Glycyrrhiza uralensis* extract containing licochalcone A, isoliquiritigenin, and liquiritigenin to diet-induced obese mice reduced body weight gain and adipose tissues depots [393,400,406]. In this case, Licochalcone A and *Glycyrrhiza uralensis* extract induced the browning phenotype in the iWAT this fat depot [393,406] as it is demonstrated by the enhanced expression of brown fat markers such as *Ucp1*, *Prdm16* and *Pgc1α* [406]. By contrast, isoliquiritigenin elevated energy expenditure by increasing the expression of thermogenic genes (*Ucp1* and *Prdm16*) as well as *Sirt1* that is linked to mitochondrial biogenesis [407] in interscapular BAT [400].

Finally, butein, besides its anti-inflammatory activity via the p38 MAPK/Nrf2/HO-1 pathway that leads to a reduction of the adipocyte hypertrophy [408] is also capable to enhance energy expenditure and increase thermogenesis. Butein induced the browning phenotype in the iWAT (upregulation of *Ucp1, Prdm16, cytochrome C oxidase 8b,* and *Cidea*) and increased the UCP1 protein levels in BAT in HFD-fed mice as well as in lean mice. The proposed molecular mechanism underlying these effects is the induction of the PR domain containing 4 (Prdm4) and the activation of the PI3Kα/Akt1/PR domain containing 4 (Prdm4) axis [409,410]. The browning effect of butein was not observed in other mice models such as ThermoMouse strain nor in methionine- and choline-deficient diet-fed mice [411]. Butein actions have also been linked to its capacity to downregulate PPARγ expression [387,410].

Finally, chalcone-rich extracts such as Safflower yellow or Ashitaba extract have also demonstrated effects in adipose tissues. Concretely, in mice fed with HFD, Safflower yellow administration exerts anti-obesity and insulin-sensitizing effects by upregulating the expression of *Pgc1α* that may indicate a browning phenotype of the scWAT as well as activating the protein levels of AKT and GSK3β in visceral WAT [412]. On its side, Ashitaba extract suppressed the HF diet-induced body weight gain and fat deposition in WAT, increased the adiponectin level and the phosphorylation AMPK, inhibited lipogenesis by downregulating *Pparγ, CCAAT/enhancer-binding protein α (C/ebpα)* and *Srebp1* [403].

9.3. Chalcones in CNS: A Potential Neuroprotective Role

The antioxidant and anti-inflammatory properties of chalcones has been linked to some of their neuroprotective effects [382,383,389] but no studies with obesity-related neuronal damage has been found. Further studies are needed to identify the potential therapeutic role of chalcones on this obesity side effect.

10. Concluding Remarks

Undoubtedly flavonoids are potential therapeutic agents against metabolic disorders such as obesity, type 2 diabetes or NAFLD. Their impact in CNS, liver, and adipose tissue has been extensively studied and the results let us to be optimistic. Several metabolic effects and signaling pathways have been described underlying the anti-obesity effects of flavonoids specially in liver, EAT and BAT but also in CNS. Globally theses effects go to control body weight, improve insulin sensitivity, reduce fat accumulation in adipose tissues as well in ectopic depots and to increase energy expenditure (Figure 1). Furthermore, the data presented in this review highlight that:

- Flavonoids are effective over a high variety of obesity and obesity-related diseases models.
- The anti-obesity effects of flavonoids are robust and consistent as they can be achieved using different sources, ways of administration and doses.
- Most of the molecular mechanisms underlying the anti-obesity effects of flavonoids are shared for the different subclasses of flavonoids (Tables 2 and 3).

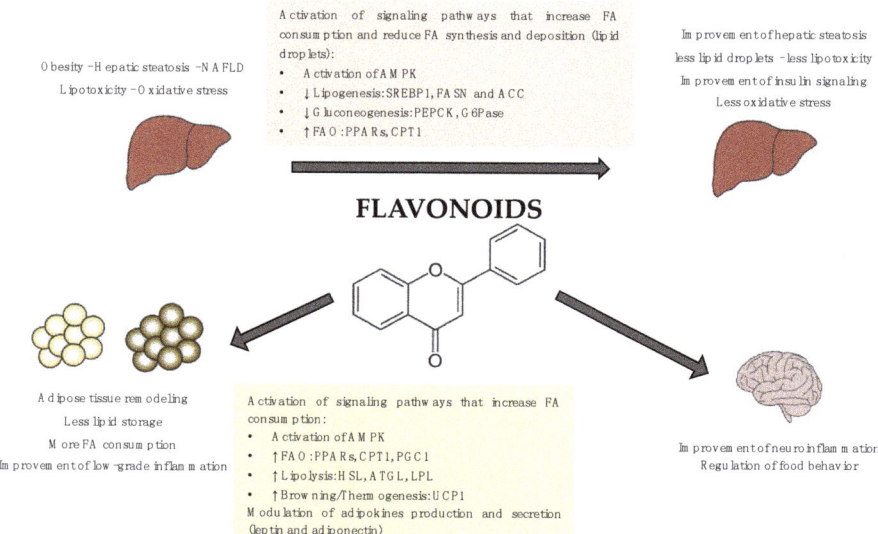

Figure 1. Summary of the metabolic and signaling pathways underlying the anti-obesity effects of flavonoids. Molecular mechanisms underlying the beneficial effects of flavonoids have been widely studied and, in many cases, involved the activation of the AMP-activated protein kinase (AMPK). AMPK is a key enzyme for the control of lipid metabolism and adipogenesis. AMPK phosphorylation and activation promote catabolic processes such as FAO, glucose uptake, or glycolysis as well as inhibits anabolic pathways such as fatty acid synthesis or gluconeogenesis.

Even so more research is needed to confirm their therapeutically functionality in humans, the doses and times needed for their effectiveness or the better combination of bioactive compounds. Nowadays is still difficult to answer some crucial questions such as what is the effective dose of polyphenols; and for how long do we need to intake them to get positive effects? It is obvious that differences among experimental diets to induce fatty liver, dosages of bioactive compounds as well as the presence of other food compounds or the use of isolated or extracted polyphenols could influence the outcomes obtained. Furthermore, the use of flavonoids as a preventive or for treatment also show different results. Usually, the doses used in published papers are much higher than the ones reached from fruits and vegetables consumed as a whole.

The Predimed study determined that Spanish adults should intake around 820 ± 323 mg of polyphones/day in a 2000 Kcal diet to get their beneficial effects [25,27] but probably these effects at this dose are closely related to the MedDiet lifestyle. It is evident that, as MedDiet, some other dietary patterns include high amounts of fruits, vegetables or polyphenols-rich beverages that make possible to reach the optimal doses of polyphenols and by extension of flavonoids. Then, the question is: Are the effects of polyphenols linked to the dietary pattern where they are included? Two recent systematic reviews analyzed if there are enough evidence to define a health promoting polyphenol-rich dietary pattern and concluded that the high variability in the experimental approaches and methods used to evaluate polyphenols intake and health outcomes make difficult to stablish specific polyphenol intake recommendations and to clarify whether total flavonoids or rather individual subclasses may exert beneficial effects [30,36].

Moreover, low is known about the effects of combining different bioactive compounds from different families. Are they going to have synergic, additive or antagonic effects? And not less important is the need to identify the role of the food matrix on polyphenols and flavonoid effects.

Table 2. Metabolic effects and signaling pathways underlying the anti-obesity effects of flavonoids in the liver.

Liver	Anthocyanins	Flavanols	Flavanones	Flavonols
Signaling pathways	Activation of the AMPK Inactivation of mTOR pathway	Activation of the AMPK. Activation of SIRT and SIRT/FoxO1 pathway. Activation of the PKB/AKT—p-GSK3α and p-PTEN Activation of PKA Inactivation of mTOR pathway Activation of the PXR/CAR-mediated phase II metabolism	Activation of the AMPK Activation of AMPK/SIRT1/PGC1α axis Activation of FGF21 signaling	Activation of the AMPK Activation of AMPK/PGC1α/ERRα axis Inactivation of LXR/SREBP1c axis Inactivation of mTOR pathway Inhibition of the PKB/AKT—downregulation of SREBP1 ↑ Adiponectin signaling
Lipid metabolism	↓ Lipogenesis and TG synthesis ↑ FA consumption (FAO) ↓ Lipid droplets	↓ Lipogenesis and TG synthesis ↑ FA consumption (FAO) ↓ Lipid droplets ↓ Cholesterol synthesis and bile acids reabsorption	↓ Lipogenesis and TG synthesis ↑ FA consumption (FAO) ↓ Lipid droplets	↓ Lipogenesis and TG synthesis ↑ FA consumption (FAO) ↓ Lipid droplets ↓ Cholesterol synthesis
Glucose metabolism	↓ Gluconeogenesis ↑ Glucose transport ↑ Glycolysis ↑ Insulin signaling	↓ Gluconeogenesis	↓ Gluconeogenesis ↓ Glucose transport ↑ Glycolysis	↑ Glucose transport ↑ Insulin signaling

LIVER	Isoflavones	Flavones	Chalcones
Signaling pathways	Activation of the AMPK Blockade of aldose reductase (AR)/polyol pathway Activation of the PKB/AKT	Activation of the AMPK. Inactivation of LXR/SREBP1c axis. Nuclear erythroid 2-related factor 2 (Nrf2) and PPARγ activity ↑ Adiponectin signaling	Activation of the AMPK Activation of AMPK/SIRT pathway Activation PI3K/AKT/PRDM4 signaling
Lipid metabolism	↓ Lipogenesis and TG synthesis ↑ FA consumption (FAO) ↓ Cholesterol synthesis	↓ Lipogenesis and TG synthesis ↑↓ FA consumption (FAO)	↓ Lipogenesis and TG synthesis ↑ FA consumption (FAO) ↓ Lipid droplets ↓ Cholesterol synthesis
Glucose metabolism	↓ Gluconeogenesis ↑ Glucose transport ↑ Insulin signaling	↓ Gluconeogenesis	↓ Gluconeogenesis ↑ Glucose transport ↑ Insulin signaling

Table 3. Metabolic effects and signaling pathways underlying the anti-obesity effects of flavonoids in the adipose tissues.

Adipose Tissue	Anthocyanins	Flavanols	Flavanones	Flavonols
Signaling pathways	Activation of the AMPK Activation of SIRT and SIRT/FoxO1 pathway Activation of the FDNC5/Irisin pathway ↑ FGF21 signaling	Activation of b-adrenergic receptor—↑ cAMP/PKA Inhibition of the PDE ↑ Adiponectin signaling		Activation of b-adrenergic receptor—↑ cAMP/PKA Activation of the AMPK/SIRT1 pathway Activation of SIRT1/PGC1α axis
Adipokines	↓ Leptin ↑ Adiponectin		↓ Leptin ↑ Adiponectin	↑ Adiponectin
Adipose tissue profile	↑ Browning and Thermogenesis ↓ Adipogenesis	↑ Browning and Thermogenesis ↓ Adipogenesis	↑ Browning and Thermogenesis	↑ Browning and Thermogenesis ↓↑ Adipogenesis
Lipid metabolism	↑ FA consumption (lipolysis and FAO) ↓↑ Lipogenesis and TG synthesis ↓ Lipid droplets	↑ FA consumption (lipolysis and FAO) ↓↑ Lipogenesis and TG synthesis	↑ FA consumption (lipolysis and FAO) ↓↑ Lipogenesis and TG synthesis	↑ FA consumption (lipolysis and FAO) ↓↑ Lipogenesis and TG synthesis
Glucose metabolism	↑ Glucose transport		↑ Glucose transport	↑ Glucose transport

ADIPOSE TISSUE	Isoflavones	Flavones		Chalcones
Signaling pathways	Activation of the AMPK Activation of the FDNC5/Irisin pathway	Activation of the AMPK Activation of the AMPK/PGC1α axis Activation of the STAT3/CD36 signaling pathway		Activation of the AMPK Activation PI3K/AKT signaling
Adipokines	↓ Leptin ↑ Adiponectin			↑ Adiponectin
Adipose tissue profile	↑ Browning and Thermogenesis	↑ Browning and Thermogenesis ↓ Adipogenesis		↑ Browning and Thermogenesis
Lipid metabolism	↑ FA consumption (lipolysis and FAO) ↓ Lipid droplets ↓↑ Lipogenesis and TG synthesis	↑ FA consumption (lipolysis and FAO) ↓ Lipid droplets ↓↑ Lipogenesis and TG synthesis		↑ FA consumption (lipolysis and FAO) ↓↑ Lipogenesis and TG synthesis
Glucose metabolism		↑ Glucose transport		

The bioavailability of polyphenols is low and not just their basic chemical structures (aglycons) are key but also the attachment of additional groups. There are described around 8000 structures of polyphenols with different physiological impact and several chemical structures, but all of them with at least one a phenolic ring with one or more hydroxyl groups attached [38,413,414]. The polyphenols absorption in human body is dose- and type-dependent and their effects are related to their bioavailability and pharmacokinetics. They show a low absorption rate and limited stability during pass through the intestinal tract where microbiome may contribute to their absorption. Once absorbed, polyphenols enter portal circulation and are metabolized in the liver. This first pass metabolism modifies the polyphenol structure and in consequence its bioavailability and bioactivity [415,416]. Finally, the conjugate metabolites reach the bloodstream and the target tissues [415–418].

Several studies have demonstrated that the bioavailability and safety of polyphenols changed when they are included in a food matrix [419–421]. Although most of the assays has been done with in vitro models of digestion [422] it seems that the food matrices protect bioactive compounds from intestinal degradation [420,423]. Finally, also cooking processes would have an impact in the polyphenols content and bioavailability of some preparations [424–426]. On the other side, it has been described that bioactive compounds with antioxidant properties are safe and beneficial but that exogenous supplementation with isolated compounds can be toxic [427].

The role of intestinal digestion and microbiota impact on polyphenols' effects must be also considered. Besides their direct action in the liver, some flavonoids may exert their metabolic effects through the gut microbiota modulation. An experimental approach with rabbits described that procyanidin b2 may downregulated fatty acid synthesis genes and protected against obesity and NAFLD by increasing the ratio of *Bacteroidetes* and *Akkermansia* [159]. Similar results were obtained with green tea oolong tea and black tea water extracts that administered to HFD-fed mice improved the glucose tolerance and reduced the weight gained caused by the HFD. Moreover, these animals showed a better hepatic lipid profile and a reduced mass of the WAT. These effects were accompanied by a reduction in plasma LPS, thus indicating less production and a significant increase in the production of short-chain fatty acids (SCFAs). A metagenomic analysis indicated that the tea extracts changed the gut microbiota's composition [428]. In the same way also flavones 'effects on obesity has been linked to gut microbiota modifications [338]. Oral hydroxysafflor yellow A (HSYA) reversed the HFD-induced gut microbiota dysbiosis and reduced the obese phenotype [429].

Author Contributions: V.S., H.S.-L., G.A. and J.R. performed the literature research and wrote the first draft of the manuscript; P.F.M., D.H. and J.R. evaluated the information, reviewed and edited the manuscript to define its last version. All authors have read and agreed to the published version of the manuscript.

Funding: This study was supported by the Ministerio de Economía y Competitividad [grants AGL2017-82417-R to PFM and DH, by the Generalitat de Catalunya [grants 2017SGR683, VS was supported by Conicyt's fellowship from the Government of Chile. The APC was funded by the University of Barcelona.

Acknowledgments: We acknowledge Jacques Truffert for the images used in Table 1 and Ursula Martínez-Garza for the images used in Figure 1. Chemical structures of flavonoids' subclasses from Table 1 have been done with Chemdraw®.

Conflicts of Interest: The authors declare no conflict of interest.

References

1. Romieu, I.; Dossus, L.; Barquera, S.; Blottiere, H.M.; Franks, P.W.; Gunter, M.; Hwalla, N.; Hursting, S.D.; Leitzmann, M.; Margetts, B.; et al. Energy balance and obesity: What are the main drivers? *Cancer Causes Control* **2017**, *28*, 247–258. [PubMed]
2. Eckel, R.H.; Kahn, S.E.; Ferrannini, E.; Goldfine, A.B.; Nathan, D.M.; Schwartz, M.W.; Smith, R.J.; Smith, S.R. Obesity and type 2 diabetes: What can be unified and what needs to be individualized? *J. Clin. Endocrinol. Metab.* **2011**, *96*, 1654–1663. [CrossRef] [PubMed]
3. O'Neill, S.; O'Driscoll, L. Metabolic syndrome: A closer look at the growing epidemic and its associated pathologies. *Obes. Rev.* **2015**, *16*, 1–12. [CrossRef] [PubMed]

4. Picone, P.; Di Carlo, M.; Nuzzo, D. Obesity and Alzheimer disease: Molecular bases. *Eur. J. Neurosci.* **2020**, 1–7. [CrossRef]
5. Mazon, J.N.; de Mello, A.H.; Ferreira, G.K.; Rezin, G.T. The impact of obesity on neurodegenerative diseases. *Life Sci.* **2017**, *182*, 22–28. [CrossRef] [PubMed]
6. Samson, S.L.; Garber, A.J. Metabolic syndrome. *Endocrinol. Metab. Clin. N. Am.* **2014**, *43*, 1–23. [CrossRef]
7. Peirce, V.; Carobbio, S.; Vidal-Puig, A. The different shades of fat. *Nature* **2014**, *510*, 76–83. [CrossRef]
8. Carobbio, S.; Pellegrinelli, V.; Vidal-Puig, A. Adipose Tissue Function and Expandability as Determinants of Lipotoxicity and the Metabolic Syndrome. *Adv. Exp. Med. Biol.* **2017**, *960*, 161–196.
9. Reagan, L.P. Insulin signaling effects on memory and mood. *Curr. Opin. Pharmacol.* **2007**, *7*, 633–637. [CrossRef]
10. Craft, S. Insulin Resistance and Alzheimers Disease Pathogenesis: Potential Mechanisms and Implications for Treatment. *Curr. Alzheimer Res.* **2007**, *4*, 147–152. [CrossRef]
11. Pugazhenthi, S.; Qin, L.; Reddy, P.H. Common neurodegenerative pathways in obesity, diabetes, and Alzheimer's disease. *Biochim. Biophys. Acta Mol. Basis Dis.* **2017**, *1863*, 1037–1045. [CrossRef] [PubMed]
12. Lustman, P.J.; Clouse, R.E. Depression in diabetic patients: The relationship between mood and glycemic control. *J. Diabetes Complicat.* **2005**, *19*, 113–122. [PubMed]
13. Samodien, E.; Johnson, R.; Pheiffer, C.; Mabasa, L.; Erasmus, M.; Louw, J.; Chellan, N. Diet-induced hypothalamic dysfunction and metabolic disease, and the therapeutic potential of polyphenols. *Mol. Metab.* **2019**, *27*, 1–10. [CrossRef] [PubMed]
14. Serra-Majem, L.; Roman, B.; Estruch, R. Scientific evidence of interventions using the Mediterranean diet: A systematic review. *Nutr. Rev.* **2006**, *64*, S27–S47. [CrossRef] [PubMed]
15. Bendall, C.L.; Mayr, H.L.; Opie, R.S.; Bes-Rastrollo, M.; Itsiopoulos, C.; Thomas, C.J. Central obesity and the Mediterranean diet: A systematic review of intervention trials. *Crit. Rev. Food Sci. Nutr.* **2018**, *58*, 3070–3084. [CrossRef]
16. Sofi, F.; Macchi, C.; Abbate, R.; Gensini, G.F.; Casini, A. Mediterranean diet and health. *BioFactors* **2013**, *39*, 335–342. [CrossRef]
17. Estruch, R.; Martinez-Gonzalez, M.A.; Corella, D.; Salas-Salvado, J.; Fito, M.; Chiva-Blanch, G.; Fiol, M.; Gomez-Gracia, E.; Aros, F.; Lapetra, J.; et al. Effect of a high-fat Mediterranean diet on bodyweight and waist circumference: A prespecified secondary outcomes analysis of the PREDIMED randomised controlled trial. *Lancet Diabetes Endocrinol.* **2019**, *7*, e6–e17. [CrossRef]
18. Tresserra-Rimbau, A.; Guasch-Ferre, M.; Salas-Salvado, J.; Toledo, E.; Corella, D.; Castaner, O.; Guo, X.; Gomez-Gracia, E.; Lapetra, J.; Aros, F.; et al. Intake of Total Polyphenols and Some Classes of Polyphenols Is Inversely Associated with Diabetes in Elderly People at High Cardiovascular Disease Risk. *J. Nutr.* **2016**, *146*, 767–777.
19. Chiva-Blanch, G.; Badimon, L.; Estruch, R. Latest evidence of the effects of the Mediterranean diet in prevention of cardiovascular disease. *Curr. Atheroscler. Rep.* **2014**, *16*, 446. [CrossRef]
20. Martínez-González, M.A.; Salas-Salvadó, J.; Estruch, R.; Corella, D.; Fitó, M.; Ros, E. Benefits of the Mediterranean Diet: Insights from the PREDIMED Study. *Prog. Cardiovasc. Dis.* **2015**, *58*, 50–60. [CrossRef]
21. Casas, R.; Sacanella, E.; Urpi-Sarda, M.; Chiva-Blanch, G.; Ros, E.; Martinez-Gonzalez, M.-A.; Covas, M.-I.; Salas-Salvado, J.; Fiol, M.; Aros, F.; et al. The effects of the mediterranean diet on biomarkers of vascular wall inflammation and plaque vulnerability in subjects with high risk for cardiovascular disease. A randomized trial. *PLoS ONE* **2014**, *9*, e100084. [CrossRef] [PubMed]
22. Amiot, M.J.; Riva, C.; Vinet, A. Effects of dietary polyphenols on metabolic syndrome features in humans: A systematic review. *Obes. Rev.* **2016**, *17*, 573–586. [CrossRef] [PubMed]
23. Castro-Barquero, S.; Lamuela-Raventós, R.M.; Doménech, M.; Estruch, R. Relationship between mediterranean dietary polyphenol intake and obesity. *Nutrients* **2018**, *10*, 1523. [CrossRef] [PubMed]
24. Schwingshackl, L.; Morze, J.; Hoffmann, G. Mediterranean diet and health status: Active ingredients and pharmacological mechanisms. *Br. J. Pharmacol.* **2019**, *177*, 1241–1257. [CrossRef] [PubMed]
25. Tresserra-Rimbau, A.; Rimm, E.B.; Medina-Remón, A.; Martínez-González, M.A.; López-Sabater, M.C.; Covas, M.I.; Corella, D.; Salas-Salvadó, J.; Gómez-Gracia, E.; Lapetra, J.; et al. Polyphenol intake and mortality risk: A re-analysis of the PREDIMED trial. *BMC Med.* **2014**, *12*, 77. [CrossRef] [PubMed]
26. Tresserra-Rimbau, A.; Rimm, E.B.; Medina-Remón, A.; Martínez-González, M.A.; de la Torre, R.; Corella, D.; Salas-Salvadó, J.; Gómez-Gracia, E.; Lapetra, J.; Arós, F.; et al. Inverse association between habitual polyphenol

intake and incidence of cardiovascular events in the PREDIMED study. *Nutr. Metab. Cardiovasc. Dis.* **2014**, *24*, 639–647. [CrossRef] [PubMed]

27. Tresserra-Rimbau, A.; Medina-Remón, A.; Pérez-Jiménez, J.; Martínez-González, M.A.; Covas, M.I.; Corella, D.; Salas-Salvadó, J.; Gómez-Gracia, E.; Lapetra, J.; Arós, F.; et al. Dietary intake and major food sources of polyphenols in a Spanish population at high cardiovascular risk: The PREDIMED study. *Nutr. Metab. Cardiovasc. Dis.* **2013**, *23*, 953–959. [CrossRef]

28. Medina-Remón, A.; Tresserra-Rimbau, A.; Pons, A.; Tur, J.A.; Martorell, M.; Ros, E.; Buil-Cosiales, P.; Sacanella, E.; Covas, M.I.; Corella, D.; et al. Effects of total dietary polyphenols on plasma nitric oxide and blood pressure in a high cardiovascular risk cohort. The PREDIMED randomized trial. *Nutr. Metab. Cardiovasc. Dis.* **2015**, *25*, 60–67. [CrossRef]

29. Manach, C.; Scalbert, A.; Morand, C.; Rémésy, C.; Jiménez, L. Polyphenols: Food sources and bioavailability. *Am. J. Clin. Nutr.* **2004**, *79*, 727–747. [CrossRef]

30. Godos, J.; Vitale, M.; Micek, A.; Ray, S.; Martini, D.; Del Rio, D.; Riccardi, G.; Galvano, F.; Grosso, G. Dietary Polyphenol Intake, Blood Pressure, and Hypertension: A Systematic Review and Meta-Analysis of Observational Studies. *Antioxidants* **2019**, *8*, 152. [CrossRef]

31. Williamson, G. The role of polyphenols in modern nutrition. *Nutr. Bull.* **2017**, *42*, 226–235. [CrossRef] [PubMed]

32. Vauzour, D.; Rodriguez-Mateos, A.; Corona, G.; Oruna-Concha, M.J.; Spencer, J.P.E. Polyphenols and human health: Prevention of disease and mechanisms of action. *Nutrients* **2010**, *2*, 1106–1131. [CrossRef] [PubMed]

33. Xing, T.; Kang, Y.; Xu, X.; Wang, B.; Du, M.; Zhu, M.J. Raspberry Supplementation Improves Insulin Signaling and Promotes Brown-Like Adipocyte Development in White Adipose Tissue of Obese Mice. *Mol. Nutr. Food Res.* **2018**, *62*, 1701035. [CrossRef] [PubMed]

34. Saibandith, B.; Spencer, J.P.E.; Rowland, I.R.; Commane, D.M. Olive Polyphenols and the Metabolic Syndrome. *Molecules* **2017**, *22*, 1082. [CrossRef]

35. Castelli, V.; Grassi, D.; Bocale, R.; d'Angelo, M.; Antonosante, A.; Cimini, A.; Ferri, C.; Desideri, G. Diet and Brain Health: Which Role for Polyphenols? *Curr. Pharm. Des.* **2018**, *24*, 227–238. [CrossRef] [PubMed]

36. Del Bo', C.; Bernardi, S.; Marino, M.; Porrini, M.; Tucci, M.; Guglielmetti, S.; Cherubini, A.; Carrieri, B.; Kirkup, B.; Kroon, P.; et al. Systematic Review on Polyphenol Intake and Health Outcomes: Is there Sufficient Evidence to Define a Health-Promoting Polyphenol-Rich Dietary Pattern? *Nutrients* **2019**, *11*, 1355.

37. Konstantinidi, M.; Koutelidakis, A.E. Functional Foods and Bioactive Compounds: A Review of Its Possible Role on Weight Management and Obesity's Metabolic Consequences. *Medicines* **2019**, *6*, 94. [CrossRef]

38. Bohn, T. Dietary factors affecting polyphenol bioavailability. *Nutr. Rev.* **2014**, *72*, 429–452. [CrossRef]

39. Lavefve, L.; Howard, L.R.; Carbonero, F. Berry polyphenols metabolism and impact on human gut microbiota and health. *Food Funct.* **2020**, *11*, 45–65. [CrossRef]

40. Eker, M.E.; Aaby, K.; Budic-Leto, I.; Brncic, S.R.; El, S.N.; Karakaya, S.; Simsek, S.; Manach, C.; Wiczkowski, W.; de Pascual-Teresa, S. A Review of Factors Affecting Anthocyanin Bioavailability: Possible Implications for the Inter-Individual Variability. *Foods* **2019**, *9*, 2. [CrossRef]

41. Xiao, J.B.; Högger, P. Dietary polyphenols and type 2 diabetes: Current insights and future perspectives. *Curr. Med. Chem.* **2015**, *22*, 23–38. [CrossRef] [PubMed]

42. Panche, A.N.; Diwan, A.D.; Chandra, S.R. Flavonoids: An overview. *J. Nutr. Sci.* **2016**, *5*, e47. [CrossRef] [PubMed]

43. Caro-Ordieres, T.; Marín-Royo, G.; Opazo-Ríos, L.; Jiménez-Castilla, L.; Moreno, J.A.; Gómez-Guerrero, C.; Egido, J. The Coming Age of Flavonoids in the Treatment of Diabetic Complications. *J. Clin. Med.* **2020**, *9*, 346. [CrossRef] [PubMed]

44. Xu, H.; Luo, J.; Huang, J.; Wen, Q. Flavonoids intake and risk of type 2 diabetes mellitus: A meta-analysis of prospective cohort studies. *Medicine* **2018**, *97*, e0686. [CrossRef]

45. Al-Ishaq, R.K.; Abotaleb, M.; Kubatka, P.; Kajo, K.; Busselberg, D. Flavonoids and Their Anti-Diabetic Effects: Cellular Mechanisms and Effects to Improve Blood Sugar Levels. *Biomolecules* **2019**, *9*, 430. [CrossRef]

46. Hussain, T.; Tan, B.; Murtaza, G.; Liu, G.; Rahu, N.; Saleem Kalhoro, M.; Hussain Kalhoro, D.; Adebowale, T.O.; Usman Mazhar, M.; Rehman, Z.U.; et al. Flavonoids and type 2 diabetes: Evidence of efficacy in clinical and animal studies and delivery strategies to enhance their therapeutic efficacy. *Pharmacol. Res.* **2020**, *152*, 104629. [CrossRef]

47. Rees, A.; Dodd, G.F.; Spencer, J.P.E. The effects of flavonoids on cardiovascular health: A review of human intervention trials and implications for cerebrovascular function. *Nutrients* **2018**, *10*, 1852. [CrossRef]
48. Kawser Hossain, M.; Abdal Dayem, A.; Han, J.; Yin, Y.; Kim, K.; Kumar Saha, S.; Yang, G.-M.; Choi, H.Y.; Cho, S.-G. Molecular Mechanisms of the Anti-Obesity and Anti-Diabetic Properties of Flavonoids. *Int. J. Mol. Sci.* **2016**, *17*, 569. [CrossRef]
49. Shin, J.H.; Jung, J.H. Non-alcoholic fatty liver disease and flavonoids: Current perspectives. *Clin. Res. Hepatol. Gastroenterol.* **2017**, *41*, 17–24. [CrossRef]
50. Salomone, F.; Godos, J.; Zelber-Sagi, S. Natural antioxidants for non-alcoholic fatty liver disease: Molecular targets and clinical perspectives. *Liver Int.* **2016**, *36*, 5–20. [CrossRef]
51. Khan, M.S.; Ikram, M.; Park, J.S.; Park, T.J.; Kim, M.O. Gut Microbiota, Its Role in Induction of Alzheimer's Disease Pathology, and Possible Therapeutic Interventions: Special Focus on Anthocyanins. *Cells* **2020**, *9*, 853. [CrossRef]
52. Reddy, V.P.; Aryal, P.; Robinson, S.; Rafiu, R.; Obrenovich, M.; Perry, G. Polyphenols in Alzheimer's Disease and in the Gut–Brain Axis. *Microorganisms* **2020**, *8*, 199. [CrossRef] [PubMed]
53. Garcia, D.; Shaw, R.J. AMPK: Mechanisms of Cellular Energy Sensing and Restoration of Metabolic Balance. *Mol. Cell* **2017**, *66*, 789–800. [CrossRef] [PubMed]
54. Petropoulos, S.A.; Sampaio, S.L.; Di Gioia, F.; Tzortzakis, N.; Rouphael, Y.; Kyriacou, M.C.; Ferreira, I. Grown to be Blue-Antioxidant Properties and Health Effects of Colored Vegetables. Part I: Root Vegetables. *Antioxidants* **2019**, *8*, 617. [CrossRef] [PubMed]
55. Di Gioia, F.; Tzortzakis, N.; Rouphael, Y.; Kyriacou, M.C.; Sampaio, S.L.; Ferreira, I.C.F.R.; Petropoulos, S.A. Grown to be Blue-Antioxidant Properties and Health Effects of Colored Vegetables. Part II: Leafy, Fruit, and Other Vegetables. *Antioxidants* **2020**, *9*, 97. [CrossRef] [PubMed]
56. Bendokas, V.; Skemiene, K.; Trumbeckaite, S.; Stanys, V.; Passamonti, S.; Borutaite, V.; Liobikas, J. Anthocyanins: From plant pigments to health benefits at mitochondrial level. *Crit. Rev. Food Sci. Nutr.* **2019**, 1–14. [CrossRef]
57. Gomes, J.V.P.; Rigolon, T.C.B.; da Silveira Souza, M.S.; Alvarez-Leite, J.I.; Della Lucia, C.M.; Martino, H.S.D.; Rosa, C.D.O.B. Antiobesity effects of anthocyanins on mitochondrial biogenesis, inflammation, and oxidative stress: A systematic review. *Nutrition* **2019**, *66*, 192–202. [CrossRef]
58. Bhaswant, M.; Shafie, S.R.; Mathai, M.L.; Mouatt, P.; Brown, L. Anthocyanins in chokeberry and purple maize attenuate diet-induced metabolic syndrome in rats. *Nutrition* **2017**, *41*, 24–31. [CrossRef]
59. Wu, T.; Gao, Y.; Guo, X.; Zhang, M.; Gong, L. Blackberry and blueberry anthocyanin supplementation counteract high-fat-diet-induced obesity by alleviating oxidative stress and inflammation and accelerating energy expenditure. *Oxid. Med. Cell. Longev.* **2018**, *2018*, 4051232. [CrossRef]
60. Wu, T.; Yu, Z.; Tang, Q.; Song, H.; Gao, Z.; Chen, W.; Zheng, X. Honeysuckle anthocyanin supplementation prevents diet-induced obesity in C57BL/6 mice. *Food Funct.* **2013**, *4*, 1654–1661. [CrossRef]
61. Huang, H.; Chen, G.; Liao, D.; Zhu, Y.; Xue, X. Effects of Berries Consumption on Cardiovascular Risk Factors: A Meta-analysis with Trial Sequential Analysis of Randomized Controlled Trials. *Sci. Rep.* **2016**, *6*, 23625. [CrossRef]
62. Wang, X.; Zhang, Z.F.; Zheng, G.H.; Wang, A.M.; Sun, C.H.; Qin, S.P.; Zhuang, J.; Lu, J.; Ma, D.F.; Zheng, Y.L. Attenuation of hepatic steatosis by purple sweet potato colour is associated with blocking Src/ERK/C/EBPβ signalling in high-fat-diet-treated mice. *Appl. Physiol. Nutr. Metab.* **2017**, *42*, 1082–1091. [CrossRef] [PubMed]
63. Tsuda, T. Recent Progress in Anti-Obesity and Anti-Diabetes Effect of Berries. *Antioxidants* **2016**, *5*, 13. [CrossRef] [PubMed]
64. Calvano, A.; Izuora, K.; Oh, E.C.; Ebersole, J.L.; Lyons, T.J.; Basu, A. Dietary berries, insulin resistance and type 2 diabetes: An overview of human feeding trials. *Food Funct.* **2019**, *10*, 6227–6243. [CrossRef] [PubMed]
65. de Pascual-Teresa, S.; Moreno, D.A.; García-Viguera, C. Flavanols and anthocyanins in cardiovascular health: A review of current evidence. *Int. J. Mol. Sci.* **2010**, *11*, 1479–1703. [CrossRef]
66. He, J.; Giusti, M.M. Anthocyanins: Natural Colorants with Health-Promoting Properties. *Annu. Rev. Food Sci. Technol.* **2010**, *1*, 163–187. [CrossRef]
67. Wood, E.; Hein, S.; Heiss, C.; Williams, C.; Rodriguez-Mateos, A. Blueberries and cardiovascular disease prevention. *Food Funct.* **2019**, *10*, 7621–7633. [CrossRef]

68. Salamone, F.; Volti, G.L.; Titta, L.; Puzzo, L.; Barbagallo, I.; La Delia, F.; Zelber-Sagi, S.; Malaguarnera, M.; Pelicci, P.G.; Giorgio, M.; et al. Moro orange juice prevents fatty liver in mice. *World J. Gastroenterol.* **2012**, *18*, 3862–3868. [CrossRef]
69. Esposito, D.; Damsud, T.; Wilson, M.; Grace, M.H.; Strauch, R.; Li, X.; Lila, M.A.; Komarnytsky, S. Black Currant Anthocyanins Attenuate Weight Gain and Improve Glucose Metabolism in Diet-Induced Obese Mice with Intact, but Not Disrupted, Gut Microbiome. *J. Agric. Food Chem.* **2015**, *63*, 6172–6180. [CrossRef]
70. Iizuka, Y.; Ozeki, A.; Tani, T.; Tsuda, T. Blackcurrant extract ameliorates hyperglycemia in type 2 diabetic mice in association with increased basal secretion of glucagon-like peptide-1 and activation of AMP-activated protein kinase. *J. Nutr. Sci. Vitaminol.* **2018**, *64*, 258–264. [CrossRef]
71. Choi, K.H.; Lee, H.A.; Park, M.H.; Han, J.-S. Mulberry (*Morus alba* L.) Fruit Extract Containing Anthocyanins Improves Glycemic Control and Insulin Sensitivity via Activation of AMP-Activated Protein Kinase in Diabetic C57BL/Ksj-db/db Mice. *J. Med. Food* **2016**, *19*, 737–745. [CrossRef]
72. Takikawa, M.; Inoue, S.; Horio, F.; Tsuda, T. Dietary Anthocyanin-Rich Bilberry Extract Ameliorates Hyperglycemia and Insulin Sensitivity via Activation of AMP-Activated Protein Kinase in Diabetic Mice. *J. Nutr.* **2010**, *140*, 527–533. [CrossRef]
73. You, Y.; Yuan, X.; Liu, X.; Liang, C.; Meng, M.; Huang, Y.; Han, X.; Guo, J.; Guo, Y.; Ren, C.; et al. Cyanidin-3-glucoside increases whole body energy metabolism by upregulating brown adipose tissue mitochondrial function. *Mol. Nutr. Food Res.* **2017**, *61*, 1700261. [CrossRef] [PubMed]
74. Nieman, D.C.; Simonson, A.; Sakaguchi, C.A.; Sha, W.; Blevins, T.; Hattabaugh, J.; Kohlmeier, M. Acute Ingestion of a Mixed Flavonoid and Caffeine Supplement Increases Energy Expenditure and Fat Oxidation in Adult Women: A Randomized, Crossover Clinical Trial. *Nutrients* **2019**, *11*, 2665. [CrossRef] [PubMed]
75. Rupasinghe, H.P.V.; Sekhon-Loodu, S.; Mantso, T.; Panayiotidis, M.I. Phytochemicals in regulating fatty acid beta-oxidation: Potential underlying mechanisms and their involvement in obesity and weight loss. *Pharmacol. Ther.* **2016**, *165*, 153–163. [CrossRef] [PubMed]
76. Solverson, P.M.; Rumpler, W.V.; Leger, J.L.; Redan, B.W.; Ferruzzi, M.G.; Baer, D.J.; Castonguay, T.W.; Novotny, J.A. Blackberry Feeding Increases Fat Oxidation and Improves Insulin Sensitivity in Overweight and Obese Males. *Nutrients* **2018**, *10*, 1048. [CrossRef] [PubMed]
77. Afzal, M.; Redha, A.; AlHasan, R. Anthocyanins Potentially Contribute to Defense against Alzheimer's Disease. *Molecules* **2019**, *24*, 4255. [CrossRef] [PubMed]
78. Burton-Freeman, B.M.; Sandhu, A.K.; Edirisinghe, I. Red Raspberries and Their Bioactive Polyphenols: Cardiometabolic and Neuronal Health Links. *Adv. Nutr.* **2016**, *7*, 44–65. [CrossRef] [PubMed]
79. Zhang, J.; Wu, J.; Liu, F.; Tong, L.; Chen, Z.; Chen, J.; He, H.; Xu, R.; Ma, Y.; Huang, C. Neuroprotective effects of anthocyanins and its major component cyanidin-3-O-glucoside (C3G) in the central nervous system: An outlined review. *Eur. J. Pharmacol.* **2019**, *858*, 172500. [CrossRef]
80. Jiang, X.; Li, X.; Zhu, C.; Sun, J.; Tian, L.; Chen, W.; Bai, W. The target cells of anthocyanins in metabolic syndrome. *Crit. Rev. Food Sci. Nutr.* **2019**, *59*, 921–946. [CrossRef]
81. Peng, C.-H.; Liu, L.-K.; Chuang, C.-M.; Chyau, C.-C.; Huang, C.-N.; Wang, C.-J. Mulberry Water Extracts Possess an Anti-obesity Effect and Ability to Inhibit Hepatic Lipogenesis and Promote Lipolysis. *J. Agric. Food Chem.* **2011**, *59*, 2663–2671. [CrossRef]
82. Sandoval, V.; Femenias, A.; Martinez-Garza, U.; Sanz-Lamora, H.; Castagnini, J.M.; Quifer-Rada, P.; Lamuela-Raventos, R.M.; Marrero, P.F.; Haro, D.; Relat, J. Lyophilized Maqui (*Aristotelia chilensis*) Berry Induces Browning in the Subcutaneous White Adipose Tissue and Ameliorates the Insulin Resistance in High Fat Diet-Induced Obese Mice. *Antioxidants* **2019**, *8*, 360. [CrossRef] [PubMed]
83. Badshah, H.; Ullah, I.; Kim, S.E.; Kim, T.H.; Lee, H.Y.; Kim, M.O. Anthocyanins attenuate body weight gain via modulating neuropeptide Y and GABAB1 receptor in rats hypothalamus. *Neuropeptides* **2013**, *47*, 347–353. [CrossRef] [PubMed]
84. Alvarez-Suarez, J.M.; Giampieri, F.; Tulipani, S.; Casoli, T.; Di Stefano, G.; González-Paramás, A.M.; Santos-Buelga, C.; Busco, F.; Quiles, J.L.; Cordero, M.D.; et al. One-month strawberry-rich anthocyanin supplementation ameliorates cardiovascular risk, oxidative stress markers and platelet activation in humans. *J. Nutr. Biochem.* **2014**, *25*, 289–294. [CrossRef] [PubMed]
85. Novotny, J.A.; Baer, D.J.; Khoo, C.; Gebauer, S.K.; Charron, C.S. Cranberry Juice Consumption Lowers Markers of Cardiometabolic Risk, Including Blood Pressure and Circulating C-Reactive Protein, Triglyceride, and Glucose Concentrations in Adults. *J. Nutr.* **2015**, *145*, 1185–1193. [CrossRef] [PubMed]

86. Yang, L.; Ling, W.; Yang, Y.; Chen, Y.; Tian, Z.; Du, Z.; Chen, J.; Xie, Y.; Liu, Z.; Yang, L. Role of Purified Anthocyanins in Improving Cardiometabolic Risk Factors in Chinese Men and Women with Prediabetes or Early Untreated Diabetes—A Randomized Controlled Trial. *Nutrients* **2017**, *9*, 1104. [CrossRef] [PubMed]
87. Valenti, L.; Riso, P.; Mazzocchi, A.; Porrini, M.; Fargion, S.; Agostoni, C. Dietary anthocyanins as nutritional therapy for nonalcoholic fatty liver disease. *Oxid. Med. Cell. Longev.* **2013**, *2013*, 145421. [CrossRef]
88. Park, S.; Cho, S.M.; Jin, B.R.; Yang, H.J.; Yi, Q.J. Mixture of blackberry leaf and fruit extracts alleviates non-alcoholic steatosis, enhances intestinal integrity, and increases Lactobacillus and Akkermansia in rats. *Exp. Biol. Med.* **2019**, *244*, 1629–1641. [CrossRef]
89. Huang, T.-W.; Chang, C.-L.; Kao, E.-S.; Lin, J.-H. Effect of Hibiscus sabdariffa extract on high fat diet-induced obesity and liver damage in hamsters. *Food Nutr. Res.* **2015**, *59*, 29018. [CrossRef]
90. Wu, T.; Qi, X.; Liu, Y.; Guo, J.; Zhu, R.; Chen, W.; Zheng, X.; Yu, T. Dietary supplementation with purified mulberry (Morus australis Poir) anthocyanins suppresses body weight gain in high-fat diet fed C57BL/6 mice. *Food Chem.* **2013**, *141*, 482–487. [CrossRef]
91. Pei, L.; Wan, T.; Wang, S.; Ye, M.; Qiu, Y.; Jiang, R.; Pang, N.; Huang, Y.; Zhou, Y.; Jiang, X.; et al. Cyanidin-3-O-β-glucoside regulates the activation and the secretion of adipokines from brown adipose tissue and alleviates diet induced fatty liver. *Biomed. Pharmacother.* **2018**, *105*, 625–632. [CrossRef]
92. Franklin, R.; Bispo, R.F.M.; Sousa-Rodrigues, C.F.; Pires, L.A.S.; Fonseca, A.J.; Babinski, M.A. Grape Leucoanthocyanidin Protects Liver Tissue in Albino Rabbits with Nonalcoholic Hepatic Steatosis. *Cells Tissues Organs* **2018**, *205*, 129–136. [CrossRef] [PubMed]
93. Overall, J.; Bonney, S.A.; Wilson, M.; Beermann, A.; Grace, M.H.; Esposito, D.; Lila, M.A.; Komarnytsky, S. Metabolic effects of berries with structurally diverse anthocyanins. *Int. J. Mol. Sci.* **2017**, *18*, 422. [CrossRef] [PubMed]
94. van der Heijden, R.A.; Morrison, M.C.; Sheedfar, F.; Mulder, P.; Schreurs, M.; Hommelberg, P.P.H.; Hofker, M.H.; Schalkwijk, C.; Kleemann, R.; Tietge, U.J.F.; et al. Effects of Anthocyanin and Flavanol Compounds on Lipid Metabolism and Adipose Tissue Associated Systemic Inflammation in Diet-Induced Obesity. *Mediat. Inflamm.* **2016**, *2016*, 2042107. [CrossRef] [PubMed]
95. Parra-Vargas, M.; Sandoval-Rodriguez, A.; Rodriguez-Echevarria, R.; Dominguez-Rosales, J.A.; Santos-Garcia, A.; Armendariz-Borunda, J. Delphinidin Ameliorates Hepatic Triglyceride Accumulation in Human HepG2 Cells, but Not in Diet-Induced Obese Mice. *Nutrients* **2018**, *10*, 1060. [CrossRef] [PubMed]
96. Yan, F.; Zheng, X. Anthocyanin-rich mulberry fruit improves insulin resistance and protects hepatocytes against oxidative stress during hyperglycemia by regulating AMPK/ACC/mTOR pathway. *J. Funct. Foods* **2017**, *30*, 270–281. [CrossRef]
97. Chang, J.-J.; Hsu, M.-J.; Huang, H.-P.; Chung, D.-J.; Chang, Y.-C.; Wang, C.-J. Mulberry Anthocyanins Inhibit Oleic Acid Induced Lipid Accumulation by Reduction of Lipogenesis and Promotion of Hepatic Lipid Clearance. *J. Agric. Food Chem.* **2013**, *61*, 6069–6076. [CrossRef]
98. Park, M.; Yoo, J.-H.; Lee, Y.-S.; Lee, H.-J. Lonicera caerulea Extract Attenuates Non-Alcoholic Fatty Liver Disease in Free Fatty Acid-Induced HepG2 Hepatocytes and in High Fat Diet-Fed Mice. *Nutrients* **2019**, *11*, 494. [CrossRef]
99. Jiang, T.; Shuai, X.; Li, J.; Yang, N.; Deng, L.; Li, S.; He, Y.; Guo, H.; Li, Y.; He, J. Protein-Bound Anthocyanin Compounds of Purple Sweet Potato Ameliorate Hyperglycemia by Regulating Hepatic Glucose Metabolism in High-Fat Diet/Streptozotocin-Induced Diabetic Mice. *J. Agric. Food Chem.* **2020**, *68*, 1596–1608. [CrossRef]
100. du Preez, R.; Wanyonyi, S.; Mouatt, P.; Panchal, S.K.; Brown, L. Saskatoon Berry Amelanchier alnifolia Regulates Glucose Metabolism and Improves Cardiovascular and Liver Signs of Diet-Induced Metabolic Syndrome in Rats. *Nutrients* **2020**, *12*, 931. [CrossRef]
101. Guo, H.; Xia, M.; Zou, T.; Ling, W.; Zhong, R.; Zhang, W. Cyanidin 3-glucoside attenuates obesity-associated insulin resistance and hepatic steatosis in high-fat diet-fed and db/db mice via the transcription factor FoxO1. *J. Nutr. Biochem.* **2012**, *23*, 349–360. [CrossRef] [PubMed]
102. Su, W.; Zhang, C.; Chen, F.; Sui, J.; Lu, J.; Wang, Q.; Shan, Q.; Zheng, G.; Lu, J.; Sun, C.; et al. Purple sweet potato color protects against hepatocyte apoptosis through Sirt1 activation in high-fat-diet-treated mice. *Food Nutr. Res.* **2020**, *64*. [CrossRef] [PubMed]
103. Li, A.; Xiao, R.; He, S.; An, X.; He, Y.; Wang, C.; Yin, S.; Wang, B.; Shi, X.; He, J. Research Advances of Purple Sweet Potato Anthocyanins: Extraction, Identification, Stability, Bioactivity, Application, and Biotransformation. *Molecules* **2019**, *24*, 3816. [CrossRef] [PubMed]

104. Chu, Q.; Zhang, S.; Chen, M.; Han, W.; Jia, R.; Chen, W.; Zheng, X. Cherry Anthocyanins Regulate NAFLD by Promoting Autophagy Pathway. *Oxid. Med. Cell. Longev.* **2019**, *2019*, 4825949. [CrossRef]
105. Ishibashi, J.; Seale, P. Beige can be slimming. *Science* **2010**, *328*, 1113–1114. [CrossRef]
106. Bartelt, A.; Heeren, J. Adipose tissue browning and metabolic health. *Nat. Rev. Endocrinol.* **2014**, *10*, 24–36. [CrossRef]
107. Barbatelli, G.; Murano, I.; Madsen, L.; Hao, Q.; Jimenez, M.; Kristiansen, K.; Giacobino, J.P.; De Matteis, R.; Cinti, S. The emergence of cold-induced brown adipocytes in mouse white fat depots is determined predominantly by white to brown adipocyte transdifferentiation. *AJP Endocrinol. Metab.* **2010**, *298*, E1244–E1253. [CrossRef]
108. Whittle, A.; Relat-Pardo, J.; Vidal-Puig, A. Pharmacological strategies for targeting BAT thermogenesis. *Trends Pharmacol. Sci.* **2013**, *34*, 347–355. [CrossRef]
109. Kim, S.Y.; Wi, H.-R.; Choi, S.; Ha, T.J.; Lee, B.W.; Lee, M. Inhibitory effect of anthocyanin-rich black soybean testa (*Glycine max* (L.) Merr.) on the inflammation-induced adipogenesis in a DIO mouse model. *J. Funct. Foods* **2015**, *14*, 623–633. [CrossRef]
110. Lee, M.; Sorn, S.R.; Park, Y.; Park, H.-K. Anthocyanin Rich-Black Soybean Testa Improved Visceral Fat and Plasma Lipid Profiles in Overweight/Obese Korean Adults: A Randomized Controlled Trial. *J. Med. Food* **2016**, *19*, 995–1003. [CrossRef]
111. Lim, S.-M.; Lee, H.S.; Jung, J.I.; Kim, S.M.; Kim, N.Y.; Seo, T.S.; Bae, J.-S.; Kim, E.J. Cyanidin-3-O-galactoside-enriched Aronia melanocarpa extract attenuates weight gain and adipogenic pathways in high-fat diet-induced obese C57BL/6 mice. *Nutrients* **2019**, *11*, 1190. [CrossRef] [PubMed]
112. Tsuda, T.; Ueno, Y.; Aoki, H.; Koda, T.; Horio, F.; Takahashi, N.; Kawada, T.; Osawa, T. Anthocyanin enhances adipocytokine secretion and adipocyte-specific gene expression in isolated rat adipocytes. *Biochem. Biophys. Res. Commun.* **2004**, *316*, 149–157. [CrossRef] [PubMed]
113. Tsuda, T.; Ueno, Y.; Yoshikawa, T.; Kojo, H.; Osawa, T. Microarray profiling of gene expression in human adipocytes in response to anthocyanins. *Biochem. Pharmacol.* **2006**, *71*, 1184–1197. [CrossRef] [PubMed]
114. Wu, T.; Jiang, Z.; Yin, J.; Long, H.; Zheng, X. Anti-obesity effects of artificial planting blueberry (Vaccinium ashei) anthocyanin in high-fat diet-treated mice. *Int. J. Food Sci. Nutr.* **2016**, *67*, 257–264. [CrossRef] [PubMed]
115. Han, X.; Guo, J.; You, Y.; Yin, M.; Liang, J.; Ren, C.; Zhan, J.; Huang, W. Vanillic acid activates thermogenesis in brown and white adipose tissue. *Food Funct.* **2018**, *9*, 4366–4375. [CrossRef] [PubMed]
116. Jayarathne, S.; Stull, A.J.; Park, O.-H.; Kim, J.H.; Thompson, L.; Moustaid-Moussa, N. Protective Effects of Anthocyanins in Obesity-Associated Inflammation and Changes in Gut Microbiome. *Mol. Nutr. Food Res.* **2019**, *63*, e1900149. [CrossRef]
117. You, Y.; Han, X.; Guo, J.; Guo, Y.; Yin, M.; Liu, G.; Huang, W.; Zhan, J. Cyanidin-3-glucoside attenuates high-fat and high-fructose diet-induced obesity by promoting the thermogenic capacity of brown adipose tissue. *J. Funct. Foods* **2018**, *41*, 62–71. [CrossRef]
118. Rocha-Rodrigues, S.; Rodriguez, A.; Gouveia, A.M.; Goncalves, I.O.; Becerril, S.; Ramirez, B.; Beleza, J.; Fruhbeck, G.; Ascensao, A.; Magalhaes, J. Effects of physical exercise on myokines expression and brown adipose-like phenotype modulation in rats fed a high-fat diet. *Life Sci.* **2016**, *165*, 100–108. [CrossRef]
119. Luna-Vital, D.; Luzardo-Ocampo, I.; Cuellar-Nunez, M.L.; Loarca-Pina, G.; Gonzalez de Mejia, E. Maize extract rich in ferulic acid and anthocyanins prevents high-fat-induced obesity in mice by modulating SIRT1, AMPK and IL-6 associated metabolic and inflammatory pathways. *J. Nutr. Biochem.* **2020**, *79*, 108343. [CrossRef]
120. Wu, T.; Tang, Q.; Yu, Z.; Gao, Z.; Hu, H.; Chen, W.; Zheng, X.; Yu, T. Inhibitory effects of sweet cherry anthocyanins on the obesity development in C57BL/6 mice. *Int. J. Food Sci. Nutr.* **2014**, *65*, 351–359. [CrossRef]
121. Fan, D.; Alamri, Y.; Liu, K.; Macaskill, M.; Harris, P.; Brimble, M.; Dalrymple-Alford, J.; Prickett, T.; Menzies, O.; Laurenson, A.; et al. Supplementation of blackcurrant anthocyanins increased cyclic glycine-proline in the cerebrospinal fluid of parkinson patients: Potential treatment to improve insulin-like growth factor-1 function. *Nutrients* **2018**, *10*, 714. [CrossRef] [PubMed]
122. Rehman, S.U.; Shah, S.A.; Ali, T.; Chung, J., II; Kim, M.O. Anthocyanins Reversed D-Galactose-Induced Oxidative Stress and Neuroinflammation Mediated Cognitive Impairment in Adult Rats. *Mol. Neurobiol.* **2017**, *54*, 255–271. [CrossRef] [PubMed]

123. Wei, J.; Zhang, G.; Zhang, X.; Xu, D.; Gao, J.; Fan, J.; Zhou, Z. Anthocyanins from Black Chokeberry (Aroniamelanocarpa Elliot) Delayed Aging-Related Degenerative Changes of Brain. *J. Agric. Food Chem.* **2017**, *65*, 5973–5984. [CrossRef] [PubMed]
124. Li, D.; Wang, P.; Luo, Y.; Zhao, M.; Chen, F. Health benefits of anthocyanins and molecular mechanisms: Update from recent decade. *Crit. Rev. Food Sci. Nutr.* **2017**, *57*, 1729–1741. [CrossRef] [PubMed]
125. Boespflug, E.L.; Eliassen, J.C.; Dudley, J.A.; Shidler, M.D.; Kalt, W.; Summer, S.S.; Stein, A.L.; Stover, A.N.; Krikorian, R. Enhanced neural activation with blueberry supplementation in mild cognitive impairment. *Nutr. Neurosci.* **2018**, *21*, 297–305. [CrossRef] [PubMed]
126. Di Lorenzo, A.; Sobolev, A.P.; Nabavi, S.F.; Sureda, A.; Moghaddam, A.H.; Khanjani, S.; Di Giovanni, C.; Xiao, J.; Shirooie, S.; Tsetegho Sokeng, A.J.; et al. Antidepressive effects of a chemically characterized maqui berry extract (*Aristotelia chilensis* (molina) stuntz) in a mouse model of Post-stroke depression. *Food Chem. Toxicol.* **2019**, *129*, 434–443. [CrossRef]
127. Pan, Z.; Cui, M.; Dai, G.; Yuan, T.; Li, Y.; Ji, T.; Pan, Y. Protective Effect of Anthocyanin on Neurovascular Unit in Cerebral Ischemia/Reperfusion Injury in Rats. *Front. Neurosci.* **2018**, *12*, 947. [CrossRef]
128. Rasmussen, S.E.; Frederiksen, H.; Struntze Krogholm, K.; Poulsen, L. Dietary proanthocyanidins: Occurrence, dietary intake, bioavailability, and protection against cardiovascular disease. *Mol. Nutr. Food Res.* **2005**, *49*, 159–174. [CrossRef]
129. Kumar, S.; Pandey, A.K. Chemistry and biological activities of flavonoids: An overview. *Sci. World J.* **2013**, *2013*, 162750. [CrossRef]
130. Scientific Opinion on the modification of the authorisation of a health claim related to cocoa flavanols and maintenance of normal endothelium-dependent vasodilation pursuant to Article 13(5) of Regulation (EC) No 1924/2006 following a request in accordan. *EFSA J.* **2016**, *12*, 3654.
131. Yu, J.; Song, P.; Perry, R.; Penfold, C.; Cooper, A.R. The effectiveness of green tea or green tea extract on insulin resistance and glycemic control in type 2 diabetes mellitus: A meta-analysis. *Diabetes Metab. J.* **2017**, *41*, 251–262. [CrossRef] [PubMed]
132. Li, X.; Wang, W.; Hou, L.; Wu, H.; Wu, Y.; Xu, R.; Xiao, Y.; Wang, X. Does tea extract supplementation benefit metabolic syndrome and obesity? A systematic review and meta-analysis. *Clin. Nutr.* **2020**, *39*, 1049–1058. [CrossRef] [PubMed]
133. Martin, M.A.; Goya, L.; Ramos, S. Protective effects of tea, red wine and cocoa in diabetes. Evidences from human studies. *Food Chem. Toxicol.* **2017**, *109*, 302–314. [CrossRef] [PubMed]
134. Akhlaghi, M.; Ghobadi, S.; Mohammad Hosseini, M.; Gholami, Z.; Mohammadian, F. Flavanols are potential anti-obesity agents, a systematic review and meta-analysis of controlled clinical trials. *Nutr. Metab. Cardiovasc. Dis.* **2018**, *28*, 675–690. [CrossRef]
135. Lin, Y.; Shi, D.; Su, B.; Wei, J.; Gaman, M.-A.; Sedanur Macit, M.; Borges do Nascimento, I.J.; Guimaraes, N.S. The effect of green tea supplementation on obesity: A systematic review and dose-response meta-analysis of randomized controlled trials. *Phytother. Res.* **2020**, 1–12. [CrossRef]
136. Payab, M.; Hasani-Ranjbar, S.; Shahbal, N.; Qorbani, M.; Aletaha, A.; Haghi-Aminjan, H.; Soltani, A.; Khatami, F.; Nikfar, S.; Hassani, S.; et al. Effect of the herbal medicines in obesity and metabolic syndrome: A systematic review and meta-analysis of clinical trials. *Phytother. Res.* **2020**, *34*, 526–545. [CrossRef]
137. Tang, G.-Y.; Meng, X.; Gan, R.-Y.; Zhao, C.-N.; Liu, Q.; Feng, Y.-B.; Li, S.; Wei, X.-L.; Atanasov, A.G.; Corke, H.; et al. Health Functions and Related Molecular Mechanisms of Tea Components: An Update Review. *Int. J. Mol. Sci.* **2019**, *20*, 6196. [CrossRef]
138. Oh, J.; Jo, S.-H.; Kim, J.S.; Ha, K.-S.; Lee, J.-Y.; Choi, H.-Y.; Yu, S.-Y.; Kwon, Y.-I.; Kim, Y.-C. Selected tea and tea pomace extracts inhibit intestinal alpha-glucosidase activity in vitro and postprandial hyperglycemia in vivo. *Int. J. Mol. Sci.* **2015**, *16*, 8811–8825. [CrossRef]
139. Ramos, S.; Martin, M.A.; Goya, L. Effects of Cocoa Antioxidants in Type 2 Diabetes Mellitus. *Antioxidants* **2017**, *6*, 84. [CrossRef]
140. Yang, C.S.; Zhang, J.; Zhang, L.; Huang, J.; Wang, Y. Mechanisms of body weight reduction and metabolic syndrome alleviation by tea. *Mol. Nutr. Food Res.* **2016**, *60*, 160–174. [CrossRef]
141. Leon-Flores, P.; Najera, N.; Perez, E.; Pardo, B.; Jimenez, F.; Diaz-Chiguer, D.; Villarreal, F.; Hidalgo, I.; Ceballos, G.; Meaney, E. Effects of Cacao By-Products and a Modest Weight Loss Intervention on the Concentration of Serum Triglycerides in Overweight Subjects: Proof of Concept. *J. Med. Food* **2020**, *23*, 745–749. [CrossRef] [PubMed]

142. Wu, E.; Zhang, T.; Tan, C.; Peng, C.; Chisti, Y.; Wang, Q.; Gong, J. Theabrownin from Pu-erh tea together with swinging exercise synergistically ameliorates obesity and insulin resistance in rats. *Eur. J. Nutr.* **2019**, *59*, 1937–1950. [CrossRef] [PubMed]
143. Zhang, Y.; Gu, M.; Wang, R.; Li, M.; Li, D.; Xie, Z. Dietary supplement of Yunkang 10 green tea and treadmill exercise ameliorate high fat diet induced metabolic syndrome of C57BL/6 J mice. *Nutr. Metab.* **2020**, *17*, 14.
144. Pezeshki, A.; Safi, S.; Feizi, A.; Askari, G.; Karami, F. The Effect of Green Tea Extract Supplementation on Liver Enzymes in Patients with Nonalcoholic Fatty Liver Disease. *Int. J. Prev. Med.* **2016**, *7*, 28.
145. Braud, L.; Battault, S.; Meyer, G.; Nascimento, A.; Gaillard, S.; de Sousa, G.; Rahmani, R.; Riva, C.; Armand, M.; Maixent, J.-M.; et al. Antioxidant properties of tea blunt ROS-dependent lipogenesis: Beneficial effect on hepatic steatosis in a high fat-high sucrose diet NAFLD obese rat model. *J. Nutr. Biochem.* **2017**, *40*, 95–104. [CrossRef]
146. Venkatakrishnan, K.; Chiu, H.-F.; Cheng, J.-C.; Chang, Y.-H.; Lu, Y.-Y.; Han, Y.-C.; Shen, Y.-C.; Tsai, K.-S.; Wang, C.-K. Comparative studies on the hypolipidemic, antioxidant and hepatoprotective activities of catechin-enriched green and oolong tea in a double-blind clinical trial. *Food Funct.* **2018**, *9*, 1205–1213. [CrossRef]
147. Li, X.; Li, S.; Chen, M.; Wang, J.; Xie, B.; Sun, Z. (-)-Epigallocatechin-3-gallate (EGCG) inhibits starch digestion and improves glucose homeostasis through direct or indirect activation of FXR/CAR-mediated phase II metabolism in diabetic mice. *Food Funct.* **2018**, *9*, 4651–4663. [CrossRef]
148. Li, Y.; Wu, S. Epigallocatechin gallate suppresses hepatic cholesterol synthesis by targeting SREBP-2 through SIRT1/FOXO1 signaling pathway. *Mol. Cell. Biochem.* **2018**, *448*, 175–185. [CrossRef]
149. Liu, C.; Guo, Y.; Sun, L.; Lai, X.; Li, Q.; Zhang, W.; Xiang, L.; Sun, S.; Cao, F. Six types of tea reduce high-fat-diet-induced fat accumulation in mice by increasing lipid metabolism and suppressing inflammation. *Food Funct.* **2019**, *10*, 2061–2074. [CrossRef]
150. Terzo, S.; Caldara, G.F.; Ferrantelli, V.; Puleio, R.; Cassata, G.; Mulè, F.; Amato, A. Pistachio Consumption Prevents and Improves Lipid Dysmetabolism by Reducing the Lipid Metabolizing Gene Expression in Diet-Induced Obese Mice. *Nutrients* **2018**, *10*, 1857. [CrossRef]
151. Chang, J.-J.; Chung, D.-J.; Lee, Y.-J.; Wen, B.-H.; Jao, H.-Y.; Wang, C.-J. Solanum nigrum Polyphenol Extracts Inhibit Hepatic Inflammation, Oxidative Stress, and Lipogenesis in High-Fat-Diet-Treated Mice. *J. Agric. Food Chem.* **2017**, *65*, 9255–9265. [CrossRef] [PubMed]
152. Tan, Y.; Kim, J.; Cheng, J.; Ong, M.; Lao, W.G.; Jin, X.L.; Lin, Y.G.; Xiao, L.; Zhu, X.Q.; Qu, X.Q. Green tea polyphenols ameliorate non-alcoholic fatty liver disease through upregulating AMPK activation in high fat fed Zucker fatty rats. *World J. Gastroenterol.* **2017**, *23*, 3805–3814. [CrossRef] [PubMed]
153. Suzuki, T.; Kumazoe, M.; Kim, Y.; Yamashita, S.; Nakahara, K.; Tsukamoto, S.; Sasaki, M.; Hagihara, T.; Tsurudome, Y.; Huang, Y.; et al. Green tea extract containing a highly absorbent catechin prevents diet-induced lipid metabolism disorder. *Sci. Rep.* **2013**, *3*, 2749. [CrossRef] [PubMed]
154. de Oliveira, P.R.B.; da Costa, C.A.; de Bem, G.F.; Cordeiro, V.S.C.; Santos, I.B.; de Carvalho, L.C.R.M.; da Conceição, E.P.S.; Lisboa, P.C.; Ognibene, D.T.; Sousa, P.J.C.; et al. Euterpe oleracea Mart.-Derived Polyphenols Protect Mice from Diet-Induced Obesity and Fatty Liver by Regulating Hepatic Lipogenesis and Cholesterol Excretion. *PLoS ONE* **2015**, *10*, e0143721. [CrossRef] [PubMed]
155. Liu, H.W.; Wei, C.C.; Chen, Y.J.; Chen, Y.A.; Chang, S.J. Flavanol-rich lychee fruit extract alleviates diet-induced insulin resistance via suppressing mTOR/SREBP-1 mediated lipogenesis in liver and restoring insulin signaling in skeletal muscle. *Mol. Nutr. Food Res.* **2016**, *60*, 2288–2296. [CrossRef] [PubMed]
156. Laplante, M.; Sabatini, D.M. An emerging role of mTOR in lipid biosynthesis. *Curr. Biol.* **2009**, *19*, R1046–R1052. [CrossRef]
157. Um, S.H.; Frigerio, F.; Watanabe, M.; Picard, F.; Joaquin, M.; Sticker, M.; Fumagalli, S.; Allegrini, P.R.; Kozma, S.C.; Auwerx, J.; et al. Absence of S6K1 protects against age- and diet-induced obesity while enhancing insulin sensitivity. *Nature* **2004**, *431*, 200–205. [CrossRef]
158. Peng, J.; Jia, Y.; Hu, T.; Du, J.; Wang, Y.; Cheng, B.; Li, K. GC-(4->8)-GCG, A Proanthocyanidin Dimer from Camellia ptilophylla, Modulates Obesity and Adipose Tissue Inflammation in High-Fat Diet Induced Obese Mice. *Mol. Nutr. Food Res.* **2019**, *63*, e1900082. [CrossRef]
159. Yin, M.; Zhang, P.; Yu, F.; Zhang, Z.; Cai, Q.; Lu, W.; Li, B.; Qin, W.; Cheng, M.; Wang, H.; et al. Grape seed procyanidin B2 ameliorates hepatic lipid metabolism disorders in db/db mice. *Mol. Med. Rep.* **2017**, *16*, 2844–2850. [CrossRef]

160. Huang, J.; Feng, S.; Liu, A.; Dai, Z.; Wang, H.; Reuhl, K.; Lu, W.; Yang, C.S. Green Tea Polyphenol EGCG Alleviates Metabolic Abnormality and Fatty Liver by Decreasing Bile Acid and Lipid Absorption in Mice. *Mol. Nutr. Food Res.* **2018**, *62*, 1700696. [CrossRef]
161. Cheng, H.; Xu, N.; Zhao, W.; Su, J.; Liang, M.; Xie, Z.; Wu, X.; Li, Q. (-)-Epicatechin regulates blood lipids and attenuates hepatic steatosis in rats fed high-fat diet. *Mol. Nutr. Food Res.* **2017**, *61*, 1–11. [CrossRef] [PubMed]
162. Chen, I.-J.; Liu, C.-Y.; Chiu, J.-P.; Hsu, C.-H. Therapeutic effect of high-dose green tea extract on weight reduction: A randomized, double-blind, placebo-controlled clinical trial. *Clin. Nutr.* **2015**, *35*, 592–599. [CrossRef] [PubMed]
163. Hibi, M.; Takase, H.; Iwasaki, M.; Osaki, N.; Katsuragi, Y. Efficacy of tea catechin-rich beverages to reduce abdominal adiposity and metabolic syndrome risks in obese and overweight subjects: A pooled analysis of 6 human trials. *Nutr. Res.* **2018**, *55*, 1–10. [CrossRef] [PubMed]
164. Kapoor, M.P.; Sugita, M.; Fukuzawa, Y.; Okubo, T. Physiological effects of epigallocatechin-3-gallate (EGCG) on energy expenditure for prospective fat oxidation in humans: A systematic review and meta-analysis. *J. Nutr. Biochem.* **2017**, *43*, 1–10. [CrossRef] [PubMed]
165. Yoneshiro, T.; Aita, S.; Kawai, Y.; Iwanaga, T.; Saito, M. Nonpungent capsaicin analogs (capsinoids) increase energy expenditure through the activation of brown adipose tissue in humans. *Am. J. Clin. Nutr.* **2012**, *95*, 845–850. [CrossRef] [PubMed]
166. Mele, L.; Bidault, G.; Mena, P.; Crozier, A.; Brighenti, F.; Vidal-Puig, A.; Del Rio, D. Dietary (Poly)phenols, Brown Adipose Tissue Activation, and Energy Expenditure: A Narrative Review. *Adv. Nutr.* **2017**, *8*, 694–704. [CrossRef]
167. Huang, J.; Wang, Y.; Xie, Z.; Zhou, Y.; Zhang, Y.; Wan, X. The anti-obesity effects of green tea in human intervention and basic molecular studies. *Eur. J. Clin. Nutr.* **2014**, *68*, 1075–1087. [CrossRef]
168. Serrano, J.; Casanova-Marti, A.; Gual, A.; Perez-Vendrell, A.M.; Blay, M.T.; Terra, X.; Ardevol, A.; Pinent, M. A specific dose of grape seed-derived proanthocyanidins to inhibit body weight gain limits food intake and increases energy expenditure in rats. *Eur. J. Nutr.* **2017**, *56*, 1629–1636. [CrossRef]
169. Yamashita, Y.; Wang, L.; Wang, L.; Tanaka, Y.; Zhang, T.; Ashida, H. Oolong, black and pu-erh tea suppresses adiposity in mice via activation of AMP-activated protein kinase. *Food Funct.* **2014**, *5*, 2420–2429. [CrossRef]
170. Varela, C.E.; Rodriguez, A.; Romero-Valdovinos, M.; Mendoza-Lorenzo, P.; Mansour, C.; Ceballos, G.; Villarreal, F.; Ramirez-Sanchez, I. Browning effects of (-)-epicatechin on adipocytes and white adipose tissue. *Eur. J. Pharmacol.* **2017**, *811*, 48–59. [CrossRef]
171. Neyrinck, A.M.; Bindels, L.B.; Geurts, L.; Van Hul, M.; Cani, P.D.; Delzenne, N.M. A polyphenolic extract from green tea leaves activates fat browning in high-fat-diet-induced obese mice. *J. Nutr. Biochem.* **2017**, *49*, 15–21. [CrossRef] [PubMed]
172. Jang, M.H.; Mukherjee, S.; Choi, M.J.; Kang, N.H.; Pham, H.G.; Yun, J.W. Theobromine alleviates diet-induced obesity in mice via phosphodiesterase-4 inhibition. *Eur. J. Nutr.* **2020**. [CrossRef] [PubMed]
173. Okla, M.; Kim, J.; Koehler, K.; Chung, S. Dietary Factors Promoting Brown and Beige Fat Development and Thermogenesis. *Adv. Nutr.* **2017**, *8*, 473–483. [CrossRef] [PubMed]
174. Silvester, A.J.; Aseer, K.R.; Yun, J.W. Dietary polyphenols and their roles in fat browning. *J. Nutr. Biochem.* **2019**, *64*, 1–12. [CrossRef] [PubMed]
175. Saito, M.; Matsushita, M.; Yoneshiro, T.; Okamatsu-Ogura, Y. Brown Adipose Tissue, Diet-Induced Thermogenesis, and Thermogenic Food Ingredients: From Mice to Men. *Front. Endocrinol.* **2020**, *11*, 222. [CrossRef]
176. Bolin, A.P.; Sousa-Filho, C.P.B.; Marinovic, M.P.; Rodrigues, A.C.; Otton, R. Polyphenol-rich green tea extract induces thermogenesis in mice by a mechanism dependent on adiponectin signaling. *J. Nutr. Biochem.* **2020**, *78*, 108322. [CrossRef]
177. Li, F.; Gao, C.; Yan, P.; Zhang, M.; Wang, Y.; Hu, Y.; Wu, X.; Wang, X.; Sheng, J. EGCG reduces obesity and white adipose tissue gain partly through AMPK activation in mice. *Front. Pharmacol.* **2018**, *9*, 1–9. [CrossRef]
178. Wang, Q.; Liu, S.; Zhai, A.; Zhang, B.; Tian, G. AMPK-Mediated Regulation of Lipid Metabolism by Phosphorylation. *Biol. Pharm. Bull.* **2018**, *41*, 985–993. [CrossRef]
179. Rodriguez Lanzi, C.; Perdicaro, D.J.; Landa, M.S.; Fontana, A.; Antoniolli, A.; Miatello, R.M.; Oteiza, P.I.; Vazquez Prieto, M.A. Grape pomace extract induced beige cells in white adipose tissue from rats and in 3T3-L1 adipocytes. *J. Nutr. Biochem.* **2018**, *56*, 224–233. [CrossRef]

180. Rodriguez Lanzi, C.; Perdicaro, D.J.; Gambarte Tudela, J.; Muscia, V.; Fontana, A.R.; Oteiza, P.I.; Vazquez Prieto, M.A. Grape pomace extract supplementation activates FNDC5/irisin in muscle and promotes white adipose browning in rats fed a high-fat diet. *Food Funct.* **2020**, *11*, 1537–1546. [CrossRef]
181. Jang, M.H.; Kang, N.H.; Mukherjee, S.; Yun, J.W. Theobromine, a Methylxanthine in Cocoa Bean, Stimulates Thermogenesis by Inducing White Fat Browning and Activating Brown Adipocytes. *Biotechnol. Bioprocess Eng.* **2018**, *23*, 617–626. [CrossRef]
182. Nakagawa, Y.; Ishimura, K.; Oya, S.; Kamino, M.; Fujii, Y.; Nanba, F.; Toda, T.; Ishii, T.; Adachi, T.; Suhara, Y.; et al. Comparison of the sympathetic stimulatory abilities of B-type procyanidins based on induction of uncoupling protein-1 in brown adipose tissue (BAT) and increased plasma catecholamine (CA) in mice. *PLoS ONE* **2018**, *13*, e0201203. [CrossRef] [PubMed]
183. Nirengi, S.; Amagasa, S.; Homma, T.; Yoneshiro, T.; Matsumiya, S.; Kurosawa, Y.; Sakane, N.; Ebi, K.; Saito, M.; Hamaoka, T. Daily ingestion of catechin-rich beverage increases brown adipose tissue density and decreases extramyocellular lipids in healthy young women. *Springerplus* **2016**, *5*, 1363. [CrossRef] [PubMed]
184. Lee, M.-S.; Shin, Y.; Jung, S.; Kim, Y. Effects of epigallocatechin-3-gallate on thermogenesis and mitochondrial biogenesis in brown adipose tissues of diet-induced obese mice. *Food Nutr. Res.* **2017**, *61*, 1325307. [CrossRef]
185. Zhou, J.; Mao, L.; Xu, P.; Wang, Y. Effects of (−)-epigallocatechin gallate (EGCG) on energy expenditure and microglia-mediated hypothalamic inflammation in mice fed a high-fat diet. *Nutrients* **2018**, *10*, 1681. [CrossRef]
186. Hursel, R.; Westerterp-Plantenga, M.S. Catechin- and caffeine-rich teas for control of body weight in humans. *Am. J. Clin. Nutr.* **2013**, *98*, 1682S–1693S. [CrossRef]
187. Dulloo, A.G.; Seydoux, J.; Girardier, L.; Chantre, P.; Vandermander, J. Green tea and thermogenesis: Interactions between catechin-polyphenols, caffeine and sympathetic activity. *Int. J. Obes. Relat. Metab. Disord. J. Int. Assoc. Study Obes.* **2000**, *24*, 252–258. [CrossRef]
188. Yoneshiro, T.; Matsushita, M.; Hibi, M.; Tone, H.; Takeshita, M.; Yasunaga, K.; Katsuragi, Y.; Kameya, T.; Sugie, H.; Saito, M. Tea catechin and caffeine activate brown adipose tissue and increase cold-induced thermogenic capacity in humans. *Am. J. Clin. Nutr.* **2017**, *105*, 873–881. [CrossRef]
189. Ibars, M.; Ardid-Ruiz, A.; Suárez, M.; Muguerza, B.; Bladé, C.; Aragonès, G. Proanthocyanidins potentiate hypothalamic leptin/STAT3 signalling and Pomc gene expression in rats with diet-induced obesity. *Int. J. Obes.* **2017**, *41*, 129–136. [CrossRef]
190. Husain, I.; Akhtar, M.; Shaharyar, M.; Islamuddin, M.; Abdin, M.Z.; Akhtar, M.J.; Najmi, A.K. High-salt- and cholesterol diet-associated cognitive impairment attenuated by tannins-enriched fraction of Emblica officinalis via inhibiting NF-kB pathway. *Inflammopharmacology* **2018**, *26*, 147–156. [CrossRef]
191. Mi, Y.; Qi, G.; Fan, R.; Qiao, Q.; Sun, Y.; Gao, Y.; Liu, X. EGCG ameliorates high-fat- and high-fructose-induced cognitive defects by regulating the IRS/AKT and ERK/CREB/BDNF signaling pathways in the CNS. *FASEB J.* **2017**, *31*, 4998–5011. [CrossRef]
192. Ettcheto, M.; Cano, A.; Manzine, P.R.; Busquets, O.; Verdaguer, E.; Castro-Torres, R.D.; Garcia, M.L.; Beas-Zarate, C.; Olloquequi, J.; Auladell, C.; et al. Epigallocatechin-3-Gallate (EGCG) Improves Cognitive Deficits Aggravated by an Obesogenic Diet Through Modulation of Unfolded Protein Response in APPswe/PS1dE9 Mice. *Mol. Neurobiol.* **2020**, *57*, 1814–1827. [CrossRef] [PubMed]
193. Macedo, R.C.; Bondan, E.F.; Otton, R. Redox status on different regions of the central nervous system of obese and lean rats treated with green tea extract. *Nutr. Neurosci.* **2019**, *22*, 119–131. [CrossRef] [PubMed]
194. Xiong, H.; Wang, J.; Ran, Q.; Lou, G.; Peng, C.; Gan, Q.; Hu, J.; Sun, J.; Yao, R.; Huang, Q. Hesperidin: A Therapeutic Agent For Obesity. *Drug Des. Devel. Ther.* **2019**, *13*, 3855–3866. [CrossRef] [PubMed]
195. Burke, A.C.; Telford, D.E.; Edwards, J.Y.; Sutherland, B.G.; Sawyez, C.G.; Huff, M.W. Naringenin Supplementation to a Chow Diet Enhances Energy Expenditure and Fatty Acid Oxidation, and Reduces Adiposity in Lean, Pair-Fed Ldlr −/− Mice. *Mol. Nutr. Food Res.* **2019**, *63*, 1–9. [CrossRef] [PubMed]
196. Barreca, D.; Gattuso, G.; Bellocco, E.; Calderaro, A.; Trombetta, D.; Smeriglio, A.; Laganà, G.; Daglia, M.; Meneghini, S.; Nabavi, S.M. Flavanones: Citrus phytochemical with health-promoting properties. *BioFactors* **2017**, *43*, 495–506. [CrossRef]
197. Li, C.; Schluesener, H. Health-promoting effects of the citrus flavanone hesperidin. *Crit. Rev. Food Sci. Nutr.* **2017**, *57*, 613–631. [CrossRef]
198. Patel, K.; Singh, G.K.; Patel, D.K. A Review on Pharmacological and Analytical Aspects of Naringenin. *Chin. J. Integr. Med.* **2018**, *24*, 551–560. [CrossRef]

199. Den Hartogh, D.J.; Tsiani, E. Antidiabetic Properties of Naringenin: A Citrus Fruit Polyphenol. *Biomolecules* **2019**, *9*, 99. [CrossRef]
200. Hernández-Aquino, E.; Muriel, P. Beneficial effects of naringenin in liver diseases: Molecular mechanisms. *World J. Gastroenterol.* **2018**, *24*, 1679–1707. [CrossRef]
201. Shirani, K.; Yousefsani, B.S.; Shirani, M.; Karimi, G. Protective effects of naringin against drugs and chemical toxins induced hepatotoxicity: A review. *Phytother. Res.* **2020**. [CrossRef] [PubMed]
202. Kannappan, S.; Anuradha, C.V. Naringenin enhances insulin-stimulated tyrosine phosphorylation and improves the cellular actions of insulin in a dietary model of metabolic syndrome. *Eur. J. Nutr.* **2010**, *49*, 101–109. [CrossRef] [PubMed]
203. Cho, K.W.; Kim, Y.O.; Andrade, J.E.; Burgess, J.R.; Kim, Y.-C. Dietary naringenin increases hepatic peroxisome proliferators-activated receptor alpha protein expression and decreases plasma triglyceride and adiposity in rats. *Eur. J. Nutr.* **2011**, *50*, 81–88. [CrossRef] [PubMed]
204. Pu, P.; Gao, D.-M.; Mohamed, S.; Chen, J.; Zhang, J.; Zhou, X.-Y.; Zhou, N.-J.; Xie, J.; Jiang, H. Naringin ameliorates metabolic syndrome by activating AMP-activated protein kinase in mice fed a high-fat diet. *Arch. Biochem. Biophys.* **2012**, *518*, 61–70. [CrossRef]
205. Assini, J.M.; Mulvihill, E.E.; Sutherland, B.G.; Telford, D.E.; Sawyez, C.G.; Felder, S.L.; Chhoker, S.; Edwards, J.Y.; Gros, R.; Huff, M.W. Naringenin prevents cholesterol-induced systemic inflammation, metabolic dysregulation, and atherosclerosis in Ldlr(-)/(-) mice. *J. Lipid Res.* **2013**, *54*, 711–724. [CrossRef]
206. Assini, J.M.; Mulvihill, E.E.; Burke, A.C.; Sutherland, B.G.; Telford, D.E.; Chhoker, S.S.; Sawyez, C.G.; Drangova, M.; Adams, A.C.; Kharitonenkov, A.; et al. Naringenin prevents obesity, hepatic steatosis, and glucose intolerance in male mice independent of fibroblast growth factor 21. *Endocrinology* **2015**, *156*, 2087–2102. [CrossRef]
207. Sui, G.-G.; Xiao, H.-B.; Lu, X.-Y.; Sun, Z.-L. Naringin Activates AMPK Resulting in Altered Expression of SREBPs, PCSK9, and LDLR to Reduce Body Weight in Obese C57BL/6J Mice. *J. Agric. Food Chem.* **2018**, *66*, 8983–8990. [CrossRef]
208. Jung, U.J.; Lee, M.-K.; Jeong, K.-S.; Choi, M.-S. The hypoglycemic effects of hesperidin and naringin are partly mediated by hepatic glucose-regulating enzymes in C57BL/KsJ-db/db mice. *J. Nutr.* **2004**, *134*, 2499–2503. [CrossRef]
209. Jung, U.J.; Lee, M.-K.; Park, Y.B.; Kang, M.A.; Choi, M.-S. Effect of citrus flavonoids on lipid metabolism and glucose-regulating enzyme mRNA levels in type-2 diabetic mice. *Int. J. Biochem. Cell Biol.* **2006**, *38*, 1134–1145. [CrossRef]
210. Mosqueda-Solis, A.; Sanchez, J.; Reynes, B.; Palou, M.; Portillo, M.P.; Palou, A.; Pico, C. Hesperidin and capsaicin, but not the combination, prevent hepatic steatosis and other metabolic syndrome-related alterations in western diet-fed rats. *Sci. Rep.* **2018**, *8*, 15100. [CrossRef]
211. Wu, H.; Liu, Y.; Chen, X.; Zhu, D.; Ma, J.; Yan, Y.; Si, M.; Li, X.; Sun, C.; Yang, B.; et al. Neohesperidin exerts lipid-regulating effects in vitro and in vivo via fibroblast growth factor 21 and AMP-activated protein kinase/sirtuin type 1/peroxisome proliferator-activated receptor gamma coactivator 1α signaling axis. *Pharmacology* **2017**, *100*, 115–126. [CrossRef] [PubMed]
212. Kwon, E.Y.; Choi, M.S. Dietary eriodictyol alleviates adiposity, hepatic steatosis, insulin resistance, and inflammation in diet-induced obese mice. *Int. J. Mol. Sci.* **2019**, *20*, 1227. [CrossRef] [PubMed]
213. Zhou, Y.; Ding, Y.-L.; Zhang, J.-L.; Zhang, P.; Wang, J.-Q.; Li, Z.-H. Alpinetin improved high fat diet-induced non-alcoholic fatty liver disease (NAFLD) through improving oxidative stress, inflammatory response and lipid metabolism. *Biomed. Pharmacother.* **2018**, *97*, 1397–1408. [CrossRef] [PubMed]
214. Cheraghpour, M.; Imani, H.; Ommi, S.; Alavian, S.M.; Karimi-Shahrbabak, E.; Hedayati, M.; Yari, Z.; Hekmatdoost, A. Hesperidin improves hepatic steatosis, hepatic enzymes, and metabolic and inflammatory parameters in patients with nonalcoholic fatty liver disease: A randomized, placebo-controlled, double-blind clinical trial. *Phyther. Res.* **2019**, *33*, 2118–2125. [CrossRef]
215. Yoshida, H.; Watanabe, H.; Ishida, A.; Watanabe, W.; Narumi, K.; Atsumi, T.; Sugita, C.; Kurokawa, M. Naringenin suppresses macrophage infiltration into adipose tissue in an early phase of high-fat diet-induced obesity. *Biochem. Biophys. Res. Commun.* **2014**, *454*, 95–101. [CrossRef]
216. Hoek-van den Hil, E.F.; van Schothorst, E.M.; van der Stelt, I.; Swarts, H.J.M.; van Vliet, M.; Amolo, T.; Vervoort, J.J.M.; Venema, D.; Hollman, P.C.H.; Rietjens, I.M.C.M.; et al. Direct comparison of metabolic health

effects of the flavonoids quercetin, hesperetin, epicatechin, apigenin and anthocyanins in high-fat-diet-fed mice. *Genes Nutr.* **2015**, *10*, 1–13. [CrossRef]
217. Tsuhako, R.; Yoshida, H.; Sugita, C.; Kurokawa, M. Naringenin suppresses neutrophil infiltration into adipose tissue in high-fat diet-induced obese mice. *J. Nat. Med.* **2020**, *74*, 229–237. [CrossRef]
218. Rebello, C.J.; Greenway, F.L.; Lau, F.H.; Lin, Y.; Stephens, J.M.; Johnson, W.D.; Coulter, A.A. Naringenin Promotes Thermogenic Gene Expression in Human White Adipose Tissue. *Obesity* **2019**, *27*, 103–111. [CrossRef]
219. Chou, Y.C.; Ho, C.T.; Pan, M.H. Immature citrus reticulata extract promotes browning of beige adipocytes in high-fat diet-induced C57BL/6 mice. *J. Agric. Food Chem.* **2018**, *66*, 9697–9703. [CrossRef]
220. Stohs, S.J.; Badmaev, V. A Review of Natural Stimulant and Non-stimulant Thermogenic Agents. *Phytother. Res.* **2016**, *30*, 732–740. [CrossRef]
221. Mosqueda-Solís, A.; Sánchez, J.; Portillo, M.P.; Palou, A.; Picó, C. Combination of capsaicin and hesperidin reduces the effectiveness of each compound to decrease the adipocyte size and to induce browning features in adipose tissue of western diet fed rats. *J. Agric. Food Chem.* **2018**, *66*, 9679–9689. [CrossRef] [PubMed]
222. Nishikawa, S.; Hyodo, T.; Nagao, T.; Nakanishi, A.; Tandia, M.; Tsuda, T. α-Monoglucosyl Hesperidin but Not Hesperidin Induces Brown-Like Adipocyte Formation and Suppresses White Adipose Tissue Accumulation in Mice. *J. Agric. Food Chem.* **2019**, *67*, 1948–1954. [CrossRef] [PubMed]
223. Ohara, T.; Muroyama, K.; Yamamoto, Y.; Murosaki, S. Oral intake of a combination of glucosyl hesperidin and caffeine elicits an anti-obesity effect in healthy, moderately obese subjects: A randomized double-blind placebo-controlled trial. *Nutr. J.* **2016**, *15*, 1–11. [CrossRef] [PubMed]
224. Sandeep, M.S.; Nandini, C.D. Influence of quercetin, naringenin and berberine on glucose transporters and insulin signalling molecules in brain of streptozotocin-induced diabetic rats. *Biomed. Pharmacother.* **2017**, *94*, 605–611.
225. Saad, M.A.; Abdel Salam, R.M.; Kenawy, S.A.; Attia, A.S. Pinocembrin attenuates hippocampal inflammation, oxidative perturbations and apoptosis in a rat model of global cerebral ischemia reperfusion. *Pharmacol. Rep.* **2015**, *67*, 115–122. [CrossRef] [PubMed]
226. Tao, J.; Shen, C.; Sun, Y.; Chen, W.; Yan, G. Neuroprotective effects of pinocembrin on ischemia/reperfusion-induced brain injury by inhibiting autophagy. *Biomed. Pharmacother.* **2018**, *106*, 1003–1010. [CrossRef] [PubMed]
227. Wang, K.; Chen, Z.; Huang, J.; Huang, L.; Luo, N.; Liang, X.; Liang, M.; Xie, W. Naringenin prevents ischaemic stroke damage via anti-apoptotic and anti-oxidant effects. *Clin. Exp. Pharmacol. Physiol.* **2017**, *44*, 862–871. [CrossRef]
228. De Lima, N.M.R.; Ferreira, E.D.O.; Fernandes, M.Y.S.D.; Lima, F.A.V.; Neves, K.R.T.; Do Carmo, M.R.S.; De Andrade, G.M. Neuroinflammatory response to experimental stroke is inhibited by boldine. *Behav. Pharmacol.* **2016**, *28*, 223–227. [CrossRef]
229. Muhammad, T.; Ikram, M.; Ullah, R.; Rehman, S.U.; Kim, M.O. Hesperetin, a citrus flavonoid, attenuates LPS-induced neuroinflammation, apoptosis and memory impairments by modulating TLR4/NF-κB signaling. *Nutrients* **2019**, *11*, 648. [CrossRef]
230. Afshin-Majd, S.; Motevalizadeh, S.-A.; Khajevand-Khazaei, M.-R.; Roghani, M.; Baluchnejadmojarad, T.; Rohani, M.; Ziaee, P. Naringenin ameliorates learning and memory impairment following systemic lipopolysaccharide challenge in the rat. *Eur. J. Pharmacol.* **2018**, *826*, 114–122.
231. Khalaj, R.; Hajizadeh Moghaddam, A.; Zare, M. Hesperetin and it nanocrystals ameliorate social behavior deficits and oxido-inflammatory stress in rat model of autism. *Int. J. Dev. Neurosci.* **2018**, *69*, 80–87. [CrossRef] [PubMed]
232. Kosari-Nasab, M.; Shokouhi, G.; Ghorbanihaghjo, A.; Abbasi, M.M.; Salari, A.A. Hesperidin attenuates depression-related symptoms in mice with mild traumatic brain injury. *Life Sci.* **2018**, *213*, 198–205. [CrossRef] [PubMed]
233. Fu, H.; Liu, L.; Tong, Y.; Li, Y.; Zhang, X.; Gao, X.; Yong, J.; Zhao, J.; Xiao, D.; Wen, K.; et al. The antidepressant effects of hesperidin on chronic unpredictable mild stress-induced mice. *Eur. J. Pharmacol.* **2019**, *853*, 236–246. [CrossRef] [PubMed]
234. Sato, M.; Okuno, A.; Suzuki, K.; Ohsawa, N.; Inoue, E.; Miyaguchi, Y.; Toyoda, A. Dietary intake of the citrus flavonoid hesperidin affects stress-resilience and brain kynurenine levels in a subchronic and mild social defeat stress model in mice. *Biosci. Biotechnol. Biochem.* **2019**, *83*, 1756–1765. [CrossRef] [PubMed]

235. Umukoro, S.; Kalejaye, H.A.; Ben-Azu, B.; Ajayi, A.M. Naringenin attenuates behavioral derangements induced by social defeat stress in mice via inhibition of acetylcholinesterase activity, oxidative stress and release of pro-inflammatory cytokines. *Biomed. Pharmacother.* **2018**, *105*, 714–723. [CrossRef]
236. Alkhalidy, H.; Wang, Y.; Liu, D. Dietary flavonoids in the prevention of T2D: An overview. *Nutrients* **2018**, *10*, 438. [CrossRef]
237. Dabeek, W.M.; Marra, M.V. Dietary quercetin and kaempferol: Bioavailability and potential cardiovascular-related bioactivity in humans. *Nutrients* **2019**, *11*, 2288. [CrossRef]
238. Batiha, G.E.-S.; Beshbishy, A.M.; Ikram, M.; Mulla, Z.S.; El-Hack, M.E.A.; Taha, A.E.; Algammal, A.M.; Elewa, Y.H.A. The Pharmacological Activity, Biochemical Properties, and Pharmacokinetics of the Major Natural Polyphenolic Flavonoid: Quercetin. *Foods* **2020**, *9*, 374. [CrossRef]
239. Hoek-van den Hil, E.F.; van Schothorst, E.M.; van der Stelt, I.; Swarts, H.J.M.; Venema, D.; Sailer, M.; Vervoort, J.J.M.; Hollman, P.C.H.; Rietjens, I.M.; Keijer, J. Quercetin decreases high-fat diet induced body weight gain and accumulation of hepatic and circulating lipids in mice. *Genes Nutr.* **2014**, *9*, 418. [CrossRef]
240. Zamora-Ros, R.; Forouhi, N.G.; Sharp, S.J.; Gonzalez, C.A.; Buijsse, B.; Guevara, M.; van der Schouw, Y.T.; Amiano, P.; Boeing, H.; Bredsdorff, L.; et al. Dietary intakes of individual flavanols and flavonols are inversely associated with incident type 2 diabetes in European populations. *J. Nutr.* **2014**, *144*, 335–343. [CrossRef]
241. Eid, H.M.; Haddad, P.S. The Antidiabetic Potential of Quercetin: Underlying Mechanisms. *Curr. Med. Chem.* **2017**, *24*, 355–364. [CrossRef] [PubMed]
242. Carrasco-Pozo, C.; Cires, M.J.; Gotteland, M. Quercetin and Epigallocatechin Gallate in the Prevention and Treatment of Obesity: From Molecular to Clinical Studies. *J. Med. Food* **2019**, *22*, 753–770. [CrossRef] [PubMed]
243. Bule, M.; Abdurahman, A.; Nikfar, S.; Abdollahi, M.; Amini, M. Antidiabetic effect of quercetin: A systematic review and meta-analysis of animal studies. *Food Chem. Toxicol.* **2019**, *125*, 494–502. [CrossRef]
244. Zhao, L.; Zhang, Q.; Ma, W.; Tian, F.; Shen, H.; Zhou, M. A combination of quercetin and resveratrol reduces obesity in high-fat diet-fed rats by modulation of gut microbiota. *Food Funct.* **2017**, *8*, 4644–4656. [CrossRef]
245. Liu, L.; Gao, C.; Yao, P.; Gong, Z. Quercetin Alleviates High-Fat Diet-Induced Oxidized Low-Density Lipoprotein Accumulation in the Liver: Implication for Autophagy Regulation. *Biomed Res. Int.* **2015**, *2015*, 607531. [CrossRef] [PubMed]
246. Xu, Y.; Han, J.; Dong, J.; Fan, X.; Cai, Y.; Li, J.; Wang, T.; Zhou, J.; Shang, J. Metabolomics Characterizes the Effects and Mechanisms of Quercetin in Nonalcoholic Fatty Liver Disease Development. *Int. J. Mol. Sci.* **2019**, *20*, 1220. [CrossRef]
247. Porras, D.; Nistal, E.; Martinez-Florez, S.; Olcoz, J.L.; Jover, R.; Jorquera, F.; Gonzalez-Gallego, J.; Garcia-Mediavilla, M.V.; Sanchez-Campos, S. Functional Interactions between Gut Microbiota Transplantation, Quercetin, and High-Fat Diet Determine Non-Alcoholic Fatty Liver Disease Development in Germ-Free Mice. *Mol. Nutr. Food Res.* **2019**, *63*, e1800930. [CrossRef]
248. Rubio-Ruiz, M.E.; Guarner-Lans, V.; Cano-Martinez, A.; Diaz-Diaz, E.; Manzano-Pech, L.; Gamas-Magana, A.; Castrejon-Tellez, V.; Tapia-Cortina, C.; Perez-Torres, I. Resveratrol and Quercetin Administration Improves Antioxidant DEFENSES and reduces Fatty Liver in Metabolic Syndrome Rats. *Molecules* **2019**, *24*, 1297. [CrossRef]
249. Aranaz, P.; Zabala, M.; Romo-Hualde, A.; Navarro-Herrera, D.; Lopez-Yoldi, M.; Vizmanos, J.L.; Martinez, J.A.; Milagro, F.I.; Gonzalez-Navarro, C.J. A combination of borage seed oil and quercetin reduces fat accumulation and improves insulin sensitivity in obese rats. *Food Funct.* **2020**. [CrossRef]
250. Qin, G.; Ma, J.; Huang, Q.; Yin, H.; Han, J.; Li, M.; Deng, Y.; Wang, B.; Hassan, W.; Shang, J. Isoquercetin Improves Hepatic Lipid Accumulation by Activating AMPK Pathway and Suppressing TGF-beta Signaling on an HFD-Induced Nonalcoholic Fatty Liver Disease Rat Model. *Int. J. Mol. Sci.* **2018**, *19*, 4126. [CrossRef]
251. Hoang, M.-H.; Jia, Y.; Lee, J.H.; Kim, Y.; Lee, S.-J. Kaempferol reduces hepatic triglyceride accumulation by inhibiting Akt. *J. Food Biochem.* **2019**, *43*, e13034. [CrossRef] [PubMed]
252. Hoang, M.H.; Jia, Y.; Mok, B.; Jun, H.J.; Hwang, K.Y.; Lee, S.J. Kaempferol ameliorates symptoms of metabolic syndrome by regulating activities of liver X receptor-β. *J. Nutr. Biochem.* **2015**, *26*, 868–875. [CrossRef] [PubMed]
253. Gaballah, H.H.; El-Horany, H.E.; Helal, D.S. Mitigative effects of the bioactive flavonol fisetin on high-fat/high-sucrose induced nonalcoholic fatty liver disease in rats. *J. Cell. Biochem.* **2019**, *120*, 12762–12774. [CrossRef] [PubMed]

254. Zeng, X.; Yang, J.; Hu, O.; Huang, J.; Ran, L.; Chen, M.; Zhang, Y.; Zhou, X.; Zhu, J.; Zhang, Q.; et al. Dihydromyricetin Ameliorates Nonalcoholic Fatty Liver Disease by Improving Mitochondrial Respiratory Capacity and Redox Homeostasis Through Modulation of SIRT3 Signaling. *Antioxid. Redox Signal.* **2019**, *30*, 163–183. [CrossRef]
255. Liu, Q.; Pan, R.; Ding, L.; Zhang, F.; Hu, L.; Ding, B.; Zhu, L.; Xia, Y.; Dou, X. Rutin exhibits hepatoprotective effects in a mouse model of non-alcoholic fatty liver disease by reducing hepatic lipid levels and mitigating lipid-induced oxidative injuries. *Int. Immunopharmacol.* **2017**, *49*, 132–141. [CrossRef]
256. Malinska, H.; Huttl, M.; Oliyarnyk, O.; Markova, I.; Poruba, M.; Racova, Z.; Kazdova, L.; Vecera, R. Beneficial effects of troxerutin on metabolic disorders in non-obese model of metabolic syndrome. *PLoS ONE* **2019**, *14*, e0220377. [CrossRef]
257. An, J.-P.; Choi, J.H.; Huh, J.; Lee, H.J.; Han, S.; Noh, J.-R.; Kim, Y.-H.; Lee, C.-H.; Oh, W.-K. Anti-hepatic steatosis activity of Sicyos angulatus extract in high-fat diet-fed mice and chemical profiling study using UHPLC-qTOF-MS/MS spectrometry. *Phytomedicine* **2019**, *63*, 152999. [CrossRef]
258. Guruvaiah, P.; Guo, H.; Li, D.; Xie, Z. Preventive Effect of Flavonol Derivatives Abundant Sanglan Tea on Long-Term High-Fat-Diet-Induced Obesity Complications in C57BL/6 Mice. *Nutrients* **2018**, *10*, 1276. [CrossRef]
259. Song, J.; Kim, Y.-S.; Kim, L.; Park, H.J.; Lee, D.; Kim, H. Anti-Obesity Effects of the Flower of Prunus persica in High-Fat Diet-Induced Obese Mice. *Nutrients* **2019**, *11*, 2176. [CrossRef]
260. Omatsu, K.-I.; Nakata, A.; Sato, K.; Mihara, Y.; Takaguri, A.; Nagashima, T.; Wakame, K. Global Liver Gene Expression Analysis on a Murine Hepatic Steatosis Model Treated with Mulberry (*Morus alba* L.) Leaf Powder. *Anticancer Res.* **2018**, *38*, 4305–4311.
261. Ezzat, S.M.; El Bishbishy, M.H.; Aborehab, N.M.; Salama, M.M.; Hasheesh, A.; Motaal, A.A.; Rashad, H.; Metwally, F.M. Upregulation of MC4R and PPAR-α expression mediates the anti-obesity activity of Moringa oleifera Lam. in high-fat diet-induced obesity in rats. *J. Ethnopharmacol.* **2020**, *251*, 112541. [CrossRef] [PubMed]
262. Nie, H.; Deng, Y.; Zheng, C.; Pan, M.; Xie, J.; Zhang, Y.; Yang, Q. A network pharmacology-based approach to explore the effects of Chaihu Shugan powder on a non-alcoholic fatty liver rat model through nuclear receptors. *J. Cell. Mol. Med.* **2020**, *24*, 5168–5184. [CrossRef] [PubMed]
263. Li, H.; Kim, U.-H.; Yoon, J.-H.; Ji, H.-S.; Park, H.-M.; Park, H.-Y.; Jeong, T.-S. Suppression of Hyperglycemia and Hepatic Steatosis by Black-Soybean-Leaf Extract via Enhanced Adiponectin-Receptor Signaling and AMPK Activation. *J. Agric. Food Chem.* **2019**, *67*, 90–101. [CrossRef] [PubMed]
264. Yamauchi, T.; Iwabu, M.; Okada-Iwabu, M.; Kadowaki, T. Adiponectin receptors: A review of their structure, function and how they work. *Best Pract. Res. Clin. Endocrinol. Metab.* **2014**, *28*, 15–23. [CrossRef]
265. Wang, T.; Wu, Q.; Zhao, T. Preventive Effects of Kaempferol on High-Fat Diet-Induced Obesity Complications in C57BL/6 Mice. *Biomed Res. Int.* **2020**, *2020*, 4532482. [CrossRef]
266. Tan, S.; Caparros-Martin, J.A.; Matthews, V.E.; Koch, H.; O'Gara, F.; Croft, K.D.; Ward, N.C. Isoquercetin and inulin synergistically modulate the gut microbiome to prevent development of the metabolic syndrome in mice fed a high fat diet. *Sci. Rep.* **2018**, *8*, 10100. [CrossRef]
267. Zhao, Y.; Chen, B.; Shen, J.; Wan, L.; Zhu, Y.; Yi, T.; Xiao, Z. The Beneficial Effects of Quercetin, Curcumin, and Resveratrol in Obesity. *Oxid. Med. Cell. Longev.* **2017**, *2017*, 1459497. [CrossRef]
268. Li, H.; Qi, J.; Li, L. Phytochemicals as potential candidates to combat obesity via adipose non-shivering thermogenesis. *Pharmacol. Res.* **2019**, *147*, 104393. [CrossRef]
269. Horvath, C.; Wolfrum, C. Feeding brown fat: Dietary phytochemicals targeting non-shivering thermogenesis to control body weight. *Proc. Nutr. Soc.* **2020**, 1–19. [CrossRef]
270. Forney, L.A.; Lenard, N.R.; Stewart, L.K.; Henagan, T.M. Dietary Quercetin Attenuates Adipose Tissue Expansion and Inflammation and Alters Adipocyte Morphology in a Tissue-Specific Manner. *Int. J. Mol. Sci.* **2018**, *19*, 895. [CrossRef]
271. Ting, Y.; Chang, W.-T.; Shiau, D.-K.; Chou, P.-H.; Wu, M.-F.; Hsu, C.-L. Antiobesity Efficacy of Quercetin-Rich Supplement on Diet-Induced Obese Rats: Effects on Body Composition, Serum Lipid Profile, and Gene Expression. *J. Agric. Food Chem.* **2018**, *66*, 70–80. [CrossRef] [PubMed]
272. Kuipers, E.N.; van Dam, A.D.; Held, N.M.; Mol, I.M.; Houtkooper, R.H.; Rensen, P.C.N.; Boon, M.R. Quercetin Lowers Plasma Triglycerides Accompanied by White Adipose Tissue Browning in Diet-Induced Obese Mice. *Int. J. Mol. Sci.* **2018**, *19*, 1786. [CrossRef] [PubMed]

273. Perdicaro, D.J.; Rodriguez Lanzi, C.; Gambarte Tudela, J.; Miatello, R.M.; Oteiza, P.I.; Vazquez Prieto, M.A. Quercetin attenuates adipose hypertrophy, in part through activation of adipogenesis in rats fed a high-fat diet. *J. Nutr. Biochem.* **2020**, *79*, 108352. [CrossRef]
274. Choi, H.; Kim, C.-S.; Yu, R. Quercetin Upregulates Uncoupling Protein 1 in White/Brown Adipose Tissues through Sympathetic Stimulation. *J. Obes. Metab. Syndr.* **2018**, *27*, 102–109. [CrossRef] [PubMed]
275. Lee, S.G.; Parks, J.S.; Kang, H.W. Quercetin, a functional compound of onion peel, remodels white adipocytes to brown-like adipocytes. *J. Nutr. Biochem.* **2017**, *42*, 62–71. [CrossRef]
276. Dong, J.; Zhang, X.; Zhang, L.; Bian, H.-X.; Xu, N.; Bao, B.; Liu, J. Quercetin reduces obesity-associated ATM infiltration and inflammation in mice: A mechanism including AMPKα1/SIRT1. *J. Lipid Res.* **2014**, *55*, 363–374. [CrossRef]
277. Arias, N.; Picó, C.; Teresa Macarulla, M.; Oliver, P.; Miranda, J.; Palou, A.; Portillo, M.P. A combination of resveratrol and quercetin induces browning in white adipose tissue of rats fed an obesogenic diet. *Obesity* **2017**, *25*, 111–121. [CrossRef]
278. Jiang, H.; Yoshioka, Y.; Yuan, S.; Horiuchi, Y.; Yamashita, Y.; Croft, K.D.; Ashida, H. Enzymatically modified isoquercitrin promotes energy metabolism through activating AMPKα in male C57BL/6 mice. *Food Funct.* **2019**, *10*, 5188–5202. [CrossRef]
279. Yuan, X.; Wei, G.; You, Y.; Huang, Y.; Lee, H.J.; Dong, M.; Lin, J.; Hu, T.; Zhang, H.; Zhang, C.; et al. Rutin ameliorates obesity through brown fat activation. *FASEB J.* **2017**, *31*, 333–345. [CrossRef]
280. Chen, N.; Lei, T.; Xin, L.; Zhou, L.; Cheng, J.; Qin, L.; Han, S.; Wan, Z. Depot-specific effects of treadmill running and rutin on white adipose tissue function in diet-induced obese mice. *J. Physiol. Biochem.* **2016**, *72*, 453–467. [CrossRef]
281. Mehanna, E.T.; El-Sayed, N.M.; Ibrahim, A.K.; Ahmed, S.A.; Abo-Elmatty, D.M. Isolated compounds from Cuscuta pedicellata ameliorate oxidative stress and upregulate expression of some energy regulatory genes in high fat diet induced obesity in rats. *Biomed. Pharmacother.* **2018**, *108*, 1253–1258. [CrossRef] [PubMed]
282. Hu, C.; Zhang, Y.; Liu, G.; Liu, Y.; Wang, J.; Sun, B. Untargeted Metabolite Profiling of Adipose Tissue in Hyperlipidemia Rats Exposed to Hawthorn Ethanol Extracts. *J. Food Sci.* **2019**, *84*, 717–725. [CrossRef] [PubMed]
283. Suganthy, N.; Devi, K.P.; Nabavi, S.F.; Braidy, N.; Nabavi, S.M. Bioactive effects of quercetin in the central nervous system: Focusing on the mechanisms of actions. *Biomed. Pharmacother.* **2016**, *84*, 892–908. [CrossRef] [PubMed]
284. Babaei, F.; Mirzababaei, M.; Nassiri-Asl, M. Quercetin in Food: Possible Mechanisms of Its Effect on Memory. *J. Food Sci.* **2018**, *83*, 2280–2287. [CrossRef]
285. Li, Y.; Tian, Q.; Li, Z.; Dang, M.; Lin, Y.; Hou, X. Activation of Nrf2 signaling by sitagliptin and quercetin combination against β-amyloid induced Alzheimer's disease in rats. *Drug Dev. Res.* **2019**, *80*, 837–845. [CrossRef]
286. Paula, P.-C.; Angelica Maria, S.-G.; Luis, C.-H.; Gloria Patricia, C.-G. Preventive Effect of Quercetin in a Triple Transgenic Alzheimer's Disease Mice Model. *Molecules* **2019**, *24*, 2287. [CrossRef]
287. Hayakawa, M.; Itoh, M.; Ohta, K.; Li, S.; Ueda, M.; Wang, M.; Nishida, E.; Islam, S.; Suzuki, C.; Ohzawa, K.; et al. Quercetin reduces eIF2α phosphorylation by GADD34 induction. *Neurobiol. Aging* **2015**, *36*, 2509–2518. [CrossRef]
288. Budzynska, B.; Faggio, C.; Kruk-Slomka, M.; Samec, D.; Nabavi, S.F.; Sureda, A.; Devi, K.P.; Nabavi, S.M. Rutin as Neuroprotective Agent: From Bench to Bedside. *Curr. Med. Chem.* **2019**, *26*, 5152–5164. [CrossRef]
289. Xia, S.-F.; Xie, Z.-X.; Qiao, Y.; Li, L.-R.; Cheng, X.-R.; Tang, X.; Shi, Y.-H.; Le, G.-W. Differential effects of quercetin on hippocampus-dependent learning and memory in mice fed with different diets related with oxidative stress. *Physiol. Behav.* **2015**, *138*, 325–331. [CrossRef]
290. Kim, J.H.; Lee, S.; Cho, E.J. Acer okamotoanum and isoquercitrin improve cognitive function via attenuation of oxidative stress in high fat diet- and amyloid beta-induced mice. *Food Funct.* **2019**, *10*, 6803–6814. [CrossRef]
291. Yang, J.; Kim, C.-S.; Tu, T.H.; Kim, M.-S.; Goto, T.; Kawada, T.; Choi, M.-S.; Park, T.; Sung, M.-K.; Yun, J.W.; et al. Quercetin Protects Obesity-Induced Hypothalamic Inflammation by Reducing Microglia-Mediated Inflammatory Responses via HO-1 Induction. *Nutrients* **2017**, *9*, 650. [CrossRef] [PubMed]
292. Maciel, R.M.; Carvalho, F.B.; Olabiyi, A.A.; Schmatz, R.; Gutierres, J.M.; Stefanello, N.; Zanini, D.; Rosa, M.M.; Andrade, C.M.; Rubin, M.A.; et al. Neuroprotective effects of quercetin on memory and anxiogenic-like

behavior in diabetic rats: Role of ectonucleotidases and acetylcholinesterase activities. *Biomed. Pharmacother.* **2016**, *84*, 559–568. [CrossRef] [PubMed]
293. Dajas, F.; Juan Andres, A.-C.; Florencia, A.; Carolina, E.; Felicia, R.-M. Neuroprotective Actions of Flavones and Flavonols: Mechanisms and Relationship to Flavonoid Structural Features. *Cent. Nerv. Syst. Agents Med. Chem.* **2013**, *13*, 30–35. [CrossRef] [PubMed]
294. McCue, P.; Shetty, K. Health benefits of soy isoflavonoids and strategies for enhancement: A review. *Crit. Rev. Food Sci. Nutr.* **2004**, *44*, 361–367. [CrossRef]
295. Dixon, R.A.; Pasinetti, G.M. Flavonoids and isoflavonoids: From plant biology to agriculture and neuroscience. *Plant Physiol.* **2010**, *154*, 453–457. [CrossRef]
296. Curtis, P.J.; Sampson, M.; Potter, J.; Dhatariya, K.; Kroon, P.A.; Cassidy, A. Chronic ingestion of flavan-3-ols and isoflavones improves insulin sensitivity and lipoprotein status and attenuates estimated 10-year CVD risk in medicated postmenopausal women with type 2 diabetes: A 1-year, double-blind, randomized, controlled trial. *Diabetes Care* **2012**, *35*, 226–232. [CrossRef]
297. Wang, S.; Wang, Y.; Pan, M.-H.; Ho, C.-T. Anti-obesity molecular mechanism of soy isoflavones: Weaving the way to new therapeutic routes. *Food Funct.* **2017**, *8*, 3831–3846. [CrossRef]
298. Cao, H.; Ou, J.; Chen, L.; Zhang, Y.; Szkudelski, T.; Delmas, D.; Daglia, M.; Xiao, J. Dietary polyphenols and type 2 diabetes: Human Study and Clinical Trial. *Crit. Rev. Food Sci. Nutr.* **2019**, *59*, 3371–3379. [CrossRef]
299. Akhlaghi, M.; Zare, M.; Nouripour, F. Effect of Soy and Soy Isoflavones on Obesity-Related Anthropometric Measures: A Systematic Review and Meta-analysis of Randomized Controlled Clinical Trials. *Adv. Nutr.* **2017**, *8*, 705–717. [CrossRef]
300. Zhou, Y.-X.; Zhang, H.; Peng, C. Puerarin: A review of pharmacological effects. *Phytother. Res.* **2014**, *28*, 961–975. [CrossRef]
301. Ganai, A.A.; Farooqi, H. Bioactivity of genistein: A review of in vitro and in vivo studies. *Biomed. Pharmacother.* **2015**, *76*, 30–38. [CrossRef] [PubMed]
302. Xin, X.; Chen, C.; Hu, Y.Y.; Feng, Q. Protective effect of genistein on nonalcoholic fatty liver disease (NAFLD). *Biomed. Pharmacother.* **2019**, *117*, 109047. [CrossRef] [PubMed]
303. Rockwood, S.; Mason, D.; Lord, R.; Lamar, P.; Prozialeck, W.; Al-Nakkash, L. Genistein diet improves body weight, serum glucose and triglyceride levels in both male and female ob/ob mice. *Diabetes. Metab. Syndr. Obes.* **2019**, *12*, 2011–2021. [CrossRef] [PubMed]
304. Marcelo, C.; Warwick, M.; Marcelo, C.; Malik, M.; Qayyum, R. The relationship between urinary genistein levels and serum alanine aminotransferase levels in adults in the USA: National Health and Nutrition Examination Survey 1999–2010. *Eur. J. Gastroenterol. Hepatol.* **2018**, *30*, 904–909. [CrossRef]
305. Hakkak, R.; Gauss, C.H.; Bell, A.; Korourian, S. Short-term soy protein isolate feeding prevents liver steatosis and reduces serum ALT and AST levels in obese female zucker rats. *Biomedicines* **2018**, *6*, 55. [CrossRef]
306. Qiu, L.-X.; Chen, T. Novel insights into the mechanisms whereby isoflavones protect against fatty liver disease. *World J. Gastroenterol.* **2015**, *21*, 1099–1107. [CrossRef]
307. Xiao, C.W.; Wood, C.M.; Weber, D.; Aziz, S.A.; Mehta, R.; Griffin, P.; Cockell, K.A. Dietary supplementation with soy isoflavones or replacement with soy proteins prevents hepatic lipid droplet accumulation and alters expression of genes involved in lipid metabolism in rats. *Genes Nutr.* **2014**, *9*, 373. [CrossRef]
308. Arunkumar, E.; Karthik, D.; Anuradha, C.V. Genistein sensitizes hepatic insulin signaling and modulates lipid regulatory genes through p70 ribosomal S6 kinase-1 inhibition in high-fat-high-fructose diet-fed mice. *Pharm. Biol.* **2013**, *51*, 815–824. [CrossRef]
309. Liu, H.; Zhong, H.; Yin, Y.; Jiang, Z. Genistein has beneficial effects on hepatic steatosis in high fat-high sucrose diet-treated rats. *Biomed. Pharmacother.* **2017**, *91*, 964–969. [CrossRef]
310. Lyons, C.L.; Roche, H.M. Nutritional Modulation of AMPK-Impact upon Metabolic-Inflammation. *Int. J. Mol. Sci.* **2018**, *19*, 3092. [CrossRef]
311. Wang, S.; Yang, F.-J.; Shang, L.-C.; Zhang, Y.-H.; Zhou, Y.; Shi, X.-L. Puerarin protects against high-fat high-sucrose diet-induced non-alcoholic fatty liver disease by modulating PARP-1/PI3K/AKT signaling pathway and facilitating mitochondrial homeostasis. *Phytother. Res.* **2019**, *33*, 2347–2359. [CrossRef] [PubMed]
312. Zheng, G.; Lin, L.; Zhong, S.; Zhang, Q.; Li, D. Effects of puerarin on lipid accumulation and metabolism in high-fat diet-fed mice. *PLoS ONE* **2015**, *10*, e0122925. [CrossRef] [PubMed]

313. Lu, Y.; Zhao, A.; Wu, Y.; Zhao, Y.; Yang, X. Soybean soluble polysaccharides enhance bioavailability of genistein and its prevention against obesity and metabolic syndrome of mice with chronic high fat consumption. *Food Funct.* **2019**, *10*, 4153–4165. [CrossRef] [PubMed]
314. Li, W.; Lu, Y. Hepatoprotective Effects of Sophoricoside against Fructose-Induced Liver Injury via Regulating Lipid Metabolism, Oxidation, and Inflammation in Mice. *J. Food Sci.* **2018**, *83*, 552–558. [CrossRef] [PubMed]
315. Duan, X.; Meng, Q.; Wang, C.; Liu, Z.; Sun, H.; Huo, X.; Sun, P.; Ma, X.; Peng, J.; Liu, K. Effects of calycosin against high-fat diet-induced nonalcoholic fatty liver disease in mice. *J. Gastroenterol. Hepatol.* **2018**, *33*, 533–542. [CrossRef] [PubMed]
316. Liu, H.; Zhong, H.; Leng, L.; Jiang, Z. Effects of soy isoflavone on hepatic steatosis in high fat-induced rats. *J. Clin. Biochem. Nutr.* **2017**, *61*, 85–90. [CrossRef]
317. Wang, W.; Chen, J.; Mao, J.; Li, H.; Wang, M.; Zhang, H.; Li, H.; Chen, W. Genistein Ameliorates Non-alcoholic Fatty Liver Disease by Targeting the Thromboxane A2 Pathway. *J. Agric. Food Chem.* **2018**, *66*, 5853–5859. [CrossRef]
318. Gan, M.; Shen, L.; Fan, Y.; Tan, Y.; Zheng, T.; Tang, G.; Niu, L.; Zhao, Y.; Chen, L.; Jiang, D.; et al. MicroRNA-451 and Genistein Ameliorate Nonalcoholic Steatohepatitis in Mice. *Int. J. Mol. Sci.* **2019**, *20*, 6084. [CrossRef]
319. Amanat, S.; Eftekhari, M.H.; Fararouei, M.; Bagheri Lankarani, K.; Massoumi, S.J. Genistein supplementation improves insulin resistance and inflammatory state in non-alcoholic fatty liver patients: A randomized, controlled trial. *Clin. Nutr.* **2018**, *37*, 1210–1215. [CrossRef]
320. Giordano, E.; Dávalos, A.; Crespo, M.C.; Tomé-Carneiro, J.; Gómez-Coronado, D.; Visioli, F. Soy isoflavones in nutritionally relevant amounts have varied nutrigenomic effects on adipose tissue. *Molecules* **2015**, *20*, 2310–2322. [CrossRef]
321. Tan, J.; Huang, C.; Luo, Q.; Liu, W.; Cheng, D.; Li, Y.; Xia, Y.; Li, C.; Tang, L.; Fang, J.; et al. Soy Isoflavones Ameliorate Fatty Acid Metabolism of Visceral Adipose Tissue by Increasing the AMPK Activity in Male Rats with Diet-Induced Obesity (DIO). *Molecules* **2019**, *24*, 2809. [CrossRef] [PubMed]
322. Jo, Y.H.; Choi, K.M.; Liu, Q.; Kim, S.B.; Ji, H.J.; Kim, M.; Shin, S.K.; Do, S.G.; Shin, E.; Jung, G.; et al. Anti-obesity effect of 6,8-diprenylgenistein, an isoflavonoid of Cudrania tricuspidata fruits in high-fat diet-induced obese mice. *Nutrients* **2015**, *7*, 10480–10490. [CrossRef] [PubMed]
323. Huang, C.-H.; Chen, C.-L.; Chang, S.-H.; Tsai, G.-J. Evaluation of Antiobesity Activity of Soybean Meal Products Fermented by Lactobacillus plantarum FPS 2520 and Bacillus subtilis N1 in Rats Fed with High-Fat Diet. *J. Med. Food* **2020**, *23*, 667–675. [CrossRef] [PubMed]
324. Zhou, L.; Xiao, X.; Zhang, Q.; Zheng, J.; Li, M.; Deng, M. A Possible Mechanism: Genistein Improves Metabolism and Induces White Fat Browning through Modulating Hypothalamic Expression of Ucn3, Depp, and Stc1. *Front. Endocrinol.* **2019**, *10*, 478. [CrossRef]
325. Palacios-González, B.; Vargas-Castillo, A.; Velázquez-Villegas, L.A.; Vasquez-Reyes, S.; López, P.; Noriega, L.G.; Aleman, G.; Tovar-Palacio, C.; Torre-Villalvazo, I.; Yang, L.J.; et al. Genistein increases the thermogenic program of subcutaneous WAT and increases energy expenditure in mice. *J. Nutr. Biochem.* **2019**, *68*, 59–68. [CrossRef]
326. Gautam, J.; Khedgikar, V.; Kushwaha, P.; Choudhary, D.; Nagar, G.K.; Dev, K.; Dixit, P.; Singh, D.; Maurya, R.; Trivedi, R. Formononetin, an isoflavone, activates AMP-activated protein kinase β-catenin signalling to inhibit adipogenesis and rescues C57BL/6 mice from high-fat diet-induced obesity and bone loss. *Br. J. Nutr.* **2017**, *117*, 645–661. [CrossRef]
327. Nie, T.; Zhao, S.; Mao, L.; Yang, Y.; Sun, W.; Lin, X.; Liu, S.; Li, K.; Sun, Y.; Li, P.; et al. The natural compound, formononetin, extracted from Astragalus membranaceus increases adipocyte thermogenesis by modulating PPARγ activity. *Br. J. Pharmacol.* **2018**, *175*, 1439–1450. [CrossRef]
328. Buhlmann, E.; Horváth, C.; Houriet, J.; Kiehlmann, E.; Radtke, J.; Marcourt, L.; Wolfender, J.-L.; Wolfrum, C.; Schröder, S. Puerariae lobatae root extracts and the regulation of brown fat activity. *Phytomedicine* **2019**, *64*, 153075. [CrossRef]
329. Shen, H.-H.; Huang, S.-Y.; Kung, C.-W.; Chen, S.-Y.; Chen, Y.-F.; Cheng, P.-Y.; Lam, K.-K.; Lee, Y.-M. Genistein ameliorated obesity accompanied with adipose tissue browning and attenuation of hepatic lipogenesis in ovariectomized rats with high-fat diet. *J. Nutr. Biochem.* **2019**, *67*, 111–122. [CrossRef]
330. Russell, A.L.; Grimes, J.M.; Cruthirds, D.F.; Westerfield, J.; Wooten, L.; Keil, M.; Weiser, M.J.; Landauer, M.R.; Handa, R.J.; Wu, T.J.; et al. Dietary Isoflavone-Dependent and Estradiol Replacement Effects on Body Weight in the Ovariectomized (OVX) Rat. *Horm. Metab. Res.* **2017**, *49*, 457–465. [CrossRef]

331. Han, F.; Li, K.; Pan, R.; Xu, W.; Han, X.; Hou, N.; Sun, X. Calycosin directly improves perivascular adipose tissue dysfunction by upregulating the adiponectin/AMPK/eNOS pathway in obese mice. *Food Funct.* **2018**, *9*, 2409–2415. [CrossRef] [PubMed]
332. Rivera, P.; Pérez-Martín, M.; Pavón, F.J.; Serrano, A.; Crespillo, A.; Cifuentes, M.; López-Ávalos, M.-D.; Grondona, J.M.; Vida, M.; Fernández-Llebrez, P.; et al. Pharmacological administration of the isoflavone daidzein enhances cell proliferation and reduces high fat diet-induced apoptosis and gliosis in the rat hippocampus. *PLoS ONE* **2013**, *8*, e64750. [CrossRef] [PubMed]
333. Ko, J.W.; Chung, Y.-S.; Kwak, C.S.; Kwon, Y.H. Doenjang, A Korean Traditional Fermented Soybean Paste, Ameliorates Neuroinflammation and Neurodegeneration in Mice Fed a High-Fat Diet. *Nutrients* **2019**, *11*, 1702. [CrossRef] [PubMed]
334. Essawy, A.E.; Abdou, H.M.; Ibrahim, H.M.; Bouthahab, N.M. Soybean isoflavone ameliorates cognitive impairment, neuroinflammation, and amyloid β accumulation in a rat model of Alzheimer's disease. *Environ. Sci. Pollut. Res.* **2019**, *26*, 26060–26070. [CrossRef]
335. Ko, Y.H.; Kwon, S.H.; Ma, S.X.; Seo, J.Y.; Lee, B.R.; Kim, K.; Kim, S.Y.; Lee, S.Y.; Jang, C.G. The memory-enhancing effects of 7,8,4'-trihydroxyisoflavone, a major metabolite of daidzein, are associated with activation of the cholinergic system and BDNF signaling pathway in mice. *Brain Res. Bull.* **2018**, *142*, 197–206. [CrossRef]
336. Lu, C.; Wang, Y.; Wang, D.; Zhang, L.; Lv, J.; Jiang, N.; Fan, B.; Liu, X.; Wang, F. Neuroprotective effects of soy isoflavones on scopolamine-induced amnesia in mice. *Nutrients* **2018**, *10*, 853. [CrossRef]
337. Seo, J.Y.; Kim, B.R.; Oh, J.; Kim, J.S. Soybean-derived phytoalexins improve cognitive function through activation of Nrf2/HO-1 signaling pathway. *Int. J. Mol. Sci.* **2018**, *19*, 268. [CrossRef]
338. Sudhakaran, M.; Doseff, A.I. The Targeted Impact of Flavones on Obesity-Induced Inflammation and the Potential Synergistic Role in Cancer and the Gut Microbiota. *Molecules* **2020**, *25*, 2477. [CrossRef]
339. Jiang, N.; Doseff, A.I.; Grotewold, E. Flavones: From Biosynthesis to Health Benefits. *Plants* **2016**, *5*, 27. [CrossRef]
340. Lin, Y.; Ren, N.; Li, S.; Chen, M.; Pu, P. Novel anti-obesity effect of scutellarein and potential underlying mechanism of actions. *Biomed. Pharmacother.* **2019**, *117*, 109042. [CrossRef]
341. Feng, X.; Yu, W.; Li, X.; Zhou, F.; Zhang, W.; Shen, Q.; Li, J.; Zhang, C.; Shen, P. Apigenin, a modulator of PPARγ, attenuates HFD-induced NAFLD by regulating hepatocyte lipid metabolism and oxidative stress via Nrf2 activation. *Biochem. Pharmacol.* **2017**, *136*, 136–149. [CrossRef]
342. Kwon, E.-Y.; Kim, S.Y.; Choi, M.-S. Luteolin-Enriched Artichoke Leaf Extract Alleviates the Metabolic Syndrome in Mice with High-Fat Diet-Induced Obesity. *Nutrients* **2018**, *10*, 979. [CrossRef]
343. Dai, J.; Liang, K.; Zhao, S.; Jia, W.; Liu, Y.; Wu, H.; Lv, J.; Cao, C.; Chen, T.; Zhuang, S.; et al. Chemoproteomics reveals baicalin activates hepatic CPT1 to ameliorate diet-induced obesity and hepatic steatosis. *Proc. Natl. Acad. Sci. USA* **2018**, *115*, E5896–E5905. [CrossRef]
344. Kim, Y.-J.; Choi, M.-S.; Woo, J.T.; Jeong, M.J.; Kim, S.R.; Jung, U.J. Long-term dietary supplementation with low-dose nobiletin ameliorates hepatic steatosis, insulin resistance, and inflammation without altering fat mass in diet-induced obesity. *Mol. Nutr. Food Res.* **2017**, *61*, 1600889. [CrossRef]
345. Inamdar, S.; Joshi, A.; Malik, S.; Boppana, R.; Ghaskadbi, S. Vitexin alleviates non-alcoholic fatty liver disease by activating AMPK in high fat diet fed mice. *Biochem. Biophys. Res. Commun.* **2019**, *519*, 106–112. [CrossRef]
346. Kwon, E.-Y.; Choi, M.-S. Luteolin Targets the Toll-Like Receptor Signaling Pathway in Prevention of Hepatic and Adipocyte Fibrosis and Insulin Resistance in Diet-Induced Obese Mice. *Nutrients* **2018**, *10*, 1415. [CrossRef]
347. Kwon, E.-Y.; Jung, U.J.; Park, T.; Yun, J.W.; Choi, M.-S. Luteolin Attenuates Hepatic Steatosis and Insulin Resistance Through the Interplay Between the Liver and Adipose Tissue in Mice with Diet-Induced Obesity. *Diabetes* **2015**, *64*, 1658–1669. [CrossRef]
348. Li, J.; Inoue, J.; Choi, J.-M.; Nakamura, S.; Yan, Z.; Fushinobu, S.; Kamada, H.; Kato, H.; Hashidume, T.; Shimizu, M.; et al. Identification of the Flavonoid Luteolin as a Repressor of the Transcription Factor Hepatocyte Nuclear Factor 4α. *J. Biol. Chem.* **2015**, *290*, 24021–24035. [CrossRef]
349. Yin, Y.; Gao, L.; Lin, H.; Wu, Y.; Han, X.; Zhu, Y.; Li, J. Luteolin improves non-alcoholic fatty liver disease in db/db mice by inhibition of liver X receptor activation to down-regulate expression of sterol regulatory element binding protein 1c. *Biochem. Biophys. Res. Commun.* **2017**, *482*, 720–725. [CrossRef]

350. Xi, Y.; Wu, M.; Li, H.; Dong, S.; Luo, E.; Gu, M.; Shen, X.; Jiang, Y.; Liu, Y.; Liu, H. Baicalin Attenuates High Fat Diet-Induced Obesity and Liver Dysfunction: Dose-Response and Potential Role of CaMKKβ/AMPK/ACC Pathway. *Cell. Physiol. Biochem.* **2015**, *35*, 2349–2359. [CrossRef]
351. Shen, K.; Feng, X.; Pan, H.; Zhang, F.; Xie, H.; Zheng, S. Baicalin Ameliorates Experimental Liver Cholestasis in Mice by Modulation of Oxidative Stress, Inflammation, and NRF2 Transcription Factor. *Oxid. Med. Cell. Longev.* **2017**, *2017*, 6169128. [CrossRef]
352. Chambel, S.S.; Santos-Gonçalves, A.; Duarte, T.L. The Dual Role of Nrf2 in Nonalcoholic Fatty Liver Disease: Regulation of Antioxidant Defenses and Hepatic Lipid Metabolism. *Biomed Res. Int.* **2015**, *2015*, 597134. [CrossRef]
353. Xu, D.; Xu, M.; Jeong, S.; Qian, Y.; Wu, H.; Xia, Q.; Kong, X. The Role of Nrf2 in Liver Disease: Novel Molecular Mechanisms and Therapeutic Approaches. *Front. Pharmacol.* **2019**, *9*, 1428. [CrossRef]
354. Zhang, X.; Ji, R.; Sun, H.; Peng, J.; Ma, X.; Wang, C.; Fu, Y.; Bao, L.; Jin, Y. Scutellarin ameliorates nonalcoholic fatty liver disease through the PPARγ/PGC-1α-Nrf2 pathway. *Free Radic. Res.* **2018**, *52*, 198–211. [CrossRef]
355. Fan, H.; Ma, X.; Lin, P.; Kang, Q.; Zhao, Z.; Wang, L.; Sun, D.; Cheng, J.; Li, Y. Scutellarin Prevents Nonalcoholic Fatty Liver Disease (NAFLD) and Hyperlipidemia via PI3K/AKT-Dependent Activation of Nuclear Factor (Erythroid-Derived 2)-Like 2 (Nrf2) in Rats. *Med. Sci. Monit.* **2017**, *23*, 5599–5612. [CrossRef]
356. Feng, X.; Weng, D.; Zhou, F.; Owen, Y.D.; Qin, H.; Zhao, J.; Huang, Y.; Chen, J.; Fu, H.; Yang, N.; et al. Activation of PPARγ by a Natural Flavonoid Modulator, Apigenin Ameliorates Obesity-Related Inflammation Via Regulation of Macrophage Polarization. *EBioMedicine* **2016**, *9*, 61–76. [CrossRef]
357. Lv, Y.; Gao, X.; Luo, Y.; Fan, W.; Shen, T.; Ding, C.; Yao, M.; Song, S.; Yan, L. Apigenin ameliorates HFD-induced NAFLD through regulation of the XO/NLRP3 pathways. *J. Nutr. Biochem.* **2019**, *71*, 110–121. [CrossRef]
358. Feng, X.; Qin, H.; Shi, Q.; Zhang, Y.; Zhou, F.; Wu, H.; Ding, S.; Niu, Z.; Lu, Y.; Shen, P. Chrysin attenuates inflammation by regulating M1/M2 status via activating PPARγ. *Biochem. Pharmacol.* **2014**, *89*, 503–514. [CrossRef]
359. Chen, J.; Liu, J.; Wang, Y.; Hu, X.; Zhou, F.; Hu, Y.; Yuan, Y.; Xu, Y. Wogonin mitigates nonalcoholic fatty liver disease via enhancing PPARalpha/AdipoR2, in vivo and in vitro. *Biomed. Pharmacother.* **2017**, *91*, 621–631. [CrossRef]
360. Pan, M.-H.; Yang, G.; Li, S.; Li, M.-Y.; Tsai, M.-L.; Wu, J.-C.; Badmaev, V.; Ho, C.-T.; Lai, C.-S. Combination of citrus polymethoxyflavones, green tea polyphenols, and Lychee extracts suppresses obesity and hepatic steatosis in high-fat diet induced obese mice. *Mol. Nutr. Food Res.* **2017**, *61*, 1601104. [CrossRef]
361. Su, T.; Huang, C.; Yang, C.; Jiang, T.; Su, J.; Chen, M.; Fatima, S.; Gong, R.; Hu, X.; Bian, Z.; et al. Apigenin inhibits STAT3/CD36 signaling axis and reduces visceral obesity. *Pharmacol. Res.* **2020**, *152*, 104586. [CrossRef]
362. Zhang, J.; Zhao, L.; Cheng, Q.; Ji, B.; Yang, M.; Sanidad, K.Z.; Wang, C.; Zhou, F. Structurally Different Flavonoid Subclasses Attenuate High-Fat and High-Fructose Diet Induced Metabolic Syndrome in Rats. *J. Agric. Food Chem.* **2018**, *66*, 12412–12420. [CrossRef]
363. Sun, Y.-S.; Qu, W. Dietary Apigenin promotes lipid catabolism, thermogenesis, and browning in adipose tissues of HFD-Fed mice. *Food Chem. Toxicol.* **2019**, *133*, 110780. [CrossRef]
364. Peng, Y.; Sun, Q.; Xu, W.; He, Y.; Jin, W.; Yuan, L.; Gao, R. Vitexin ameliorates high fat diet-induced obesity in male C57BL/6J mice via the AMPKα-mediated pathway. *Food Funct.* **2019**, *10*, 1940–1947. [CrossRef]
365. Zhang, L.; Han, Y.-J.; Zhang, X.; Wang, X.; Bao, B.; Qu, W.; Liu, J. Luteolin reduces obesity-associated insulin resistance in mice by activating AMPKα1 signalling in adipose tissue macrophages. *Diabetologia* **2016**, *59*, 2219–2228. [CrossRef]
366. Xu, N.; Zhang, L.; Dong, J.; Zhang, X.; Chen, Y.-G.; Bao, B.; Liu, J. Low-dose diet supplement of a natural flavonoid, luteolin, ameliorates diet-induced obesity and insulin resistance in mice. *Mol. Nutr. Food Res.* **2014**, *58*, 1258–1268. [CrossRef]
367. Sanchez-Gurmaches, J.; Tang, Y.; Jespersen, N.Z.; Wallace, M.; Martinez Calejman, C.; Gujja, S.; Li, H.; Edwards, Y.J.K.; Wolfrum, C.; Metallo, C.M.; et al. Brown Fat AKT2 Is a Cold-Induced Kinase that Stimulates ChREBP-Mediated De Novo Lipogenesis to Optimize Fuel Storage and Thermogenesis. *Cell Metab.* **2018**, *27*, 195–209. [CrossRef]
368. Mottillo, E.P.; Balasubramanian, P.; Lee, Y.-H.; Weng, C.; Kershaw, E.E.; Granneman, J.G. Coupling of lipolysis and de novo lipogenesis in brown, beige, and white adipose tissues during chronic β3-adrenergic receptor activation. *J. Lipid Res.* **2014**, *55*, 2276–2286. [CrossRef]

369. Zhang, X.; Zhang, Q.-X.; Wang, X.; Zhang, L.; Qu, W.; Bao, B.; Liu, C.-A.; Liu, J. Dietary luteolin activates browning and thermogenesis in mice through an AMPK/PGC1α pathway-mediated mechanism. *Int. J. Obes.* **2016**, *40*, 1841–1849. [CrossRef]
370. Min, W.; Wu, M.; Fang, P.; Yu, M.; Shi, M.; Zhang, Z.; Bo, P. Effect of Baicalein on GLUT4 Translocation in Adipocytes of Diet-Induced Obese Mice. *Cell. Physiol. Biochem.* **2018**, *50*, 426–436. [CrossRef]
371. Jack, B.U.; Malherbe, C.J.; Mamushi, M.; Muller, C.J.F.; Joubert, E.; Louw, J.; Pheiffer, C. Adipose tissue as a possible therapeutic target for polyphenols: A case for Cyclopia extracts as anti-obesity nutraceuticals. *Biomed. Pharmacother.* **2019**, *120*, 109439. [CrossRef]
372. Pan, M.-H.; Li, M.-Y.; Tsai, M.-L.; Pan, C.-Y.; Badmaev, V.; Ho, C.-T.; Lai, C.-S. A mixture of citrus polymethoxyflavones, green tea polyphenols and lychee extracts attenuates adipogenesis in 3T3-L1 adipocytes and obesity-induced adipose inflammation in mice. *Food Funct.* **2019**, *10*, 7667–7677. [CrossRef]
373. Liu, Y.; Fu, X.; Lan, N.; Li, S.; Zhang, J.; Wang, S.; Li, C.; Shang, Y.; Huang, T.; Zhang, L. Luteolin protects against high fat diet-induced cognitive deficits in obesity mice. *Behav. Brain Res.* **2014**, *267*, 178–188. [CrossRef]
374. Shanmugasundaram, J.; Subramanian, V.; Nadipelly, J.; Kathirvelu, P.; Sayeli, V.; Cheriyan, B.V. Anxiolytic-like activity of 5-methoxyflavone in mice with involvement of GABAergic and serotonergic systems—In vivo and in silico evidences. *Eur. Neuropsychopharmacol.* **2020**, *36*, 100–110. [CrossRef]
375. Wang, L.; Li, C.; Sreeharsha, N.; Mishra, A.; Shrotriya, V.; Sharma, A. Neuroprotective effect of Wogonin on Rat's brain exposed to gamma irradiation. *J. Photochem. Photobiol. B* **2020**, *204*, 111775. [CrossRef]
376. Wu, C.; Xu, Q.; Chen, X.; Liu, J. Delivery luteolin with folacin-modified nanoparticle for glioma therapy. *Int. J. Nanomed.* **2019**, *14*, 7515–7531. [CrossRef]
377. Guo, Y.; Yu, X.-M.; Chen, S.; Wen, J.-Y.; Chen, Z.-W. Total flavones of Rhododendron simsii Planch flower protect rat hippocampal neuron from hypoxia-reoxygenation injury via activation of BK(Ca) channel. *J. Pharm. Pharmacol.* **2020**, *72*, 111–120. [CrossRef]
378. Yu, C.-I.; Cheng, C.-I.; Kang, Y.-F.; Chang, P.-C.; Lin, I.-P.; Kuo, Y.-H.; Jhou, A.-J.; Lin, M.-Y.; Chen, C.-Y.; Lee, C.-H. Hispidulin Inhibits Neuroinflammation in Lipopolysaccharide-Activated BV2 Microglia and Attenuates the Activation of Akt, NF-κB, and STAT3 Pathway. *Neurotox. Res.* **2020**, *38*, 163–174. [CrossRef]
379. Cazarolli, L.H.; Kappel, V.D.; Zanatta, A.P.; Suzuki, D.O.H.; Yunes, R.A.; Nunes, R.J.; Pizzolatti, M.G.; Silva, F.R.M.B. Chapter 2—Natural and Synthetic Chalcones: Tools for the Study of Targets of Action—Insulin Secretagogue or Insulin Mimetic? In *Studies in Natural Products Chemistry*; Atta-ur-Rahman, Ed.; Elsevier: Amsterdam, The Netherlands, 2013; Volume 39, pp. 47–89. ISBN 1572-5995.
380. Bak, E.-J.; Choi, K.-C.; Jang, S.; Woo, G.-H.; Yoon, H.-G.; Na, Y.; Yoo, Y.-J.; Lee, Y.; Jeong, Y.; Cha, J.-H. Licochalcone F alleviates glucose tolerance and chronic inflammation in diet-induced obese mice through Akt and p38 MAPK. *Clin. Nutr.* **2016**, *35*, 414–421. [CrossRef]
381. Karimi-Sales, E.; Mohaddes, G.; Alipour, M.R. Chalcones as putative hepatoprotective agents: Preclinical evidence and molecular mechanisms. *Pharmacol. Res.* **2018**, *129*, 177–187. [CrossRef]
382. Iwasaki, M.; Izuo, N.; Izumi, Y.; Takada-Takatori, Y.; Akaike, A.; Kume, T. Protective Effect of Green Perilla-Derived Chalcone Derivative DDC on Amyloid β Protein-Induced Neurotoxicity in Primary Cortical Neurons. *Biol. Pharm. Bull.* **2019**, *42*, 1942–1946. [CrossRef] [PubMed]
383. Bai, P.; Wang, K.; Zhang, P.; Shi, J.; Cheng, X.; Zhang, Q.; Zheng, C.; Cheng, Y.; Yang, J.; Lu, X.; et al. Development of chalcone-O-alkylamine derivatives as multifunctional agents against Alzheimer's disease. *Eur. J. Med. Chem.* **2019**, *183*, 111737. [CrossRef] [PubMed]
384. Padmavathi, G.; Roy, N.K.; Bordoloi, D.; Arfuso, F.; Mishra, S.; Sethi, G.; Bishayee, A.; Kunnumakkara, A.B. Butein in health and disease: A comprehensive review. *Phytomedicine* **2017**, *25*, 118–127. [CrossRef] [PubMed]
385. Legette, L.L.; Moreno Luna, A.Y.; Reed, R.L.; Miranda, C.L.; Bobe, G.; Proteau, R.R.; Stevens, J.F. Xanthohumol lowers body weight and fasting plasma glucose in obese male Zucker fa/fa rats. *Phytochemistry* **2013**, *91*, 236–241. [CrossRef]
386. Costa, R.; Rodrigues, I.; Guardão, L.; Rocha-Rodrigues, S.; Silva, C.; Magalhães, J.; Ferreira-de-Almeida, M.; Negrão, R.; Soares, R. Xanthohumol and 8-prenylnaringenin ameliorate diabetic-related metabolic dysfunctions in mice. *J. Nutr. Biochem.* **2017**, *45*, 39–47. [CrossRef]
387. Prabhu, D.S.; Rajeswari, V.D. PPAR-Gamma as putative gene target involved in Butein mediated anti-diabetic effect. *Mol. Biol. Rep.* **2020**. [CrossRef]

388. Johnson, R.; de Beer, D.; Dludla, P.V.; Ferreira, D.; Muller, C.J.; Joubert, E. Aspalathin from Rooibos (Aspalathus linearis): A Bioactive C-glucosyl Dihydrochalcone with Potential to Target the Metabolic Syndrome. *Planta Med.* **2018**, *84*, 568–583. [CrossRef]
389. Zhu, X.; Liu, J.; Chen, S.; Xue, J.; Huang, S.; Wang, Y.; Chen, O. Isoliquiritigenin attenuates lipopolysaccharide-induced cognitive impairment through antioxidant and anti-inflammatory activity. *BMC Neurosci.* **2019**, *20*, 41. [CrossRef]
390. Cardozo, C.M.L.; Inada, A.C.; Cardoso, C.A.L.; Filiú, W.F.D.O.; Farias, B.B.D.; Alves, F.M.; Tatara, M.B.; Croda, J.H.R.; Guimarães, R.D.C.A.; Hiane, P.A.; et al. Effect of Supplementation with Hydroethanolic Extract of Campomanesia xanthocarpa (Berg.) Leaves and Two Isolated Substances from the Extract on Metabolic Parameters of Mice Fed a High-Fat Diet. *Molecules* **2020**, *25*, 2693. [CrossRef]
391. Hsieh, C.-T.; Chang, F.-R.; Tsai, Y.-H.; Wu, Y.-C.; Hsieh, T.-J. 2-Bromo-4′-methoxychalcone and 2-Iodo-4′-methoxychalcone Prevent Progression of Hyperglycemia and Obesity via 5′-Adenosine-Monophosphate-Activated Protein Kinase in Diet-Induced Obese Mice. *Int. J. Mol. Sci.* **2018**, *19*, 2763. [CrossRef]
392. Iniguez, A.B.; Zhu, M.-J. Hop bioactive compounds in prevention of nutrition-related noncommunicable diseases. *Crit. Rev. Food Sci. Nutr.* **2020**, 1–14. [CrossRef] [PubMed]
393. Liou, C.-J.; Lee, Y.-K.; Ting, N.-C.; Chen, Y.-L.; Shen, S.-C.; Wu, S.-J.; Huang, W.-C. Protective Effects of Licochalcone A Ameliorates Obesity and Non-Alcoholic Fatty Liver Disease Via Promotion of the Sirt-1/AMPK Pathway in Mice Fed a High-Fat Diet. *Cells* **2019**, *8*, 447. [CrossRef] [PubMed]
394. Jalalvand, F.; Amoli, M.M.; Yaghmaei, P.; Kimiagar, M.; Ebrahim-Habibi, A. Acarbose versus trans-chalcone: Comparing the effect of two glycosidase inhibitors on obese mice. *Arch. Endocrinol. Metab.* **2015**, *59*, 202–209. [CrossRef] [PubMed]
395. Dorn, C.; Kraus, B.; Motyl, M.; Weiss, T.S.; Gehrig, M.; Schölmerich, J.; Heilmann, J.; Hellerbrand, C. Xanthohumol, a chalcon derived from hops, inhibits hepatic inflammation and fibrosis. *Mol. Nutr. Food Res.* **2010**, *54*, S205–S213. [CrossRef]
396. Takahashi, K.; Osada, K. Effect of Dietary Purified Xanthohumol from Hop (*Humulus lupulus* L.) Pomace on Adipose Tissue Mass, Fasting Blood Glucose Level, and Lipid Metabolism in KK-Ay Mice. *J. Oleo Sci.* **2017**, *66*, 531–541. [CrossRef]
397. Mahli, A.; Seitz, T.; Freese, K.; Frank, J.; Weiskirchen, R.; Abdel-Tawab, M.; Behnam, D.; Hellerbrand, C. Therapeutic Application of Micellar Solubilized Xanthohumol in a Western-Type Diet-Induced Mouse Model of Obesity, Diabetes and Non-Alcoholic Fatty Liver Disease. *Cells* **2019**, *8*, 359. [CrossRef]
398. Son, M.J.; Minakawa, M.; Miura, Y.; Yagasaki, K. Aspalathin improves hyperglycemia and glucose intolerance in obese diabetic ob/ob mice. *Eur. J. Nutr.* **2013**, *52*, 1607–1619. [CrossRef]
399. Mazibuko-Mbeje, S.E.; Dludla, P.V.; Roux, C.; Johnson, R.; Ghoor, S.; Joubert, E.; Louw, J.; Opoku, A.R.; Muller, C.J.F. Aspalathin-Enriched Green Rooibos Extract Reduces Hepatic Insulin Resistance by Modulating PI3K/AKT and AMPK Pathways. *Int. J. Mol. Sci.* **2019**, *20*, 633. [CrossRef]
400. Lee, Y.; Kwon, E.-Y.; Choi, M.-S. Dietary Isoliquiritigenin at a Low Dose Ameliorates Insulin Resistance and NAFLD in Diet-Induced Obesity in C57BL/6J Mice. *Int. J. Mol. Sci.* **2018**, *19*, 3281. [CrossRef]
401. Bao, L.D.; Wang, Y.; Ren, X.H.; Ma, R.L.; Lv, H.J.; Agula, B. Hypolipidemic effect of safflower yellow and primary mechanism analysis. *Genet. Mol. Res.* **2015**, *14*, 6270–6278. [CrossRef]
402. Ohnogi, H.; Hayami, S.; Kudo, Y.; Deguchi, S.; Mizutani, S.; Enoki, T.; Tanimura, Y.; Aoi, W.; Naito, Y.; Kato, I.; et al. Angelica keiskei Extract Improves Insulin Resistance and Hypertriglyceridemia in Rats Fed a High-Fructose Drink. *Biosci. Biotechnol. Biochem.* **2012**, *76*, 928–932. [CrossRef] [PubMed]
403. Zhang, T.; Yamashita, Y.; Yasuda, M.; Yamamoto, N.; Ashida, H. Ashitaba (Angelica keiskei) extract prevents adiposity in high-fat diet-fed C57BL/6 mice. *Food Funct.* **2015**, *6*, 135–145. [CrossRef] [PubMed]
404. Karkhaneh, L.; Yaghmaei, P.; Parivar, K.; Sadeghizadeh, M.; Ebrahim-Habibi, A. Effect of trans-chalcone on atheroma plaque formation, liver fibrosis and adiponectin gene expression in cholesterol-fed NMRI mice. *Pharmacol. Reports* **2016**, *68*, 720–727. [CrossRef]
405. Nozawa, H. Xanthohumol, the chalcone from beer hops (*Humulus lupulus* L.), is the ligand for farnesoid X receptor and ameliorates lipid and glucose metabolism in KK-Ay mice. *Biochem. Biophys. Res. Commun.* **2005**, *336*, 754–761. [CrossRef] [PubMed]

406. Lee, H.E.; Yang, G.; Han, S.-H.; Lee, J.-H.; An, T.-J.; Jang, J.-K.; Lee, J.Y. Anti-obesity potential of Glycyrrhiza uralensis and licochalcone A through induction of adipocyte browning. *Biochem. Biophys. Res. Commun.* **2018**, *503*, 2117–2123. [CrossRef]
407. Strycharz, J.; Rygielska, Z.; Swiderska, E.; Drzewoski, J.; Szemraj, J.; Szmigiero, L.; Sliwinska, A. SIRT1 as a Therapeutic Target in Diabetic Complications. *Curr. Med. Chem.* **2018**, *25*, 1002–1035. [CrossRef]
408. Wang, Z.; Ka, S.-O.; Lee, Y.; Park, B.-H.; Bae, E.J. Butein induction of HO-1 by p38 MAPK/Nrf2 pathway in adipocytes attenuates high-fat diet induced adipose hypertrophy in mice. *Eur. J. Pharmacol.* **2017**, *799*, 201–210. [CrossRef]
409. Song, N.-J.; Choi, S.; Rajbhandari, P.; Chang, S.-H.; Kim, S.; Vergnes, L.; Kwon, S.-M.; Yoon, J.-H.; Lee, S.; Ku, J.-M.; et al. Prdm4 induction by the small molecule butein promotes white adipose tissue browning. *Nat. Chem. Biol.* **2016**, *12*, 479–481. [CrossRef]
410. Song, N.-J.; Chang, S.-H.; Kim, S.; Panic, V.; Jang, B.-H.; Yun, U.J.; Choi, J.H.; Li, Z.; Park, K.-M.; Yoon, J.-H.; et al. PI3Kα-Akt1-mediated Prdm4 induction in adipose tissue increases energy expenditure, inhibits weight gain, and improves insulin resistance in diet-induced obese mice. *Cell Death Dis.* **2018**, *9*, 876. [CrossRef]
411. Hemmeryckx, B.; Vranckx, C.; Bauters, D.; Lijnen, H.R.; Scroyen, I. Does butein affect adipogenesis? *Adipocyte* **2019**, *8*, 209–222. [CrossRef]
412. Zhu, H.; Wang, X.; Pan, H.; Dai, Y.; Li, N.; Wang, L.; Yang, H.; Gong, F. The Mechanism by Which Safflower Yellow Decreases Body Fat Mass and Improves Insulin Sensitivity in HFD-Induced Obese Mice. *Front. Pharmacol.* **2016**, *7*, 127. [CrossRef]
413. Del Rio, D.; Rodriguez-Mateos, A.; Spencer, J.P.E.; Tognolini, M.; Borges, G.; Crozier, A. Dietary (poly)phenolics in human health: Structures, bioavailability, and evidence of protective effects against chronic diseases. *Antioxid. Redox Signal.* **2013**, *18*, 1818–1892. [CrossRef] [PubMed]
414. Cory, H.; Passarelli, S.; Szeto, J.; Tamez, M.; Mattei, J. The Role of Polyphenols in Human Health and Food Systems: A Mini-Review. *Front. Nutr.* **2018**, *5*, 1–9. [CrossRef] [PubMed]
415. Kim, Y.A.; Keogh, J.B.; Clifton, P.M. Polyphenols and glycémie control. *Nutrients* **2016**, *8*, 17. [CrossRef] [PubMed]
416. Schön, C.; Wacker, R.; Micka, A.; Steudle, J.; Lang, S.; Bonnländer, B. Bioavailability study of maqui berry extract in healthy subjects. *Nutrients* **2018**, *10*, 1720. [CrossRef] [PubMed]
417. Monagas, M.; Urpi-Sarda, M.; Sánchez-Patán, F.; Llorach, R.; Garrido, I.; Gómez-Cordovés, C.; Andres-Lacueva, C.; Bartolomé, B. Insights into the metabolism and microbial biotransformation of dietary flavan-3-ols and the bioactivity of their metabolites. *Food Funct.* **2010**, *1*, 233–253. [CrossRef]
418. Cardona, F.; Andr??s-Lacueva, C.; Tulipani, S.; Tinahones, F.J.; Queipo-Ortu?o, M.I. Benefits of polyphenols on gut microbiota and implications in human health. *J. Nutr. Biochem.* **2013**, *24*, 1415–1422. [CrossRef]
419. Mandalari, G.; Vardakou, M.; Faulks, R.; Bisignano, C.; Martorana, M.; Smeriglio, A.; Trombetta, D. Food Matrix Effects of Polyphenol Bioaccessibility from Almond Skin during Simulated Human Digestion. *Nutrients* **2016**, *8*, 568. [CrossRef]
420. Pineda-Vadillo, C.; Nau, F.; Dubiard, C.G.; Cheynier, V.; Meudec, E.; Sanz-Buenhombre, M.; Guadarrama, A.; Tóth, T.; Csavajda, É.; Hingyi, H.; et al. In vitro digestion of dairy and egg products enriched with grape extracts: Effect of the food matrix on polyphenol bioaccessibility and antioxidant activity. *Food Res. Int.* **2016**, *88*, 284–292. [CrossRef]
421. Dufour, C.; Loonis, M.; Delosière, M.; Buffière, C.; Hafnaoui, N.; Santé-Lhoutellier, V.; Rémond, D. The matrix of fruit & vegetables modulates the gastrointestinal bioaccessibility of polyphenols and their impact on dietary protein digestibility. *Food Chem.* **2018**, *240*, 314–322.
422. Wojtunik-Kulesza, K.; Oniszczuk, A.; Oniszczuk, T.; Combrzyński, M.; Nowakowska, D.; Matwijczuk, A. Influence of In Vitro Digestion on Composition, Bioaccessibility and Antioxidant Activity of Food Polyphenols-A Non-Systematic Review. *Nutrients* **2020**, *12*, 1401. [CrossRef] [PubMed]
423. Tarko, T.; Duda-Chodak, A. Influence of Food Matrix on the Bioaccessibility of Fruit Polyphenolic Compounds. *J. Agric. Food Chem.* **2020**, *68*, 1315–1325. [CrossRef] [PubMed]
424. Rinaldi de Alvarenga, J.F.; Quifer-Rada, P.; Francetto Juliano, F.; Hurtado-Barroso, S.; Illan, M.; Torrado-Prat, X.; Lamuela-Raventós, R.M. Using Extra Virgin Olive Oil to Cook Vegetables Enhances Polyphenol and Carotenoid Extractability: A Study Applying the sofrito Technique. *Molecules* **2019**, *24*, 1555. [CrossRef] [PubMed]

425. Beltrán Sanahuja, A.; De Pablo Gallego, S.L.; Maestre Pérez, S.E.; Valdés García, A.; Prats Moya, M.S. Influence of Cooking and Ingredients on the Antioxidant Activity, Phenolic Content and Volatile Profile of Different Variants of the Mediterranean Typical Tomato Sofrito. *Antioxidants* **2019**, *8*, 551. [CrossRef] [PubMed]
426. Rinaldi de Alvarenga, J.F.; Quifer-Rada, P.; Westrin, V.; Hurtado-Barroso, S.; Torrado-Prat, X.; Lamuela-Raventós, R.M. Mediterranean sofrito home-cooking technique enhances polyphenol content in tomato sauce. *J. Sci. Food Agric.* **2019**, *99*, 6535–6545. [CrossRef] [PubMed]
427. Bouayed, J.; Bohn, T. Exogenous antioxidants—Double-edged swords in cellular redox state: Health beneficial effects at physiologic doses versus deleterious effects at high doses. *Oxid. Med. Cell. Longev.* **2010**, *3*, 228–237. [CrossRef]
428. Liu, J.; Hao, W.; He, Z.; Kwek, E.; Zhao, Y.; Zhu, H.; Liang, N.; Ma, K.Y.; Lei, L.; He, W.-S.; et al. Beneficial effects of tea water extracts on the body weight and gut microbiota in C57BL/6J mice fed with a high-fat diet. *Food Funct.* **2019**, *10*, 2847–2860. [CrossRef]
429. Liu, J.; Yue, S.; Yang, Z.; Feng, W.; Meng, X.; Wang, A.; Peng, C.; Wang, C.; Yan, D. Oral hydroxysafflor yellow A reduces obesity in mice by modulating the gut microbiota and serum metabolism. *Pharmacol. Res.* **2018**, *134*, 40–50. [CrossRef]

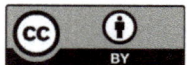

© 2020 by the authors. Licensee MDPI, Basel, Switzerland. This article is an open access article distributed under the terms and conditions of the Creative Commons Attribution (CC BY) license (http://creativecommons.org/licenses/by/4.0/).

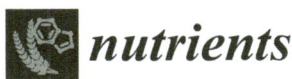

Review

Antidiabetic Effects of Flavan-3-ols and Their Microbial Metabolites

Estefanía Márquez Campos, Linda Jakobs and Marie-Christine Simon *

Department of Nutrition and Food Sciences, Nutrition and Microbiota, University of Bonn, 53115 Bonn, Germany; estefania.marquezc@gmail.com (E.M C.); ljakobs@uni-bonn.de (L.J.)
* Correspondence: marie-christine.simon@uni-bonn.de; Tel.: +49-228-73-36-80

Received: 25 April 2020; Accepted: 26 May 2020; Published: 29 May 2020

Abstract: Diet is one of the pillars in the prevention and management of diabetes mellitus. Particularly, eating patterns characterized by a high consumption of foods such as fruits or vegetables and beverages such as coffee and tea could influence the development and progression of type 2 diabetes. Flavonoids, whose intake has been inversely associated with numerous negative health outcomes in the last few years, are a common constituent of these food items. Therefore, they could contribute to the observed positive effects of certain dietary habits in individuals with type 2 diabetes. Of all the different flavonoid subclasses, flavan-3-ols are consumed the most in the European region. However, a large proportion of the ingested flavan-3-ols is not absorbed. Therefore, the flavan-3-ols enter the large intestine where they become available to the colonic bacteria and are metabolized by the microbiota. For this reason, in addition to the parent compounds, the colonic metabolites of flavan-3-ols could take part in the prevention and management of diabetes. The aim of this review is to present the available literature on the effect of both the parent flavan-3-ol compounds found in different food sources as well as the specific microbial metabolites of diabetes in order to better understand their potential role in the prevention and treatment of the disease.

Keywords: polyphenol; diabetes; flavonoids; catechins

1. Introduction

Diabetes can be classified into type 1 diabetes (T1D), type 2 diabetes (T2D), and gestational diabetes mellitus (GDM). Its prevalence has increased over the last decade, with 463 million people registered as suffering from it in 2019 (9.3% of the global population) [1]. In the case of T2D, whose prevalence constitutes around 90% of the total number of diabetes cases, its increase is directly related to ageing, increased urbanization, and obesogenic environments [1]. A rising prevalence of T1D has also been observed, but in this case the causes are not completely clear [2].

In general terms, glucose homeostasis involves glucose absorption in the intestine, glucose uptake and metabolism by organs and tissues, and glucose hepatic production [3]. In T2D, peripheral glucose uptake, mainly in muscle, is decreased. This, together with an increased endogenous glucose production, leads to a hyperglycemic status. Moreover, lipolysis is increased and the resulting free fatty acids (FFAs) and intermediary lipid metabolites all lead to a more pronounced glucose output, decreased glucose utilization, and impaired activity of beta cells. Pancreatic beta cells are stimulated to compensate the hyperglycemic state by secreting insulin, but this function deteriorates over time. Glucagon secretion by pancreatic alpha cells is, moreover, impaired. A deterioration in the incretin effect could be the cause of both the impaired insulin and glucagon secretion since there is an inadequate release of, or response to, the gastrointestinal incretin hormones post-prandially. Moreover, renal tubular glucose reabsorption is increased [3].

Due to the adverse effects that the most commonly used antidiabetic drugs can have [4], finding natural substances for preventing or treating T2D has become an attractive potential alternative.

Flavan-3-ols, the most commonly ingested flavonoids [5], have been related to different health promoting outcomes such as the prevention of cardiovascular disease [6] and cancer [7]. Regarding their effects on T2D, epidemiological data show that some foods rich in flavan-3-ols, such as green tea, could lower the risk of the disease [8–10].

This review presents in vitro, in vivo, and clinical studies regarding the effects of flavan-3-ols on diabetes both in their original form and their microbial metabolites in order to better comprehend the underlying molecular mechanisms on diabetes prevention.

2. Search Criteria

A literature search was performed in Medline via PubMed for in vitro, in vivo, and human intervention trials published between 2005 and 2019 investigating the protective role of flavan-3-ols and their colonic metabolites on diabetes. Search terms included flavan-3-ol, flavanol, catechin, epicatechin, epigallocatechin, gallocatechin, procyanidin, theaflavin, γ-valerolactone, valeric acid, 3,4-dihydroxyphenyl propionic acid, 3-hydroxyphenyl propionic acid, 3-hydroxyphenylacetic acid, 3,4-dihydroxyphenylacetic acid, homovanillic acid, protocatechuic acid, 3-hydroxybenzoic acid, green tea, grape seed extract, cacao, diabetes, glucose, insulin, insulin resistance, beta cell, pancreas, glucagon, incretin effect, and vasodilation. In vitro and in vivo studies included both diabetic models and non-diabetic models. Only human trials with a study population presenting an impaired glucose metabolism (type 1 or type 2 diabetes mellitus, gestational diabetes, or pre-diabetes) were considered. The focus was on studies that primarily investigated effects on glucose metabolism.

3. Flavan-3-ols: Intake and Metabolism

Flavan-3-ols constitute a flavonoid subclass naturally present in food as monomers (catechin (C) and epicatechin (EC)), oligomers, polymers (proanthocyanidins), and other derived compounds (such as theaflavins and thearubigins) [11].

Monomeric forms of flavan-3-ols are commonly present in cocoa beans, nuts, and fruits such as berries, stone fruits, apples, and pears [12]. Cocoa, berries, and nuts are also rich in proanthocyanidins [12]. Green tea is rich in gallocatechins while fermented black and oolong teas are sources of theaflavins and thearubigins [13].

The mean flavan-3-ol intake seems to range between 77 mg/day and 182 mg/day depending on the region, representing a much higher intake than that of other polyphenols [5]. Although the intake of flavan-3-ols is the highest among other polyphenols, the amount as well as the subtype ingested differ among countries. For example, the UK was shown to be the country with the highest total flavan-3-ol consumption in Europe, which is probably due to the widespread and high consumption of tea [14]. Therefore, monomer (especially epigallocatechin-3-gallate (EGCG)) and theaflavin (TF) intake were the highest in the UK [5,14]. Nevertheless, proanthocyanidin intake was statistically higher in Mediterranean countries, with the main sources there being stone and pome fruits [5,14].

After ingestion, the monomeric forms of the flavan-3-ols are absorbed directly in the small intestine by passive diffusion before undergoing reactions lead by the phase II enzymes [11]. These enzymatic reactions, which first take place in the enterocyte and later in the liver, are performed by uridine-5′-diphosphate glucuronosyltransferases (UGT), catechol-O-methyltransferases (COMT), and sulfotransferases (SULT). The conjugated metabolites (glucuronides, O-methyl-esters, and sulphates, respectively) are then released [11]. The conjugated metabolites are water-soluble and can circulate through the human body via the systemic blood stream or be removed from the body in the urine and bile [11,15,16]. When the conjugated metabolites are eliminated via the bile, they can be recycled because they can be transported to the duodenum, where they will undergo enzymatic modifications and be reabsorbed [15].

The remaining unabsorbed ingested oligomeric and polymeric forms of flavan-3-ols, as well as a fraction of the structures already absorbed in the small intestine, go to the colon [11]. There, the microbiota can perform metabolic transformations of the flavan-3-ols aided by hydrolysis reactions

(O-deglycosylation and ester hydrolysis), cleavage (C-ring cleavage, delactonization, demethylation), and reductions (dehydroxylation and double bond reduction) [17,18]. Specific colonic metabolites for flavan-3-ols are γ-valerolactones, while further phenolic compounds are also common after the microbial catabolism of other flavonoids [11].

After absorption, flavan-3-ols' colonic metabolites go through phase II metabolism in the liver and their conjugated forms reach the organs and tissues, where they exert their potential positive effects [11]. Since the microbial metabolites could be the active substances with beneficial physiological effects in addition to their precursor compounds, flavan-3-ol-derived metabolites formed by the colonic microbiota have been given significant attention [11].

4. Antidiabetic Effects of Flavan-3-ols: In Vitro and In Vivo Studies

Flavan-3-ols and their colonic metabolites can modulate the molecular mechanisms involved in the pathogenesis of diabetes, including the glucose absorption rate in the gut, glucose peripheral uptake, glucose secretion, the modulation of beta cell function, the modulation of insulin secretion, and the modulation of the incretin effect (Figure 1).

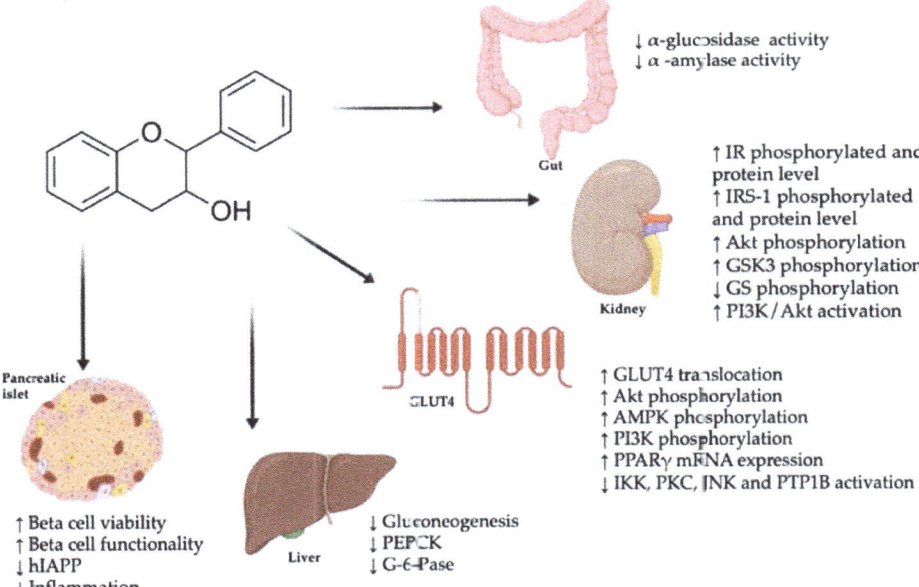

Figure 1. Potential molecular mechanisms underlying the antidiabetic properties of flavan-3-ols. ↑: increase; ↓: decrease; Akt: protein kinase B; AMPK: 5′ adenosine monophosphate-activated protein kinase; G-6-Pase: glucose-6-phosphatase; GLUT4: glucose transporter type 4; GS: glycogen synthase; GSK3: glycogen synthase kinase 3; hIAPP: human islet amyloid polypeptide; IKK: IκB kinase; IR: insulin receptor; IRS-1: insulin receptor substrate 1. JNK: c-Jun N-terminal kinases; mRNA: messenger RNA; PEPCK: phosphoenolpyruvate carboxykinase; PI3K: phosphoinositide 3-kinase; PKC: protein kinase C; PPARγ: peroxisome proliferator-activated receptor-γ; PTP1B: protein-tyrosine phosphatase 1B.

4.1. Glucose Absorption in the Gut

The first factor contributing to the postprandial glycemic level in the plasma is the absorption of glucose in the gastrointestinal tract. This process is regulated by key enzymes such as α-glucosidase, which releases glucose from complex carbohydrates. Inhibition of α-glucosidase activity by a green tea water extract, a green tea polyphenol mixture, and EGCG has been shown to be stronger than by acarbose (half maximal inhibitory concentration (IC_{50}) values were 4.421 ± 0.018, 10.019 ± 0.017, and 5.272 ± 0.009 µg/mL for flavan-3-ols, respectively, and 4822.783 ± 26.042 µg/mL for acarbose) [19] (Table 1). In addition, grape seed extract (GSE) (86% gallic acid equivalents) inhibited α-glucosidase activity ($IC_{50} = 1.2 \pm 0.2$ µg/mL) more strongly than acarbose ($IC_{50} = 91.0 \pm 10.8$ µg/mL), and of the individual catechin 3-gallates, EGCG was the one with the strongest inhibitory effect ($IC_{50} = 0.3 \pm 0.1$ µg/mL) [20].

Table 1. In vitro studies on antidiabetic effect of flavan-3-ols and their microbial metabolites [1].

In Vitro Test	Flavan-3-ol	Concentration/Dose	Results	Ref.
Glucose absorption in the gut				
Inhibition of α-glucosidase and α-amylase activity	GTE, GTP, EGCG	α-amylase: IC$_{50}$ = 1370.812 ± 59.081–1849.612 ± 73.475 µg/mL α-glucosidase: IC$_{50}$ = 4.421 ± 0.018–10.019 ± 0.017 µg/mL	Inhibition of α-glucosidase by GTE was stronger than by acarbose (IC$_{50}$ = 4822.783 ± 26.042 µg/mL) and the other compounds but had no effect on α-amylase.	[19]
			Combination of GTE, GTP, EGCG, and acarbose at low concentrations had synergistic suppressive effects on α-glucosidase.	
			α-amylase was inhibited at high concentrations of GTP and EGCG, but lower than that of acarbose (IC$_{50}$ = 2715.654 ± 24.709 µg/mL).	
			α-amylase was only inhibited by GTE extract similarly to acarbose.	
Inhibition of α-amylase and α-glucosidase activity	GSE, tea extracts, C, EC, EGC, EGCG, GCG, ECG	α-amylase: IC$_{50}$ = 8.7 ± 0.8–378 ± 134 µg/L α-glucosidase: IC$_{50}$ = 0.3 ± 0.1–31 µg/L	α-glucosidase was significantly inhibited by all compounds except C, EC following this order: Teavigo® > FCxG$_i$ > GTE> GSF > GCG > WTF > FCG	[20]
Inhibition of α-glucosidase activity	EGCG, ECG, EGCG3″Me, ECG3″Me	IC$_{50}$ = 8.1–61.1 µM	Inhibition of α-glucosidase EGCG3″Me > EGCG > ECG3″Me > ECG	[21]
α-glucosidase inhibition assay	C	IC$_{50}$ = 87.55 µg/mL	The α-glucosidase inhibitory potency was greater than acarbose (IC$_{50}$ = 199.53 µg/mL).	[22]
Inhibition of α-glucosidase activity	Procyanidins B2, B5 and C1	IC$_{50}$ = 4.7 ± 0.2, 5.5 ± 0.1 and 3.8 ± 0.2 µg/mL	Trimeric procyanidin (C1) exerted the strongest inhibitory activity. Inhibitory effect was stronger than for acarbose (130.0 ± 20.0 µg/mL).	[23]
Insulin signaling pathways and glucose peripheral uptake				
Glucose uptake assay and insulin signaling pathway in HepG2 cells treated with PA	Theaflavin mixture (TF, TF-3-G, TF-3′-G, and TFDG)	2.5–10 µg/mL	Increased 2-NBDG uptake. Increased membrane bound GLUT4 protein level and Akt phosphorylation. Decreased IRS-1 phosphorylation at Ser307. Increase of mtDNA copy number. Downregulation of PGC-1β mRNA level and increase of PRC mRNA expression.	[24]
GLUT1-mediated uptake of 3-O-methylglucose in human red blood cells	EGCG and ECG	-	Uptake of 0.1 mM 3MG was dose-dependently inhibited.	[25]
Glucose uptake, GLUT4 translocation, and JNK phosphorylation in insulin resistant 3T3-L1 adipocytes	EGCG	0.1–5 µM	At 5 µM, increased glucose uptake. Dose-dependent reversion of Dex- and TNFα-induced JNK phosphorylation. At 1 µM, increased GLUT4 translocation	[26]
GLUT4 translocation in L6 skeletal muscle cells	5-(3,5-dihydroxyphenyl)-γ-VL	1 and 3 µM	3 µM promoted the strongest effect on GLUT4 translocation. AMPK phosphorylation increased.	[27]

Table 1. Cont.

In Vitro Test	Flavan-3-ol	Concentration/Dose	Results	Ref.
Glucose transport in human and murine 3T3-L1 adipocytes stimulated or not with insulin	PCA	100 µmol/L	Reversion of oxLDL-induced decrease in glucose uptake and GLUT4 translocation. Reversion of oxLDL-induced decrease of adiponectin mRNA expression and secretion, and of PPARγ mRNA expression and activity.	[28]
Insulin signaling, glucose uptake, and glucose production in rat renal NRK-52E cells	EC, 2,3-DHB, 3,4-DHPA, 3-HPP and VA	5–20 µM	Glucose uptake, glucose production, and PEPCK reduced after treatment with EC (5–20 µM) and 2,3-DBH (20 µM). IR and IRS-1 phosphorylated and total protein levels increased at 10 µM EC and 20 µM 2,3-DHB. Increased phosphorylation of Akt and GSK3. The inhibition of the PI3K/Akt pathway was restrained.	[29]
Insulin signaling and glucose uptake and production in rat renal NRK-52E cells treated with high glucose	EC, 3,4-DHPA, 2,3-DHB and 3-HPP	5–20 µM	The altered glucose uptake and production caused by high glucose was prevented by EC (5–20 µM) and 3,4-DHPA (10–20 µM). At 10 µM, tyrosine phosphorylated, and total levels of IR increased. The PI3K/Akt pathway and AMPK were activated and the PEPCK expression was reduced.	[30]
Beta cell viability and function				
GSIS in INS-1 cell. [Ca2+] oscillations induced by glucose in INS-1 cells	EGCG, GCG, EC, C, EGC, GC, ECG, CG	10–100 µM	GSIS was decreased by 10 and 30 µM EGCG. GSIS was terminated by 100 µM EGCG and 100 µM GCG. EGC nearly abolished GSIS at 100 µM, GC and ECG partly inhibited it. EC, C, and CG did not show any effect. 100 µM EGCG decreased the oscillation of intracellular calcium.	[31]
GSIS in SFA-treated INS-1 cell; ROS production in high-glucose and H2O2-treated INS-1 cell	EC	0.3 µmol/L 30 µmol/L	Increase of GSIS. Reversion of SFA-induced inhibition of CaMKII phosphorylation. Reduced ROS production.	[32]
Insulin production in iron-loaded RINm5F pancreatic cells. Iron and ROS levels in RINm5F pancreatic cells	GTE	1–20 µM EGCG 1–10 µM EGCG	Dose-dependent increase of insulin secretion. Dose-dependent decrease of iron and ROS levels.	[33]
Cell viability and GSIS in PA- and H2O2-treated INS-1 pancreatic beta cells. H2O2-stimulated ROS production	Cinnam-tannin B1, procyanidin C1, cinnam-tannin D1	12.5–100 µmol/L	Dose-dependent increase of cell viability. GSIS increase at 25 µmol/L. Decreased ROS production.	[34]
Inhibition of hIAPP aggregation and molecular mechanism	EGCG	-	Blockage of inter-peptide hydrophobic/aromatic interactions and intra-peptide interactions. Abolishment of β-hairpin-containing three-stranded β-sheet conformation. Shift of hIAPP dimer toward loosely packed coil-rich conformations.	[35]

Table 1. Cont.

In Vitro Test	Flavan-3-ol	Concentration/Dose	Results	Ref.
Amyloid formation by IAPP and disaggregation of amyloid fibrils with thioflavin-T binding assay and TEM. Cell viability in mixture IAPP:EGCG on rat INS-1	EGCG	3.2–32 µM	At 32 µM, inhibition of amyloid formation by IAPP. IAPP:EGCG (3.2 µM) complex did not seed amyloid formation by IAPP. Disaggregation of IAPP. Increased cell viability of INS-1 cells to 77%.	[36]
hIAPP fibrillation and aggregation	EGCG	2–32 µM	Inhibition of hIAPP fibrillation. Formation of amorphous aggregates instead of ordered fibrils.	[37]
Beta cell function of rat INS-1E pancreatic beta cells and rat pancreatic islets	3,4-DHPA, 2,3-DHB and 3-HPP	1–5 µM	3,4-DHPA and 3-HPP enhanced GSIS (5 and 1 µM, respectively). Under oxidative stress, 3,4-DHPA and 3-HPP reduced ROS and carbonyl group production, and GSIS returned to control levels. PKC and ERKs phosphorylation improved.	[38]
Beta cell function of Min6 pancreatic beta cells incubated with cholesterol	3,4-DHPA	10–250 µM	3,4-DHPA reversed the diminished insulin secretion induced by cholesterol. It protected beta cells against apoptosis, oxidative stress, and mitochondrial dysfunction.	[39]
Beta cell function and glucose utilization in rat INS-1 beta cells and human skeletal muscle	EC, IIA, IIVA and 5-PVA	5–100 µM	EC (10 and 25 µM), HA, and 5-PVA (25 µM) provoked glucose oxidation in skeletal muscle. After oxidative insult, skeletal mitochondrial function was conserved. In beta cells, EC (100 µM) and metabolites (5–100 µM) stimulated GSIS.	[40]
Endogenous glucose production				
Glucose production and PEPCK/G-6-Pase gene expression in H4IIE rat hepatoma cells incubated with pyruvate and lactate	EGCG	12.5–100 µM	At 25 µM, glucose production was repressed comparable to that of insulin. Dose-dependent reduction of PEPCK mRNA as well as G-6-Pase. PI3K inhibitor LY 294,002 reversed the repression of EGCG on PEPCK and G-6-Pase gene expression. NAC and SOD reversed the increased protein-tyrosine phosphorylation and reversed PEPCK and G-6-Pase gene repression.	[41]
Gluconeogenesis and PEPCK/G-6-Pase gene expression in mouse cAMP-Dex-stimulated hepatocytes	EGCG	0.25–1 µM	Dose-dependent attenuation of gluconeogenesis. Expression of PEPCK and G-6-Pase genes was blocked. Activation of AMPK mediated by CaMKK and ROS-dependent.	[42]
Gluconeogenesis pathway in palmitate-induced insulin resistant HepG2 cells	EGCG	40 µM	Expression of PEPCK and G-6-Pase was reduced by 53% and 67%, respectively. Glucose production was reduced by 50%.	[43]

211

Table 1. Cont.

In Vitro Test	Flavan-3-ol	Concentration/Dose	Results	Ref.
		Incretin effect		
Plasma membrane potential and GLP-1 secretion in STC-1 cells under basal and nutrient-stimulated conditions	GSPE	0.05–50 mg/L	At 0.05 and 0.5 mg/L, membrane depolarization. At 50 mg/L, hyperpolarization and suppression of GLP-1 secretion. Under nutrient-stimulation, 50 mg/L limited membrane depolarization and reduced GLP-1 secretion.	[44]
Insulin-stimulated glycogen synthesis and lipogenesis in high-glucose treated human hepatoma HepG2 cells	GTP (60% EGCG)	0.1–10 µM	Enhanced glycogen synthesis, increased phosphorylation of Ser9 GSK3β and Ser641 GS. Inhibition of lipogenesis through enhanced expression of phosphorylated AMPKα and acetyl CoA carboxylase.	[45]
		Inflammation		
TNFα-induced activation of NF-κB, MAPKs, AP-1, and PPARγ in differentiated white 3T3-L1 adipocytes	EC	0.5–10 µM	Dose-dependent decrease of JNK, ERK1/2, and p-38 phosphorylation, and nuclear AP-1-DNA binding. Inhibition of NF-κB signaling cascade activation, preventing p65 nuclear transport and nuclear NF-κB-DNA binding. Altered transcription of genes (MCP-1, IL-6, TNFα, resistin, PTP1B). Attenuation of decreased PPARγ expression.	[46]
		Vasodilation		
Vasodilation of pre-contracted isolated rat aortic rings	3-PP, 4-HPP, 3,4-DHPP, 4-HPA, 3,4-DHPA, HVA, 3-HB, PhG, 4-MC, m-CoA, 3-HPP and 3-HPA	100 nM	3-HPP had the strongest vasodilatory activity, which was NO and endothelium-dependent.	[47]
NO production by human aortic endothelial cells under glucotoxic conditions	3-HPP	1 µM	Insulin-stimulated increase in NO production was preserved, as well as phosphorylation of Akt and eNOS. The increase in ROS and RNS was prevented.	[48]
Endothelial function in human EA.hy926 endothelial cells	3,4-DHPA, 2,3-DHB and 3-HPP	10–12 µM	3,4-DHPA and a mixture of the metabolites increased the NO generation and phosphorylation of eNOS, Akt, and AMPK. Under oxidative stress, cell viability was improved by the metabolites and reduced eNOS phosphorylation was reversed. ROS generation and phosphorylation of ERK and JNK were reversed.	[49]

Table 1. Cont.

In Vitro Test	Flavan-3-ol	Concentration/Dose	Results	Ref.
		Antiglycative activity		
AGEs formation in BSA/glucose system and glyoxal trapping ability	PG, 3,4-DHPP, DHFA, 3-HPA, 3,4-DHPA and HVA	2–50 µmol/L	DHFA at 10 µmol/L significantly inhibited albumin glycation. At 2 µmol/L, a mix of 3-HPA, 3,4-DHPA, and HVA inhibited glycation. PG, 3,4-DHPP, and 3,4-DHPA had a glyoxal trapping ability of 60%, 90%, and 65%, respectively.	[50]
AGEs formation in BSA/glucose and BSA/MGO systems	3,4-DHPA, 3-HPA and HVA	1 mM	The order of AGEs' inhibition ability was: rutin > quercetin > 3,4-DHPA > aminoguanidine > 3-HPA > HVA	[51]

^{1} 2-NBDG: 2-(N-(7-nitrobenz-2-oxa-1,3-diazol-4-yl)amino)-2-deoxyglucose; Akt: protein kinase B; AMPK: 5′ adenosine monophosphate-activated protein kinase; AP-1: activator protein 1; CaMK: Ca^{2+}/calmodulin-dependent protein kinase; CaMKK: calcium/calmodulin-dependent protein kinase kinase; cAMP: cyclic adenosine monophosphate; Dex: dexamethasone; ERK: extracellular signal-regulated kinases; G-6-Pase: glucose-6-phosphatase; GLP-1: glucagon-like peptide-1; GLUT1: glucose transporter type 1; GLUT4: glucose transporter type 4; GSE: grape seed extract; GS: glycogen synthase; GSIS: glucose-stimulated insulin secretion; GSK3β: glycogen synthase kinase 3 beta; GSPE: grape seed procyanidin extract; GTE: green tea extract; GTP: green tea polyphenol mixture; hIAPP: human islet amyloid polypeptide; IAPP: islet amyloid polypeptide; IC$_{50}$: half maximal inhibitory concentration; IL: interleukin; IR: insulin receptor; IRS-1: insulin receptor substrate 1; JNK: c-Jun N-terminal kinases; MAPK: mitogen-activated protein kinase; MCP-1: monocyte chemoattractant protein 1; mtDNA: mitochondrial DNA; NAC: N-acetylcysteine; NF-κB: nuclear factor kappa-light-chain-enhancer of activated B cells; oxLDL: oxidized LDL; PA: palmitic acid; PEPCK: phosphoenolpyruvate carboxykinase; PGC-1: peroxisome proliferator-activated receptor coactivator-1; PI3K: phosphoinositide 3-kinase; PKC: protein kinase C; PPARγ: peroxisome proliferator-activated receptor-γ; PRC: PGC-1-related coactivator; PTP1B: protein-tyrosine phosphatase 1B; ROS: reactive oxygen species; SFA: saturated fatty acid; SOD: superoxide dismutase; STC: secretin tumor cell; TEM: transmission electron microscopy; TNFα: tumor necrosis factor; WTE: white tea extract. Flavan-3-ols and microbial metabolites. 2,3 DHB: 2,3 dihydroxybenzoic acid; 3-HB: 3-hydroxybenzoic acid; 3-HPA: 3-hydroxyphenylacetic acid; 3-HPP: 3-hydroxyphenyl propionic acid; 3-PP: 3-phenylpropionic acid; 3,4-DHPA: 3,4-dihydroxyphenylacetic-acid; 3,4-DHPP: 3,4-dihydroxyphenyl propionic acid; 4-HPA: 4-hydroxyphenylacetic acid; 4-MC: 4-methylcatechol; 5-PVA: 5-phenylvaleric acid; C: catechin; CG: catechin gallate; DHFA: dihydroferulic acid; EC: epicatechin; ECG: epicatechin gallate; ECG3″Me: epicatechin-3-O-(3-O-methyl) gallate; EGC: epigallocatechin; EGCG: epigallocatechin gallate; EGCG3″Me: epigallocatechin-3-O-(3-O-methyl) gallate; GC: gallocatechin; GCG: gallocatechin gallate; HA: hippuric acid; HVA: homovanillic acid; m-CoA: m-coumaric acid; PCA: protocatechuic acid; PhG: phloroglucinol; PG: pyrogallol; TF: theaflavin; TF-3-G: theaflavin-3-gallate; TF-3′-G: theaflavin-3′-gallate; TFDG: theaflavin-3,3′-digallate; VA: valeric acid; VL: valerolactone.

Similarly, epicatechin-3-O-(3-O-methyl) gallate (ECG3"Me), epigallocatechin-3-O-(3-O-methyl) gallate (EGCG3"Me), EGCG, and epicatechin-3-O-gallate (ECG) inhibited α-glucosidase, and in this case EGCG3"Me had the strongest effect. Their IC_{50} values were 14.7, 8.1, 13.3, and 61.1 µM respectively [21]. C was also shown to inhibit α-glucosidase stronger than acarbose (IC_{50} = 87.55 µg/mL vs. 199.53 ± 1.12 µg/mL, respectively) [22].

Interestingly, isolated procyanidins B2, B5 (dimeric), and C1 (trimeric) also had stronger α-glucosidase inhibitory activities than acarbose (IC_{50} = 4.7 ± 0.2, 5.5 ± 0.1, and 3.8 ± 0.2 µg/mL, versus IC_{50} = 130.0 ± 20.0 µg/mL, respectively), suggesting that the inhibitory activity could be correlated to the molecular weight of the compound [23].

For α-amylase, another digestive enzyme responsible for starch hydrolysis, GSE (86% gallic acid equivalents) inhibited its activity (IC_{50} = 8.7 ± 0.8 µg/mL), with the same potency as acarbose (IC_{50} = 6.9 ± 0.8 µg/mL) [20]. However, α-amylase was not strongly inhibited by tea extracts and individual catechin 3-gallates [20].

These effects have also been observed in mice fed with proanthocyanidins with different degrees of polymerization [52] (Table 2). Mice fed with proanthocyanidins with a high degree of polymerization showed a stronger inhibition of α-amylase activity both in the small intestine and in the pancreas than those fed with a low degree of polymerization proanthocyanidins. The rates of inhibition compared to the control group were 41% in the small intestine and 45% in the pancreas for high degree of polymerization proanthocyanidins, and 21% and 26% for low degree of polymerization proanthocyanidins [52].

Table 2. In vivo studies on antidiabetic effects of flavan-3-ols and their microbial metabolites [2].

In Vivo Model	Treatment	Dose/Route/Period	Results	Ref.
Glucose absorption in the gut				
Inhibition of α-amylase activity in mice.	High vs. low DP proanthocyanidins	150 mg/kg/day. Oral. 56 days.	High DP proanthocyanidins had a stronger inhibition rate of digestive enzyme activity than the low DP group (0.20 ± 0.03 vs. 0.27 ± 0.06 U mg/prot in small intestine, 0.26 ± 0.04 vs. 0.35 ± 0.04 U mg/prot in pancreas)	[52]
Insulin signaling pathways and glucose peripheral uptake				
GLUT4 translocation in ICR mice. GLUT4 translocation in C57BL/6 mice.	CLP (EC, C, procyanidin)	250 mg/kg. Oral. Single dose. Diet with 0.5% (w/w). Oral. 7 days.	Enhanced GLUT4 translocation in skeletal muscle of ICR mice after a single dose following glucose load. Enhanced GLUT4 translocation in skeletal muscle of C57BL/6 mice after consecutive administration of CLP.	[53]
GLUT-4 expression and JNK phosphorylation in KK-Ay mice.	GTP	150–300 mg/kg/day. Oral. 4 weeks.	Decreased glucose levels and enhanced glucose tolerance. JNK phosphorylation in adipose tissues was reduced and GLUT4 expression was increased. ROS content was reduced.	[26]
OGTT and GLUT4 translocation in skeletal muscle of ICR mice. AMPK activation in ICR mice.	CLP and high vs. low DP pro-cyanidins	10 mg/kg. Oral. Single dose.	Reduction of plasma glucose levels after OGTT. Promotion of GLUT4 translocation by high and low DP procyanidins. Activation of AMPK-signaling pathway. Increased phosphorylation of IRβ, IRS-1, and PI3K in muscle. Low-DP increased phosphorylation of Akt. Increased insulin secretion in plasma.	[54]
GLUT4 translocation in skeletal muscle of ICR mice. Activation of insulin and AMPK signaling pathways in ICR mice soleus muscle.	EC, Procyanidin B2, Procya-nidin C1, PA4-1 and cinnamtannin A2	10 μg/kg. Oral. Single dose.	Reduction of hyperglycemia after an OGTT. Increase of GLUT4 translocation. Promotion of AMPK, PI3K, and Akt phosphorylation.	[55]
Glucose uptake in STZ-induced T1D Wistar/ST rats. Glucose uptake in KK-Ay mice	GTE (C, EC, GC, EGC, CG, ECG, GCG, EGCG and caffeine)	2 g/L. Oral. 12 d. 2 g/L. Oral. 63 days vs. 42 days.	Significantly lower blood glucose level after OGTT. Increased GLUT4 translocation. Reduction in STZ-induced increase in plasma fructosamine and HbA1c. Significantly lower blood glucose level after OGTT. Increased GLUT4 translocation. Reduced fructosamine and HbA1c concentration.	[56]
Glucose intolerance of HFD-induced obese and diabetic C57BL/6 mice.	EGCG	75 mg/kg. Oral. Single dose.	Blood glucose increased until 15 min (30 min in control), and rapidly decreased thereafter. It was significantly lower than in control group.	[56]
Insulin sensitivity in HFD-induced obese and diabetic C57BL/6 mice.	EC	20 mg/kg. Oral. 15 weeks.	Increase of insulin was prevented. Phosphorylation of IRS-1 and Akt was increased, while that of PKC, JNK, IKK, and PTP1B was downregulated.	[57]

Table 2. Cont.

In Vivo Model	Treatment	Dose/Route/Period	Results	Ref.
IRes and effect on insulin signaling cascade in HFr-fed rats.	EC	20 mg/kg. Oral. 8 weeks.	Reversion of impaired activation of IR, IRS-1, Akt, and ERK1/2 induced by HFr diet. Reversion of upregulation of PKC, IKK, JNK, and PTP1B induced by HFr. Inhibition of HFr-induced increase of expression and activation of NADPH oxidase, expression of cytokines and chemokines, and activation of redox-sensitive signals.	[58]
Plasma glucose level in ICR mice during OGTT and GLUT4 translocation of soleus muscle.	5-(3,5-dihydroxy-phenyl)-γ-VL32 mg/kg. Oral. Single dose.		Suppression of postprandial hyperglycemia at 15 and 30 min after OGTT. Increased GLUT4 translocation. Increased phosphorylation of AMPK.	[27]
Beta cell viability and function				
Glycemia, insulin, and HbA1c glycation on nicotinamide and STZ-induced diabetic rats.	EGCG	2 mg/kg. Oral. 15 days.	Glucose, HbA1c, and HOMA-IR decreased. Insulin increased.	[59]
Insulin synthesis and apoptosis in male Wistar cafeteria-induced obese rats.	GSPE	25 mg/kg. Oral. 21 days.	Decreased HOMA-IR and HOMA-β. Decreased expression of Cpe. Increase in Bax protein levels.	[60]
IRes, insulin clearance, and serum lipids in NAFLD C57BL/6 mice.	EGCG	10, 20, 40 mg/kg/day. i.p. 4 weeks.	Reduction of fasting blood glucose and serum insulin. Decrease of GSIS was dose-dependently reversed. Metabolic clearance rate of insulin and IDE increased. Dose-dependent decrease of serum TC, TG, and LDL. Dose-dependent increase of serum HDL.	[61]
Antidiabetic effects in a *db/db* diabetic mouse model.	EGCG	10 g/kg diet, 1% (w/w). Oral. 10 weeks.	After an OGTT, fasting blood glucose levels decreased similarly to rosiglitazone. No changes in HOMA-IR or QUICKI. Increase in number and size of pancreatic islets comparable to rosiglitazone.	[62]
hIAPP amyloidogenesis in hIAPP transgenic mice	EGCG	0.4 mg/mL. Oral. 3 weeks.	Reduction of amyloid fibril intensity of hIAPP in the pancreas of non-diabetic transgenic mice.	[63]
Development of T1D and protective effect on pancreatic islets in NOD mice.	EGCG	0.05% in drinking water. Oral. 32 weeks.	Delayed onset of T1D. Increased plasma insulin levels compared to control. Decreased HbA1c. Increased concentration of cytokine IL-10 level. Increased islet viability when exposed to pro-inflammatory cytokines.	[64]
Immunity modulation and prevention of T1D in NOD mice.	EC	0.5% in drinking water. Oral. Single dose.	Prevention of T1D onset. Blood glucose levels decreased within the first 60 min of OGTT. HbA1c concentration reduced compared to control group. Plasma insulin levels were higher than in untreated group. Pancreatic islet mass improved. High proportion of immune cell-free islets. Enhanced plasma IL-10 and IL-12 levels	[65]

Table 2. Cont.

In Vivo Model	Treatment	Dose/Route/Period	Results	Ref.
Incretin effect				
Plasma GLP-1 in ICR mice.	High vs. low DP pro-cyanidins	10 mg/kg. Oral. Single dose.	Increased GLP-1 secretion in plasma.	[54]
GLP-1 and plasma insulin levels in male ICR mice.	Cinnam-tannin A2	10 µg/kg. Oral. Single dose.	Increase of plasma insulin level. Increase of GLP-1 secretion levels in plasma 60 min after administration. Increased phosphorylation of IRβ and IRS-1 in vitro in skeletal muscle.	[66]
Oxidative stress				
Oxidative damage and serum lipid profile in STZ-induced diabetic rats.	C	20–80 mg/kg/day. i.p. 4 weeks.	Dose-dependent decrease of blood glucose levels. Dose-dependent increase of SOD, GST, and CAT activity. Dose-dependent decrease of TC, TG, LDL, and apoB. Dose-dependent increase of HDL and apo A-I.	[67]
Serum glucose levels and serum and hepatic biomarkers of oxidative stress in STZ-induced diabetic rats.	GTE	100 and 200 mg/kg. Oral. 4 weeks.	Decreased serum glucose levels, as well as serum and hepatic MDA concentration with 200 µg/kg for 4 weeks. TAC increased.	[68]

2 Akt: protein kinase B; AMPK: 5′ adenosine monophosphate-activated protein kinase; Apo: apoprotein; Bax: Bcl-2-associated X protein; bw: body weight; CAT: catalase; CLP: cacao liquor procyanidin; Cpe: carboxypeptidase E; d: day; DP: degree of polymerization; ERK: extracellular signal–regulated kinases; GLP-1: glucagon-like peptide-1; GLUT4: glucose transporter type 4; GSIS: glucose-stimulated insulin secretion; GSPE: grape seed procyanidin extract; GST: glutathione-S-transferase; GTE: green tea extract; GTP: green tea polyphenol mixture; HbA1c: glycated hemoglobin; HDL: high density lipoprotein-cholesterol; hIAPP: human islet amyloid polypeptide; HFD: high fat diet; HFr: high fructose; HOMA-IR: homeostasis model assessment of insulin resistance; HOMA-β: homeostasis model assessment of beta cell function; i.p.: intraperitoneal; ICR: Institute of Cancer Research; IDE: insulin-degrading enzyme; IL: interleukin; IKK: IκB kinase; IR: insulin receptor; IRes: insulin resistance; IRS-1: insulin receptor substrate 1; JNK: c-Jun N-terminal kinases; LDL: low density lipoprotein-cholesterol; MDA: malondialdehyde; NAFLD: non-alcoholic fatty liver disease; NADPH: nicotinamide adenine dinucleotide phosphate; NOD: non-obese diabetic; OGTT: oral glucose tolerance test; PI3K: phosphoinositide 3-kinase; PKC: protein kinase C; PTP1B: protein-tyrosine phosphatase 1B; SOD: superoxide dismutase; STZ: streptozotocin; TAC: total antioxidant capacity; T1D: type 1 diabetes; TC: total cholesterol; TG: triglycerides; QUICKI: quantitative insulin sensitivity check index; w: week. Flavan-3-ols and their microbial metabolites: C: catechin; CG: catechin gallate; EC: epicatechin; ECG: epicatechin gallate; EGC: epigallocatechin; EGCG: epigallocatechin gallate; GC: gallocatechin; GCG: gallocatechin gallate; PA4-1: EC-(4β-6)-EC-(4β-8)-EC-(4β-8)-EC; VL: valerolactone.

4.2. Insulin Signaling Pathways and Glucose Peripheral Uptake

Due to the polar nature of glucose, its transport into the cell requires the use of transporter proteins in the cell membrane. These glucose transporters have different tissue distributions and a specific affinity for carbohydrates [69]. The insulin-regulatable glucose transporter type 4 (GLUT4) is found in insulin-sensitive tissues: skeletal muscle, cardiomyocytes, and adipocytes. Under physiological conditions, the insulin-mediated translocation of intracellular GLUT4 from the cytoplasm to the plasma membrane results in the uptake of glucose. This process is influenced by phosphoinositide 3-kinase (PI3K), protein kinase B (PKB or Akt), and protein kinase C zeta type (PKCζ). In short, insulin binding to insulin receptor (IR) leads to the phosphorylation of the beta subunit which, at the same time, phosphorylates the insulin receptor substrate (IRS). Upon tyrosine phosphorylation, which could be inhibited by serine phosphorylation of insulin receptor substrate 1 (IRS-1), PI3K binds to IRS and activates the Akt/PKB and the PKCζ cascades. Activated Akt induces glycogen synthesis via the inhibition of glycogen synthase kinase (GSK-3). Eventually, the Rab GTPase-activating protein AS160 (Akt substrate of 160 kDa) is activated, leading to the translocation of GLUT4 to the plasma membrane and glucose uptake [70].

When the translocation of intracellular GLUT4 to the plasma membrane is impaired, insulin resistance (IRes) takes place. T2D develops when both IRes and defects in insulin secretion occur [3].

Since approximately 80% of insulin-stimulated glucose uptake in the postprandial state takes place in the skeletal muscle, this tissue plays a key role in maintaining glucose homeostasis; therefore, many studies have focused on the effect of flavan-3-ols on GLUT4 translocation in skeletal muscle.

In vitro, a cacao liquor procyanidin (CLP) extract (1–10 µg/mL), consisting of EC, C, and other procyanidins, dose-dependently enhanced glucose uptake and promoted GLUT4 translocation to the plasma membrane of L6 myotubes after 15 min of incubation [53].

A mixture of TF, theaflavin-3-gallate (TF-3-G), theaflavin-3′-gallate (TF-3′-G), and theaflavin-3,3′-digallate (TFDG) (2.5–10 µg/mL, 24 h treatment) improved IRes induced by palmitic acid in HepG2 cells, as measured by the increase in 2-(N-(7-nitrobenz-2-oxa-1,3-diazol-4-yl)amino)-2-deoxyglucose (2-NBDG) uptake using metformin as a positive control [24]. Total GLUT4 and protein levels of GLUT4 bound to the membrane were increased by theaflavins in a dose-dependent manner [24]. They reversed the reduction of the phosphorylation level of Akt induced by palmitic acid and led to an increased phosphorylation of IRS-1 (Ser307) in HepG2 cells [24].

Interestingly, Ojelabi et al. showed that EGCG and ECG dose-dependently inhibited sugar uptake by glucose transporter type 1 (GLUT1), which was measured using 3-O-methylglucose uptake. It was found that low concentrations of the flavan-3-ols activated sugar uptake, while higher concentrations inhibited sugar uptake and noncompetitively inhibited sugar exit [25].

Glucose uptake in induced insulin-resistant 3T3-L1 adipocytes significantly increased after incubation with EGCG at 5 µM. Moreover, EGCG dose-dependently reversed the dexamethasone (Dex) and tumor necrosis factor (TNFα)-induced increase of c-Jun N-terminal kinases (JNK) phosphorylation levels and promoted GLUT4 translocation (1 µM) [26].

In vivo studies showed similar results. KK-Ay mice, when supplemented with green tea catechins (98% pure) at a low as well as at high concentrations (150 mg/kg/day and 300 mg/kg/day), showed a reduced JNK phosphorylation in adipose tissues when compared to untreated animals and an increased GLUT4 content in the plasma membrane [26].

Yamashita et al. administered a CLP extract as a single dose (250 mg/kg) to mice at the Institute of Cancer Research (ICR). After carbohydrate ingestion, CLP suppressed the hyperglycemic response and improved GLUT4 translocation in skeletal muscle [53]. In fact, the GLUT4 translocation was approximately 3.9-fold higher in comparison with the control group, who were only administered water and no glucose [53]. These results were further confirmed by a consecutive administration of a CLP-supplemented (0.5%) diet to C57BL/6 mice for 7 days, which had the same effects on skeletal muscle GLUT4 after glucose load [53]. Similarly, procyanidins (both low and high degree of polymerization, 10 mg/kg) from a CLP extract prevented hyperglycemia through the promotion of GLUT4 translocation in the skeletal muscle of ICR mice [54]. This could be explained by the significantly increased phosphorylation of 5' adenosine monophosphate-activated protein kinase (AMPK), ß-subunit of IR (IRβ), IRS-1, and PI3K by procyanidins with both low and high degrees of polymerization [54].

After the oral administration of EC, procyanidin B2, procyanidin C1, EC-(4β–6)-EC-(4β–8)-EC-(4β–8)-EC (PA4-1), and cinnamtannin A2 (PA4–2) (10 μg/kg) to ICR mice, GLUT4 translocation in skeletal muscle significantly increased compared to in control mice [55]. Trimeric and tetrameric procyanidins significantly promoted phosphorylation of PI3K, and PA4-1 was able to significantly induce phosphorylation of Akt1 at both serine 473 and threonine 308 [55]. The latter compound was the only one able to significantly promote the phosphorylation of IRS-1 as well as increase the insulin plasma level. Similarly, all compounds significantly induced phosphorylation of AMPK [55].

In a model of T1D, streptozotocin (STZ)-induced rats were administered a green tea extract (GTE) for 12 days composed of the following catechins: C, EC, (−)-gallocatechin (GC), (−)-epigallocatechin (EGC), (−)-catechin gallate (CG), ECG, (−)-gallocatechin gallate (GCG), EGCG, and caffeine [56]. After an oral glucose tolerance test (OGTT), high blood glucose induced by STZ was significantly reduced with the GTE treatment when compared to the control group. When the possible mechanisms were investigated, the authors found that the GTE treatment increased the translocation of GLUT4 in the skeletal muscle to a normal level when compared to untreated rats. In contrast, the level of the IRß was not changed. These results imply that the green tea improved hyperglycemia in T1D rats without having an influence on insulin secretion from pancreatic beta cells, by promoting GLUT4 translocation in skeletal muscle. In addition to these findings, the degree of protein glycation induced by STZ measured by fructosamine and glycated hemoglobin (HbA1c) significantly decreased after the treatment with the GTE. This result suggests not only a protective role of green tea against the manifestation of diabetic complications but also an ability to improve those already presenting [56].

In a parallel experiment, an OGTT in KK-Ay mice was also performed, but in this case, mice were treated with GTE for 63 days (one group) or for 42 days directly after the appearance of hyperglycemia (another group). The authors found that the blood glucose after green tea intake was significantly lower when compared to the control and GLUT4 translocation in the skeletal muscle was significantly increased when compared to the control, but the level of IRß remained unaltered [56]. Another result from this experiment is the significant reduction of protein glycation and triacylglycerol by green tea [56].

In a study from Cremonini et al., EC supplementation (20 mg/kg) in high-fat-diet-induced obese and diabetic C57BL/6 mice improved insulin sensitivity and glucose homeostasis when compared to non-supplemented and control mice. The impairment of the insulin signaling cascade in the liver and the adipose tissue induced by the high-fat diet was prevented and the upregulation/activation of proteins which inhibit the insulin pathway (IκB kinase (IKK), protein kinase C (PKC), JNK, and protein-tyrosine phosphatase 1B (PTP1B)) was prevented [57].

Bettaieb et al. found that the supplementation of the diet of high-fructose-fed rats with EC (20 mg/kg) for 8 weeks mitigated the IRes induced by the high fructose concentrations, and it reversed both the impaired activation of the insulin signaling cascade (IR, IRS-1, Akt, and extracellular signal–regulated kinases 1/2 (ERK1/2)) as well as the upregulation of negative regulators (PKC, IKK, JNK, and PTP1B) in the liver and adipose tissue [58].

Glucose uptake has been shown to be promoted not only by the flavan-3-ols in their original form but also by some of their microbial metabolites. Specifically, 5-(3,5-dihydroxyphenyl)-γ-valerolactone promoted GLUT4 translocation in L6 skeletal muscle cells and soleus muscle by phosphorylation of the AMP-activated protein kinase (AMPK) signaling pathway both in vitro and in vivo at concentrations of 1–3 μM and 32 mg/kg, respectively [27]. At 32 mg/kg it caused suppression of hyperglycemia after an OGTT, while a higher dosage of 64 mg/kg only influenced AMPK phosphorylation [27].

Other microbial metabolites unspecific to flavan-3-ols have also been shown to modulate molecular mechanisms related to diabetes. Scazzocchio et al. investigated whether protocatechuic acid exerted an effect on glucose transport in adipocytes [28]. Incubation of the metabolite at 100 µM for 18 h with human and murine adipocytes treated with oxidized low density lipoprotein (oxLDL) significantly improved glucose uptake, GLUT4 translocation, and adiponectin secretion. These effects were observed after stimulation with insulin and also without it [28]. Glucose uptake was significantly and dose-dependently enhanced in non-oxLDL-treated human and murine adipocytes without the presence of insulin up to 40% and 60%, respectively [28]. These results indicate an insulin-like activity. A reversion of the oxLDL-induced diminishment of mRNA expression and activity of the peroxisome proliferator-activated receptor-γ (PPARγ) was also observed, and its inhibition impeded both the adiponectin and GLUT4 upregulation suggesting its implication in the insulin-like activity [28].

Both EC at 10 µM and 2,3-dihydroxybenzoic acid (2,3-DHB) at 20 µM increased IR and IRS-1 tyrosine phosphorylated and total protein levels in rat renal NRK-52E cells. In addition, phosphorylated levels of Akt and GSK-3 increased and those of glycogen synthase (GS) decreased [29]. Similarly, after treatment of renal tubular NRK-52E cells with high glucose levels and either EC at 5–20 µM or 3,4-dihydroxyphenylacetic-acid (3,4-DHPA) at 10–20 µM, the induced impairment of glucose uptake was restored. At 10 µM, EC and 3,4-DHPA increased tyrosine phosphorylated levels and total levels of IR, reversed the inhibition of the PI3K/Akt pathway involved in the insulin signaling cascade, and prevented the high-glucose-induced downregulation of AMPK phosphorylation [30].

4.3. Beta Cell Viability and Function

In the situation of IRes, pancreatic beta cells try to maintain glucose levels by enhancing insulin production and increasing islet size and beta cell mass. However, an increased insulin response does not mean that beta cells are functioning normally. In fact, beta cells in this situation are kept under a high workload which, when maintained over time, results in functional exhaustion, dedifferentiation, and eventually beta cell death [71]. Apoptosis of beta cells is mainly induced by glucotoxicity, lipotoxicity, and deposits of islet amyloid polypeptide (IAPP) [72,73].

Glucose-stimulated insulin secretion (GSIS) in the beta cell line INS-1D after treatment with catechins was studied by Kaneko et al. [31]. Both EGCG at 10 µM as well as GCG at 30 µM significantly inhibited the GSIS. Furthermore, at 100 µM they almost eliminated GSIS. EC and C did not modify GSIS at concentrations up to 100 µM. At 10 µM, EGC nearly eliminated GSIS, while GC and ECG partially inhibited it. CG did not alter GSIS at concentrations up to 100 µM. Apart from this, EGCG, and not EC, inhibited the variation of intracellular Ca^{2+} concentration. These results suggest that, at concentrations higher than physiological levels, some catechins have an inhibitory effect on GSIS, which is induced by the structure-dependent inhibition of voltage-dependent Ca^{2+}-channels [31].

Supporting these results, a treatment with EC at a physiological dose of 0.3 µmol/L but not at 30 µmol/L improved GSIS of saturated fatty acid (SFA)-impaired INS-1 cells [32]. This was thought to be due to a modulation of the cell secretory capacity via the activation of the Ca^{2+}/calmodulin-dependent protein kinase II (CaMKII) pathway and possibly through the GPR40 receptor [32].

In humans and animals, beta cell functionality can be measured by several methods. Some of the most commonly used methods include the homeostasis model assessment (HOMA), OGTT or intravenous glucose tolerance tests and the hyperglycemic clamp procedure [74]. The ability of flavan-3-ols to affect these has been as well assessed. In a study from Othman et al., treatment of diabetic rats with EGCG (2 mg/kg) every other day over one month significantly decreased the HOMA of insulin resistance (HOMA-IR) value and increased insulin levels when compared to untreated diabetic rats [59].

In a model where male Wistar rats were contrived to be obese through a cafeteria diet, a 21-day treatment with grape seed procyanidin extract (GSPE) at 25 mg/kg (defined composition) improved IRes measured by HOMA-IR [60]. The HOMA of beta cell function (HOMA-β) index also decreased. Insulin gene expression in the pancreas tended to decrease in treated rats, and a significant decrease in the expression of carboxypeptidase E (Cpe) was also shown [60]. On the other hand, treatment with GSPE enhanced the increase in the Bcl-2-associated X protein (Bax) levels induced by the cafeteria diet, which suggests an increased apoptosis in the pancreas in contrast to results from other studies [60].

Gan et al. suggested that EGCG dose-dependently improved IRes in high-fat diet non-alcoholic fatty liver disease (NAFLD) mice by enhancing the insulin clearance of the hepatic insulin degrading enzyme (IDE) [61]. In this study, NAFLD mice were administered 10, 20, and 40 mg/kg EGCG intraperitoneally. Hyperglycemia, hyperinsulinemia, and IRes observed in mice fed a high-fat diet without EGCG were reversed by the polyphenol [61].

Insulin deficiency and IRes have been described in ß-thalassemia patients with iron overload, which is probably a secondary effect of a diminished pancreatic beta cell function. The incubation of iron-loaded rat insulinoma pancreatic β-cells with a GTE (2.29 µg EGCG equivalent) increased insulin secretion levels 2.5-fold and decreased cellular levels of iron and reactive oxygen species (ROS) [33].

The effect of flavan-3-ols directly on beta cell viability was also assessed. Cinnamtannin B1, procyanidin C1, and cinnamtannin D1 from cinnamon extracts were shown to dose-dependently protect INS-1 cells from palmitic acid and H_2O_2-induced reduction in terms of cell viability [34]. At 25 µmol/L, they enhanced insulin secretion in lipotoxic INS-1 cells [34]. However, the flavan-3-ols EC and procyanidin B2 had no significant effects [34].

In *db/dayb* mice, treatment with EGCG (10 g/kg diet, 1% (*w/w*)) for 10 weeks improved glucose tolerance and additionally increased GSIS similarly to rosiglitazone, although no significant effect was found in IRes (HOMA-IR and quantitative insulin sensitivity check index (QUICKI)). This effect may be mediated by changes in pancreatic islets, since the number and size of pancreatic islets increased, together with a reduction of islet endoplasmic reticulum stress markers ex vivo [62].

The literature suggests that human islet amyloid polypeptide (hIAPP) fibril formation contributes to T2D by causing beta cell dysfunction and apoptosis. For this reason, the inhibition of the formation of toxic hIAPP oligomers and fibrils may be a good therapeutic strategy for the management of T2D. Some authors have therefore tried to elucidate the role of flavan-3-ols in the prevention of their formation. In hemizygous non-diabetic hIAPP transgenic mice treated with EGCG (0.4 mg/mL) for three weeks, EGCG reduced amyloid fiber intensity suggesting a beneficial effect on pancreatic amyloid fibrils in vivo [63]. However, there was no effect on diabetic hIAPP transgenic mice. This, therefore, suggests that EGCG would be effective as an early therapeutic method.

Mo et al. went further and examined the molecular process by which EGCG could inhibit hIAPP aggregation [35]. The authors found that in vitro EGCG could block the inter-peptide hydrophobic/aromatic interactions responsible for inter-peptide β-sheet formation and the intra-peptide interaction related to ß-hairpin formation. Thus, the three-stranded β-sheet structures were removed and loosely packed coil-rich conformations were formed. This EGCG-induced conformational shift of the hIAPP dimer was related to hydrophobic, aromatic stacking, cation-π, and H-bonding interactions [35].

Adding to these results, Meng et al. proved that EGCG inhibited in vitro amyloid formation by IAPP and disaggregated IAPP amyloid fibrils. At the same time, EGCG protected cultured rat INS-1 cells against IAPP-induced toxicity at 30 µM [36]. EGCG (2–32 µM) was also shown to inhibit the nucleation and fibrillation of hIAPP by forming hIAPP amorphous aggregates instead of ordered fibrils [37]. Moreover, a complex of Al(III)/ECCG was able to inhibit hIAPP fibrillation more effectively than the flavan-3-ol alone [37].

T-cell-mediated destruction of pancreatic beta cells leads to insulin deficiency in T1D. In addition, inflammation is known to play a role in the pathogenesis of T1D [3]. In this regard, EGCG prevented the onset of T1D in non-obese diabetic (NOD) mice when administered at 0.05% in drinking water (60–90 mg/kg body weight (b.w.), equivalent to 4.5–6.8 g/day by a 75 kg person) for 32 weeks [64]. Compared to control mice, plasma insulin levels were higher, HbA1c concentrations were lower, and circulating anti-inflammatory cytokine interleukin 10 (IL-10) levels were increased. However, no effect on pancreatic insulitis was observed. When human pancreatic islets were incubated with inflammatory cytokines, addition of EGCG (1 and 10 µM) promoted islet viability [64]. Similarly, the administration of EC at 0.5% in drinking water (equivalent to an intake of 250 g dark chocolate containing 6% EC) for 32 weeks also delayed the development of T1D [65]. Importantly, pancreatic islet mass was preserved and the lymphatic infiltration into islets was lower meaning an improvement in the insulitis. Anti-inflammatory cytokine IL-10 levels increased [65]. HbA1c concentrations were, in this case, significantly lower and plasma insulin levels were significantly higher in mice treated with EC than in untreated mice [65].

The effect of low molecular weight phenolics produced after colonic metabolism of flavan-3-ols on beta cell functionality and viability has also been assessed. Fernández-Millán et al. found out a significant increase in GSIS in INS-1E pancreatic beta cells and isolated rat islets after treatment with 3,4-DHPA and 3-hydroxyphenyl propionic acid (3-HPP) at low concentrations (5 and 1 µM, respectively) [38]. Under oxidative stress induced by tert-butyl hydroperoxide (t-BOOH), both metabolites restored GSIS to control levels and significantly decreased cell death [38]. PKC and ERK could play a role in producing the observed effect, since their phosphorylation levels increased after treatment [38].

3,4-DHPA (250 µM) could also prevent the diminished insulin secretion induced by high cholesterol on Min6 pancreatic beta cells [39]. Moreover, it dose-dependently prevented cholesterol-induced cytotoxicity and apoptosis. Oxidative stress and mitochondrial dysfunction were also prevented [39].

5-Phenylvaleric acid, hippuric acid and homovanillic acid improved GSIS in beta cells more effectively than EC at concentrations up to 100 µM [40]. In addition to stimulating beta cell function, the microbial metabolites enhanced glucose utilization in skeletal muscle [40].

4.4. Endogenous Glucose Production

The liver's inability to perceive insulin signals directly after glucose ingestion leads to the continuing production of glucose and, therefore, importantly contributes to a hyperglycemic status [3]. The maintained glucose output by the liver can be a consequence of two processes: gluconeogenesis and glycogenolysis [3]. However, the latter has a less important role in the increased glucose production of T2D patients [75]. The mechanisms responsible for the increase in hepatic gluconeogenesis include hyperglucagonemia, higher circulating levels of gluconeogenic precursors (lactate, alanine, and glycerol), elevated FFA oxidation, enhanced sensitivity to glucagon, and reduced sensitivity to insulin [3].

Increased activity of insulin-influenced phosphoenolpyruvate carboxykinase 1 (PCK1) and glucose-6-phosphatase (G-6-Pase) seems to contribute to the accelerated rate of hepatic glucose production [3]. In this sense, studies have shown how flavan-3-ols affect the expression of key regulators of the gluconeogenesis pathway.

Waltner-Law et al. studied the effects of green tea compounds on insulin signaling pathways, gene expression, and glucose production [41]. The authors found that EGCG had insulin-like activities in hepatoma cells. At 25 µM, EGCG reduced glucose production to basal levels in a similar way to insulin (10 nM) and these effects were already significant at lower concentrations (12.5 µM). When studying the impact of the flavan-3-ol on the expression of genes encoding gluconeogenic enzymes, EGCG reduced phosphoenolpyruvate carboxykinase (PEPCK) mRNA in a dose-dependent manner (12.5–100 µM) and both PEPCK mRNA and G-6-Pase in a phosphoinositide 3-kinase (PI3K)-dependent manner [41]. In addition, 50 µM EGCG could activate PI3K within 10 min, similar to insulin (10 nM), but the activation of other kinases such as PKB and p70s6k was much slower and not significant. The authors suggested that EGCG has a similar mechanism to insulin in reducing glucose production and expressing the PEPCK and G-6-Pase genes by modulation of the redox state of the cell [41].

Smaller amounts of EGCG (0.25–1 µM) suppressed gluconeogenesis in mouse cyclic adenosine monophosphate dexamethasone (cAMP-Dex)-stimulated hepatocytes and blocked the expression of the PEPCK and G-6-Pase genes [42]. However, no effect on the stimulation of tyrosine phosphorylation of IRS-1 or Akt, nor an influence of the PI3K inhibitor LY294002, was found suggesting an independent mechanism to the insulin signaling pathway [42]. The other known suppressor of hepatic gluconeogenesis, apart from the insulin signaling, is AMPK. In this case, EGCG increased the AMPK and acetyl-CoA carboxylase (ACC) phosphorylation in a time- and dose-dependent manner, and the suppression of AMPK resulted in the reversion of the effect of EGCG on the expression of the PEPCK and G-6-Pase genes in a calcium/calmodulin-dependent protein kinase kinase (CaMKK)- and ROS-dependent manner [42].

Yadollah et al. showed that 40 µM EGCG significantly reduced the expression of PEPCK and G-6-Pase in insulin-resistant HepG2 cells by 53% and 67%, respectively [43]. This effect was similar to that of 10 µM pioglitazone, which is a medication used to treat T2D. A combination of EGCG and pioglitazone induced a stronger reduction in the expression of PEPCK and G-6-Pase. The authors also proved that glucose production in HepG2 cells was significantly reduced by 50% by EGCG, by 55% by pioglitazone, and by 69% by a combination of both EGCG and pioglitazone [43].

Aside from the liver, the kidneys are also involved in glucose homeostasis and gluconeogenesis. EC (5–20 µM) and 2,3-DHB (20 µM) reduced cellular glucose uptake in rat renal NRK-52E cells similarly to the sodium-glucose cotransporter-2 (SGLT-2) antagonist phlorizin, leaving the expression of SGLT-2 and glucose transporter type 2 (GLUT2) unaltered [29]. A reduction in glucose production and PEPCK levels was also observed [29]. Moreover, the authors showed that Akt was involved in the modulation of both PEPCK levels and glucose production in NRK-52E cells [29].

Treatment of renal tubular NRK-52E cells with EC (10–20 µM) and 3,4-DHPA (10 µM) separately alleviated the alterations in glucose production and the upregulation of PEPCK induced by high glucose [30]. However, the protective effect disappeared when Akt and AMPK were inhibited. Therefore, both Akt and AMPK seem to be key molecules in the modulation of the glucose homeostasis and the preservation of renal tubular functionality [30].

4.5. Incretin Effect

Incretin hormones include glucose-dependent insulinotropic polypeptide (GIP) and glucagon-like peptide-1 (GLP-1). They are gut peptides secreted after the intake of nutrients, such as glucose, and are responsible for the incretin effect, which is the increased stimulation of insulin secretion by oral glucose rather than by intravenous glucose infusion. This effect is impaired in patients with T2D due to the reduced insulinotropic effect of GIP and GLP-1 [76]. In addition to the insulinotropic activity, the incretin hormones work together to regulate glucagon secretion: GIP stimulates glucagon secretion while GLP-1 inhibits glucagon secretion by alpha cells. In diabetic patients, glucagon secretion is altered since it is not inhibited in hyperglycemic conditions [70].

Yamashita et al. studied if isolated dimeric, trimeric, and tetrameric procyanidins from cacao liquor administered as a single-dose (10 µg/kg) in mice could influence GLP-1 and insulin levels in plasma [66]. The tetrameric procyanidin cinnamtannin A2 was the only compound able to increase the plasma insulin level without a glucose load as well as significantly increase the GLP-1 secretion levels in plasma 60 min after oral administration [66]. In vitro experiments revealed an increased phosphorylation of proteins IRß and IRS-1 in the soleus muscle as a result of the action of insulin. Procyanidins (low and high degree of polymerization, 10 mg/kg) from a CLP-rich extract increased GLP-1 secretion with or without glucose load in mice [54].

González-Abuín et al. evaluated the modulation of the mechanisms that have an influence on GLP-1 secretion in STC-1 cells by GSPE [44]. The authors found out that 0.05 mg/L GSPE induced depolarization, while 50 mg/L induced hyperpolarization in enteroendocrine cells [44]. This high extract concentration suppressed GLP-1 secretion by around 40%. Under nutrient-stimulated conditions, 50 mg/L GSPE reduced the membrane depolarization induced by nutrients and reduced GLP-1 secretion by 20% in glucose- and proline-stimulated cells. These results indicate the importance of the GSPE concentration in depolarization and GLP-1 secretion by STC-1 cells, as well as the influence that nutrients have on GLP-1 secretion by enteroendocrine cells [44].

Glycogen synthesis is also one of the functions of incretin hormones. Its secretion rate in muscle is controlled by GS, which is also enhanced by insulin. Therefore, this stimulates a cascade of phosphorylation-dephosphorylation reactions [3]. Glycogen synthase phosphatase (PP1) is activated by the phosphorylation of serine phosphorylation site 1 in the regulatory subunit (G) of PP1 by insulin and this phosphorylation is catalyzed by insulin-stimulated protein kinase 1 (ISPK-1). Phosphorylation of site 2 by cAMP-dependent kinase (PKA) leads, on the contrary, to its inactivation [3].

Some authors have studied how flavan-3-ols influence glycogen synthesis. Kim et al. showed that green tea polyphenols consisting of 68% EGCG were able to enhance glycogen synthesis by up to a factor of 2 (10 µM) in high glucose treated HepG2 cells under 100 nM insulin stimulation [45]. The molecular mechanism can involve the regulation of enzymes such as glycogen synthase kinase 3-beta (GSK3β) and GS since expression of phospho-GSK3β (Ser9) and phospho-GS (Ser461) were enhanced by EGCG [45].

4.6. Other Mechanisms

The production of cellular oxidants may affect insulin sensitivity via the negative regulation of insulin signaling pathways (JNK, IKK), the promotion of sustained chronic inflammation, and oxidative stress. Flavan-3-ols are known to have antioxidative functions, and these could exert a protective effect against diabetes and its complications via controlling the oxidative stress. Cinnamtannin B1, procyanidin C1, and cinnamtannin D1 (12.5–50 µmol/L) from cinnamon extracts inhibited H_2O_2-induced ROS generation as well as increased cell viability of INS-1 cells [34]. Similarly, under t-BOOH-induced oxidative stress, the microbial metabolites 3,4-DHPA and 3-HPP (5 and 1 µM, respectively) significantly decreased rat pancreatic beta cell death and ROS and carbonyl group production [38]. While EC at a low dose of 0.3 µmol/L, but not at a higher dose of 30 µmol/L, improved GSIS of SFA-impaired INS-1 cells, only the highest dose of EC significantly reduced ROS after treatment with H_2O_2 and high glucose [32].

Bettaieb et al. found that the supplementation of high-fructose-fed rats with EC (20 mg/kg) for 8 weeks, mitigated the IRes induced by high fructose concentrations. EC supplementation (20 mg/kg) in high-fructose-fed rats showed an ability to inhibit the expression and activity of NADPH oxidase and the activation of redox-sensitive signals [58].

Treatment of STZ-induced diabetic rats with C (20 and 40 mg/kg/day) significantly decreased glucose levels, while superoxide dismutase (SOD), catalase (CAT), and glutathione S-transferase (GST) levels increased in a concentration-dependent manner, especially after treatment with 80 mg/kg/day [67].

Haidari et al. showed that a GTE given to STZ-induced diabetic rats at 200 mg/kg for 4 weeks, significantly decreased their serum glucose levels as well as the serum and hepatic malondialdehyde (MDA) concentration when compared to the diabetic control group. Total antioxidant capacity (TAC) was significantly increased after treatment [68].

Plasma glucose levels could also be controlled by the modulation of lipid digestion and the reduction of hyperlipidemia [77]. C treatment of STZ-induced diabetic rats dose-dependently decreased the serum levels of total cholesterol (TC), triglycerides, LDL, apoprotein B, and glucose levels, while it increased the serum levels of high density lipoprotein (HDL) and apoprotein A-I (20–80 mg/kg) [67]. EGCG dose-dependently reversed increased serum lipid levels including TC, TG, and LDL, and increased HDL in high-fat diet NAFLD mice compared with control mice [61]. EC (20 mg/kg body weight) prevented the high-fat-diet-induced increase in plasma TG and FFA in C57BL/6 mice [57]. Treatment of HepG2 cells with 100 nM insulin and 0.1–10 µM EGCG reduced lipogenesis to 65% compared to cells treated with insulin alone through increased expressions of phosphor-AMPKα and phosphor-ACC [45].

Inflammation contributes to impaired glucose management by adipocytes, hepatocytes, and muscle cells and interferes with insulin production and insulin signaling [78]. TNFα plays an important role in the activation of signaling cascades in adipocytes related to inflammation and IRes. In this context, EC (0.5–10 µM) has been shown to dose-dependently reduce TNFα-mediated JNK, ERK1/2, and p-38 phosphorylation, and nuclear AP-1-DNA binding in 3T3-L1 adipocytes [46]. It also inhibited the activation of the nuclear factor kappa-light-chain-enhancer of activated B cells (NF-κB) signaling cascade preventing the p65 nuclear transport and nuclear NF-κB-DNA binding. Moreover, EC reversed the TNFα-mediated downregulation of PPARγ expression and reduced nuclear DNA binding. The altered transcription of genes involved in inflammation and insulin signaling (monocyte chemoattractant protein 1 (MCP-1), IL-6, TNFα, resistin and protein-tyrosine phosphatase 1B) mediated by TNFα was inhibited by EC [46].

EC supplementation (20 mg/kg) in high-fructose-fed rats inhibited the expression of NF-κB regulated pro-inflammatory cytokines and chemokines [58].

The colonic metabolites of flavan-3-ols have also been shown to exert beneficial effects in diabetes other than those directly related to glycemia. One of them is the positive effect on vascular function, which is known to be directly linked to diabetes [79]. As reported in several studies, low molecular weight phenolics such as 2,3-dihydroxybenzoic acid (2,3-DHB), 3-HPP, and 3,4-DHPA could exert vasodilatory activities by stimulating NO production [47–49]. Apart from this, dihydroferulic acid, 3-hydroxyphenylacetic acid (3-HPA), 3,4-DHPA, and homovanillic acid could reduce the formation of advanced glycation end-products (AGEs) [50,51], which are thought to be linked to the development of diabetes and insulin resistance and to the occurrence of diabetic complications [80].

5. Antidiabetic Effects of Flavan-3-ols: Clinical Intervention Trials

Some authors have studied the effect of the supplementation of pure flavan-3-ols on antidiabetic effects in order to exclude potential interactions with other compounds and with other flavonoids present in flavan-3-ol-rich food. Zhang et al. investigated the effects of a daily intake of EGCG (500 mg/day) in women with a diagnosed GDM at the beginning of the third quarter of pregnancy (29 weeks). HOMA-IR, HOMA-β fasting blood glucose and insulin levels decreased whereas the insulin sensitivity as measured by QUICKI increased due to the intervention. Furthermore, neonatal complications at birth, such as low birth weight or hypoglycemia, were significantly reduced in the intervention group [81] (Table 3).

Table 3. Human clinical trials on antidiabetic effect of flavan-3-ols [3].

Intervention	Study Design	Population	Duration	Parameter	Results	Ref.
Single polyphenols						
500 mg EGCG/day (one capsule/day) Control: 500 mg starch powder/day (one capsule/day)	CT, pc, d-b	n = 326 (women, GDM, 3rd trimester of pregnancy, Chinese, 25–34 years, ≈ 26kg/m²)	Until child's birth	FBG, INS, HOMA-IR, QUICKI, HOMA-β, BW, BMI, neonatal complications at birth (LBW, hypoglycemia, RD, macrosomia, 1 and 5 min Apgar scores)	↓FBG *#, ↓INS *#, ↓HOMA-IR *#, ↑QUICKI *#, ↓HOMA-β *#, ↓Neonatal complications at birth	[81]
Chocolate						
FRC dark (100 g/day in 2 half-bar doses, 1008 mg TP, 36.12 g C), Control: FFWC	RCT, co	n = 19 (women 8, men 11, IGT + hypertension, 44.8 ± 8.0 years, 26.5 ± 1.9 kg/m²)	15 days (+ 7-day run-in and 7-day washout phase)	FBG, INS, 3-h-PBG, 3-h-PINS, HOMA-IR, β-cell function (CIR$_{120}$), QUCIKI, ISI, lipids (TC, LDL, HDL, TG), SPB und DBP (clinical + 24-h ABMP), FMD, hsCRP, plasma homo-cysteine, electrolytes, uric acid, fibrinogen	↓HOMA-IR *#, ↑QUICKI *#, ↑ISI *#, ↑ISI$_0$ *#, ↑β-cell function (CIR$_{120}$) *# → affected 3-h-PBG and 3-h-PINS ↓SBP *# +DBP #, ↓24-h ABMP *#, ↑FMD *#, ↓TC *#, ↓LDL *#	[82]
27 g/day FRC (2 × 13.5 g, 850 mg flavan-3-ols (90 mg EC) and 100 mg IsoF	RCT, pd, pc	n = 93 (women, postmeno-pausal, T2D, standard therapy; receiving TC-lowering therapy, UK, ≈ 62 years, ≈ 32 kg/m²)	1 year	FBG, INS, HOMA-IR, HbA1c, QUICKI, lipids (TC, LDL, HDL, TG), 2-h ABPM, BW, 10-y total CHD risk	↓INS *# ↓HOMA-IR *#, ↑QUICKI *#, ↓TC:HDL ratio *#, ↓LDL *#, ↑HDL:LDL ratio *# ↑CHD risk * but ↓CHD risk #	[83]
GTE						
1500 mg decaffeinated GTE (3 × 500 mg/day, 856 mg EGCG	RCT, pc, d-b	n = 68 (women 44, men 24, obese T2D, Taiwanese, 51.3 ± 9.2 years, 29.7 ± 4.0 kg/m²)	16 weeks	FBG, INS, HOMA-IR, HbA1c, leptin, ghrelin, adiponectin, lipids (TG, TC, LDL, HDL), SPB, DBP, creatinine, ALT, uric acid, BW, BMI, WC	↓HbA1c *, ↓HOMA-IR *, ↓INS *, ↑ghrelin * (placebo too), ↓WC *	[84]
340 mL green tea + GTE/day (582.8 mg catechins/day) Control: 340 mL green tea + GTE/day (96.3 mg catechins/day)	CT, pd, d-b	n = 43 (women 25, men 18, T2D, no INS therapy, hypoglycemic drugs (n = 35))	12 weeks (+ 4-week run-in, 4-week follow-up period)	FBG, INS, HbA1c, lipids (TG, TC, FFAs), total keton bodies, remnant-like lipoprotein C, adiponectin, enzymes, total protein, albumin, urea nitrogen, uric acid, creatinine, electrolytes, hematology analysis, SBP, DBP, BW, BMI, WC, HC, WHR, FM (%)	At wk 12: ↑INS *#, ↑adiponectin *, ↓TC *, ↓FFAs *, ↓total ketone Bodies *, ↓WC *#, ↓WHR *# At wk 8: ↓SBP *	[85]
GTE powder (one packet/day, 544 mg PP, 456 mg C)	RCT, co	n = 60 (women 11, men 49; glucose abnormalities, T2D medication (n = 16), 71% IRes, Japanese, ≈ 54 years, ≈ 26 kg/m²)	2 months/inter-vention	FBG, INS, HOMA-IR, HbA1c, lipids (TC, LDL, HDL, TG), hsCRP, SPB, DBP, BW, BMI, FM	↓HbA1c *	[86]

Table 3. Cont.

Intervention	Study Design	Population	Duration	Parameter	Results	Ref.
GTE powder (one packet/day, 544 mg PP, 456 mg C)	RCT, pd	$n = 66$ (women 13, men 53; (borderline) T2D, Japanese, ≈ 54 years, ≈ 26 kg/m^2)	2 months	FBG, INS, HOMA-IR, HbA1c, hsCRP, SPB, DBP, BW, BMI	↓ FBG, ↓ INS, ↓ HOMA-IR, ↓ HbA1c *, ↓ SPB * and DBP *, ↓ BW * and BMI *	[87]
900 mL green tea (9 g) Control: water	CT, co	$n = 55$ (women 24, men 32, T2D, 53.9 ± 7.7 years, 25.0 ± 2.2 kg/m^2)	4 weeks	FBG, INS, HOMA-IR, adiponectin, lipids (TC, LDL, HDL, TG), hsCRP, IL-6, arterial stiffness	No effects	[88]
GSE						
600 mg GSE/day (2 × 300 mg/day)	RCT, co, pc, d-b	$n = 32$ (women 16, men 16, T2D at high CV risks, oral glucose-lowering therapy ($n = 19$), UK, 61.8 ± 6.36 years, 30.2 ± 5.92 kg/m^2)	4 weeks/intervention (+2-week washout)	FBG, INS, HOMA-IR, HbA1c (only at baseline), fructosamine, lipids (TC, LDL, HDL, TG), liver function, hsCRP, endothelial function, oxidative stress (TAOS, GSH, GSSG), ACR	↓ TC *, ↓ hsCRP *, ↓ fructosamine *, ↑ GSH *	[89]
Cacao						
Cacao capsules (2.5 g/day ACTICOA™ cacao powder, 207.5 mg Fla)	RCT, pc, pd, d-b	$n = 35$ (women 17, men 18, T2D + hypertension, dietetic and/or pharmacological treatment, 64.2 ± 1.5 years, ≈ 29 kg/m^2)	12 weeks	FBG, INS, HOMA-IR, HbA1c, lipids (TC, LDL, HDL, TG), SBP, DBD, creatinine, BW, BMI, WC, WHR, FM	↓ WC ↓ WHR *	[90]
Cacao beverages (2 × 28 g Cacao powder/day, 180, 400 or 900 mg Fla/day) Control: cacao beverages (30 mg Fla/day)	Exploratory randomized study, co	$n = 19$ (women 10, men 9, obese at risk for IRes, IGT ($n = 6$), 46 ± 2.3 years, 36.8 ± 1.0 kg/m^2)	5 days (10 days washout)	FBG, INS, TG, hsCRP, ICAM, IL-6, total 8-isoprostane, SBP, DBP, BW, BMI, WC, FM After OGTT: AUC-BG, AUC-INS, 2h-PBG, 2h-PINS, 2h-TG, 2h-hsCRP, 2h-ICAM, 2h-IL-6, total 8-isoprostane (1h and 1,5h), fibrinogen (1h and 1,5h), HOMA-IR, QUICKI, ISI	↓ 8-isoprostane *, ↓ hsCRP *, IL-6 * (as the dose of Fla increased)	[91]
Cacao beverage (960 mg PP, 480 mg Fla) with high-fat breakfast (766 kcal, 50 g fat)	RCT, pc, co, d-b (1 week washout phase)	$n = 18$ (women 14, men 4, T2D, no insulin therapy, 56 ± 3.2 years, 35.3 ± 2.0 kg/m^2)	Single dose (6-h study: 0, 1, 2, 3, 4, 5, 6 h)	Fasting + post-prandial: BG, INS, HOMA-IR, lipids (TC, LDL, HDL, TG), hsCRP, SBP, DBP, SAE, LAE; fasting: BW, BMI, WC	↑ HDL# (1 h and 4 h, 6 h-AUC, overall Δ:1.5 ± 0.8 mg/dL), ↑ Ins# (4 h, overall Δ: 5.2 ± 3.2 mU/L), ↑ HOMA-IR# (4 h, 4 h-AUC, no overall), ↓ LAE# (2 h, overall Δ: −1.6 ± 0.7 mL/mm Hg)	[92]

Table 3. Cont.

Intervention	Study Design	Population	Duration	Parameter	Results	Ref.
2.5 g cacao (5 capsules: 0.5 g ACTICOA™ cacao powder, 40.4 mg EC) with diabetic-suitable breakfast. Control: cellulose	RCT, pc, co, d-b	$n = 12$ (women 3, men 9; T2D + overweight/obesity + hypertension, no insulin therapy; 68.0 ± 9.0 years)	Single dose (4-h study: 0, 2, 4h) (≥2 week wash-out)	Fasting & post-prandial: BG, INS, HOMA-IR, lipids (TC, LDL, HDL, TG), SBP, DBP, fasting: BW, WC, HC, WHR, FM	No effects	[93]

* compared with the baseline values. # compared with the control group; ³ ABPM: ambulatory blood pressure monitoring; ACR: (urinary) albumin:creatinine ratio; ALT: alanine aminotransferase; AUC: area under the curve; BW: body weight; co: cross-over; CV: cardiovascular; BG: blood glucose; BMI: body mass index; CHD: coronary heart disease; CIR: corrected insulin response; CT: clinical trial; d: day; d-b: double-blind; DBP: diastolic blood pressure; FBG: fasting blood glucose; FFAs: free fatty acids; FFWC: flavanol-free white chocolate; Fla: flavanols; FM: fat mass; FMD: flow-mediated dilation; FRC: flavanol-rich chocolate; GDM: gestational diabetes mellitus; GSE: grape seed extract; GSH: reduced glutathione; GSSG: oxidized glutathione; GTE: green tea extract; HbA1c: glycated hemoglobin; HC: hip circumference; HDL: high density lipoprotein cholesterol; HOMA-IR: homeostasis model assessment for insulin resistance; hsCRP: high-sensitivity C-reactive protein; ICAM: intercellular adhesion molecule-1; IGT: impaired glucose tolerance; IL-6: interleukin-6; INS: insulin; IRes: insulin resistance; ISI: insulin sensitivity index; IsoF: isoflavones; LAE: large artery elasticity; LBW: low birth weight; LDL: low density lipoprotein cholesterol; m: men; mo: month; OGTT: oral glucose tolerance test; PBG: postprandial blood glucose; pc: placebo-controlled; pd: parallel group design; PINS: postprandial insulin concentration; PP: polyphenols; QUICKI: quantitative insulin sensitivity check index; RCT: randomized controlled trial; RD: respiratory distress; SAE: small artery elasticity; SBP: systolic blood pressure; TAOS: total antioxidant status; TC: total cholesterol; TG: triglycerides; TP: total phenols; T2D: type 2 diabetes; w: women; sig-: significant; WC: waist circumference; WHR: waist to hip ratio; wk: week; y: year. Flavan-3-ols and their microbial metabolites: EC: epicatechin; EGCG: epigallocatechin gallate.

Hsu et al. found no statistical differences in several parameters (fasting glucose, insulin, HOMA-IR, HbA1c, lipoproteins, hormones (leptin, ghrelin, adiponectin), blood pressure, anthropometrics) between a decaffeinated GTE-supplemented group (3 × 500 mg/day; 856 mg EGCG) of T2D obese patients and the placebo group. However, 16 weeks of treatment led to a significant reduction of HbA1c, HOMA-IR index and the insulin level from the baseline to the end of the treatment (within-group changes) [84].

A randomized controlled trial (RCT) assessed the effect of a daily consumption of 100 g of flavanol-rich dark chocolate (FRC; 1008 mg total phenols and 36.12 g C) for 15 days on IRes and showed a significant reduction of HOMA-IR, an enhancement of the insulin sensitivity and an increase in the beta cell activity in hypertensive individuals with impaired glucose tolerance [82]. Furthermore, the consumption of FRC decreased TC and LDL when compared to the baseline values and the control, but it did not affect HDL and TG. High-sensitivity C-reactive protein (hsCRP) did not change either [82]. Similarly, the daily consumption of 27 g FRC (850 mg flavan-3-ols and 90 mg EC) and 100 mg isoflavones for one year reduced HOMA-IR, LDL, and the TC:HDL ratio and increased QUICKI and the HDL:LDL ratio in postmenopausal women with T2D. These metabolic improvements resulted in a lower 10-year total coronary heart disease (CHD) risk compared to the control [83].

A clinical trial investigating the effects of the daily intake of green tea (340 mL) and GTE (582.8 mg catechins/day) for 12 weeks showed an increased insulin level and an increase in the adiponectin level (only within-group changes) in subjects with T2D. Furthermore, there was a reduction of FFA compared to the baseline and a decrease of the TC level when compared to the control. Fasting blood glucose and HbA1c remained unchanged [85].

The daily supplementation with a GTE (one packet/day; 544 mg polyphenols, 456 mg C) for two months improved the HbA1c value in individuals with glucose abnormalities when compared to the baseline. No other parameters of glucose metabolism (fasting blood glucose, insulin, HOMA-IR) or lipid metabolism (TC, LDL, HDL, TG) were affected by the intervention [85]. Furthermore, the daily intake of a GTE powder did not improve the hsCRP level [86]. In individuals with borderline T2D or T2D, GTE (544 mg polyphenols, 456 mg C) decreased the IRes, as measured by HOMA-IR, the fasting blood glucose, the insulin levels and the HbA1c when compared to the baseline. No significant differences between the intervention and the control were observed [87].

However, not all studies showed unambiguous protective effects against diabetes. A daily intake of 9 g green tea in 900 mL hot water for four weeks did not affect the IRes, the fasting blood glucose or the insulin concentration in subjects suffering from T2D. Furthermore, no beneficial effects on the lipid metabolism, hsCRP or IL-6 were shown [88]. Similarly, daily supplementation of GSE (2 × 300 mg/day) for four weeks did not improve the IRes [89]. Fasting blood glucose, insulin level, and HOMA-IR remained unchanged in individuals with T2D and a high cardiovascular risk. Moreover, the supplementation did not result in an improved lipoprotein status apart from a decrease in TC level. However, the regular intake of the GSE significantly decreased fructosamine concentration, decreased hsCRP, and increased the reduced glutathione (GSH) compared to the baseline value. Total antioxidant status (TAOS) and the concentration of oxidized glutathione (GSSG) remained unchanged [89].

A daily intake of 2.5 g cacao powder (ACTICOA TM; 207.5 mg flavanols) for 12 weeks did not enhance the glucose or lipid metabolism in T2D hypertensive patients [90]. The consumption of two cacao beverages per day (2 × 28 g cacao powder/day) containing 180 mg, 400 mg or 900 mg flavanols on five consecutive days did not affect fasting and postprandial glucose parameters in obese individuals who were at risk of IRes either. However, hsCRP, 8-isoprostane, and IL-6 decreased as the dose of flavanols increased. These effects were only significant when compared to the baseline values but not when compared to the control [91].

Acute cacao studies also showed no distinct improvement of postprandial glycemia and the insulin response in participants with T2D. The acute supplementation of a cacao beverage (960 mg polyphenols; 480 mg flavanols) with a high-fat fast-food-style breakfast (766 kcal, 50 g fat) elicited a higher insulin response and a decreased IRes, as measured by HOMA-IR. HDL increased while the concentration of TC, LDL, TG, and hsCRP remained unchanged [92]. No effects could be observed after an acute supplementation of 2.5 g cacao powder (ACTICOA™; 40.4 mg EC) with a diabetic-suitable breakfast in hypertensive, overweight or obese subjects with T2D [93].

6. Concluding Remarks

Increasing evidence suggests that flavan-3-ols are responsible for the protective role of certain foods, such as green tea, against diabetes. Possible molecular mechanisms by which they could prevent or treat diabetes include the promotion of beta cell functionality and viability, the amelioration of glucose transport in muscle and adipose tissue by the promotion of the insulin signaling pathway, the enhancement of the incretin effect, and the decrease of endogenous glucose production.

Microbial metabolites of flavan-3-ols are suggested to be the actual active form by which these compounds exert their potential health benefits, such as the antidiabetic effect. However, the evidence regarding this is still scarce and only few studies assessed the effects of flavan-3-ol specific microbial metabolites.

One of the determinants of the possible antidiabetic effect of flavan-3-ols seems to be their concentration. In this regard, when interpreting the results of in vitro studies, it is necessary to consider not only the bioavailability of the compounds investigated but also their physiological plasma concentration after absorption. Some of the studies used higher concentrations than those found in human plasma after ingestion. Conjugated flavan-3-ols have been detected in plasma in low nanomolar ranges [94,95]. Their colonic metabolites phenyl-γ-valerolactones and phenylvaleric acids have been detected in plasma at concentrations under 1 µM [95–99]. The lower weight phenolics are usually found in plasma at concentrations lower than 0.5 µM [96–99], although phenylacetic acid, protocatechuic acid, and hippuric acid were also detected at concentrations ≈ 40 µmol/L [96–100].

Although many studies used physiological concentrations of the compound and microbial metabolites, some tested higher concentrations and suggested that, in some cases, supraphysiological ranges could induce an opposite response to that from lower ranges. A careful evaluation of the flavan-3-ol dose would, therefore, be needed when used as nutraceutical.

Under physiological concentrations, flavan-3-ols and their microbial metabolites exert different biological activities at varying concentrations. The concentration needed to exert a specific function by a particular compound might not be the same than the one needed to exert another biological activity. For example, 3,4-DHPA IC_{50} on vasodilation is lower than on AGEs formation [101,102]. In the prevention and management of diabetes, low concentrations of flavan-3-ols and their microbial metabolites could influence determined molecular mechanisms while higher concentrations could be needed to positively influence other mechanisms, as shown in many of the presented studies.

Although increasing evidence supports the stated mechanisms of action, the results of many studies are inconclusive, with some of them exhibiting contradictory outcomes or even negative effects. Possible reasons for the varying results could be not only the different compound concentrations used, but also the different methodologies used in each study. As for the in vitro and animal studies, a variety of models for diabetes was used. In the literature described in this review, the most frequent in vitro techniques used insulin-secreting cell line INS-1 and pancreatic beta cell lines, and they also included in vitro studies on glucose uptake mainly in skeletal muscle cells but also in 3T3-L1 adipocytes. In addition, assays on α-amylase inhibition and inhibition of α-glucosidase activity were performed. In vivo studies included spontaneous diabetic obese animal models, mice genetically predisposed to obesity and T2D, and others used chemicals to induce the disease, mainly streptozotocin. However, not all models were specific for diabetes mellitus. Therefore, although many of these studies showed positive effects on diabetic parameters, concluding that they are beneficial for the treatment of diabetes mellitus would not be appropriate. For the proper elucidation of the effect of a substance regarding diabetes management suitable models are required. For this reason, more in vitro and animal studies using the adequate models for the disease should be performed.

Moreover, it is worth mentioning that some of the used treatment samples often include other bioactive components. Therefore, the flavan-3-ol fraction does not always represent the exclusive component present in the sample, which must be taken into account when attributing positive effects to these compounds.

In the case of human clinical trials, the compliance of the patients to the treatment was not measured in all cases and the diet during the intervention was not always recorded. In addition, other confounders, such as body composition, were often insufficiently registered. Therefore, these factors could have influenced the studies' results. Moreover, not only the concentration of the flavan-3-ols might be a determinant of the possible antidiabetic effect, but also, the duration of the intervention could be a determinant. Further methodological weaknesses in some of the human trials presented are the absence of a wash-out phase, or not choosing the dietary restrictions of the control groups appropriately.

It is known that the individual gut microbiota composition has an influence on both the bioavailability and the metabolization of flavan-3-ols [3]. However, none of the included clinical trials investigated the bioavailability and the metabolization of the ingested flavan-3-ols in the study population. Therefore, no conclusion can be reached about whether there is a positive association between the blood concentration of the flavan-3-ols or their metabolites, the administered dose, and the putative effect. That is, it is not possible to know to what extent different metabolic effects are related to a different bioavailability and metabolization of the flavan-3-ols by individuals. In order to better understand the effects of flavan-3-ols and their metabolites on the prevention and management of diabetes, it is relevant to record not only metabolic parameters after treatment but also the pharmacokinetics of these substances.

For all these reasons, the use of homogeneous and more appropriate methods is essential for the clarification of flavan-3-ol's antidiabetic effect and mechanisms of action.

Author Contributions: E.M.C., L.J., and M.-C.S. wrote the paper; M.-C.S. conceived and supervised the project. All authors have read and agreed to the published version of the manuscript.

Funding: This work was funded by the Department of Nutrition and Food Sciences, Nutrition and Microbiota, University of Bonn and supported by the grant no 01EA1707 of the German Federal Ministry of Education and Research.

Acknowledgments: The authors would like to thank Katherine Macmillan for the professional English editing service.

Conflicts of Interest: The authors declare no conflicts of interest.

References

1. Saeedi, P.; Petersohn, I.; Salpea, P.; Malanda, B.; Karuranga, S.; Unwin, N.; Colagiuri, S.; Guariguata, L.; Motala, A.A.; Ogurtsova, K.; et al. Global and regional diabetes prevalence estimates for 2019 and projections for 2030 and 2045: Results from the International Diabetes Federation Diabetes Atlas, 9th ed. *Diabetes Res. Clin. Prac.* **2019**, *157*, 107843.
2. Patterson, C.C.; Dahlquist, G.G.; Gyürüs, E.; Green, A.; Soltész, G.; EURODIAB Study Group. Incidence trends for childhood type 1 diabetes in Europe during 1989–2003 and predicted new cases 2005–2020: A multicentre prospective registration study. *Lancet* **2009**, *373*, 2027–2033. [PubMed]
3. Cersosimo, E.; Triplitt, C.; Solis-Herrera, C.; Mandarino, L.J.; DeFronzo, R.A. Pathogenesis of Type 2 Diabetes Mellitus. In *Endotext [Internet]*; Feingold, K.R., Anawalt, B., Boyce, A., Chrousos, G., Dungan, K., Grossman, A., Hershman, J.M., Kaltsas, G., Koch, C., Kopp, P., et al., Eds.; MDText.com, Inc.: South Dartmouth, MA, USA, 2018. Available online: https://www.ncbi.nlm.nih.gov/books/NBK279115/ (accessed on 27 February 2018).
4. Stein, S.A.; Lamos, E.M.; Davis, S.N. A review of the efficacy and safety of oral antidiabetic drugs. *Expert Opin. Drug Saf.* **2013**, *12*, 153–175. [CrossRef]
5. Vogiatzoglou, A.; Mulligan, A.A.; Lentjes, M.A.H.; Luben, R.N.; Spencer, J.P.E.; Schroeter, H.; Khaw, K.-T.; Kuhnle, G.G.C. Flavonoid Intake in European Adults (18 to 64 Years). *PLoS ONE* **2015**, *10*, e0128132. [CrossRef]
6. Wang, X.; Ouyang, Y.Y.; Liu, J.; Zhao, G. Flavonoid intake and risk of CVD: A systematic review and meta-analysis of prospective cohort studies. *Br. J. Nutr.* **2014**, *111*, 1–11. [CrossRef]

7. Lei, L.; Yang, Y.; He, H.; Chen, E.; Du, L.; Dong, J.; Yang, J. Flavan-3-ols consumption and cancer risk: A meta-analysis of epidemiologic studies. *Oncotarget* **2016**, *7*, 73573–73592. [PubMed]
8. Iso, H.; Date, C.; Wakai, K.; Fukui, M.; Tamakoshi, A.; JACC Study Group. The Relationship between Green Tea and Total Caffeine Intake and Risk for Self-Reported Type 2 Diabetes among Japanese Adults. *Ann. Intern. Med.* **2006**, *144*, 554–562. [CrossRef] [PubMed]
9. The InterAct Consortium. Tea consumption and incidence of type 2 diabetes in Europe: The EPIC-InterAct case-cohort study. *PLoS ONE* **2012**, *7*, e36910. [CrossRef]
10. Nguyen, C.T.; Lee, A.H.; Pham, N.M.; Do, V.V.; Ngu, N.D.; Tran, B.Q.; Binns, C. Habitual tea drinking associated with a lower risk of type 2 diabetes in Vietnamese adults. *Asia Pac. J. Clin. Nutr.* **2018**, *27*, 701–706. [CrossRef]
11. Monagas, M.; Urpi-Sarda, M.; Sánchez-Patán, F.; Llorach, R.; Garrido, I.; Gómez-Cordovés, C.; Andres-Lacueva, C.; Bartolomé, B. Insights into the metabolism and microbial biotransformation of dietary flavan-3-ols and the bioactivity of their metabolites. *Food Funct.* **2010**, *1*, 233–253. [CrossRef]
12. Hellstrom, J.K.; Torronen, A.R.; Mattila, P.H. Proanthocyanidins in common food products of plant origin. *J. Agric. Food Chem.* **2009**, *57*, 7899–7906. [CrossRef] [PubMed]
13. *Fruit and Vegetable Phytochemicals: Chemistry Nutritional Value and Stability*, 1st ed.; De la Rosa, L.A.; Alvarez-Parrilla, E.; Gonzalez-Aguilar, G.A. (Eds.) Wiley-Blackwell: Ames, IA, USA, 2009.
14. Knaze, V.; Zamora-Ros, R.; Lujan-Barroso, L.; Romieu, I.; Scalbert, A.; Slimani, N.; Riboli, E.; Van Rossum, C.; Bueno-De-Mesquita, H.B.; Trichopoulou, A.; et al. Intake estimation of total and individual flavan-3-ols, proanthocyanidins and theaflavins, their food sources and determinants in the European Prospective Investigation into Cancer and Nutrition (EPIC) study. *Br. J. Nutr.* **2011**, *108*, 1095–1108. [CrossRef]
15. Manach, C.; Scalbert, A.; Morand, C.; Rémésy, C.; Jiménez, L. Polyphenols: Food sources and bioavailability. *Am. J. Clin. Nutr.* **2004**, *79*, 727–747. [CrossRef] [PubMed]
16. Crozier, A.; Del Rio, D.; Clifford, M.N. Bioavailability of dietary flavonoids and phenolic compounds. *Mol. Asp. Med.* **2010**, *31*, 446–467. [CrossRef]
17. Selma, M.V.; Espín, J.C.; Tomás-Barberán, F.A. Interaction between Phenolics and Gut Microbiota: Role in Human Health. *J. Agric. Food Chem.* **2009**, *57*, 6485–6501. [CrossRef] [PubMed]
18. Espín, J.C.; González-Sarrías, A.; Tomás-Barberán, F.A. The gut microbiota: A key factor in the therapeutic effects of (poly)phenols. *Biochem. Pharmacol.* **2017**, *139*, 82–93. [CrossRef] [PubMed]
19. Gao, J.; Xu, P.; Wang, Y.; Wang, Y.; Hochstetter, D. Combined Effects of Green Tea Extracts, Green Tea Polyphenols or Epigallocatechin Gallate with Acarbose on Inhibition against α-Amylase and α-Glucosidase in Vitro. *Molecules* **2013**, *18*, 11614–11623. [CrossRef] [PubMed]
20. Yilmazer-Musa, M.; Griffith, A.M.; Michels, A.J.; Schneider, E.; Frei, B. Inhibition of α-Amylase and α-Glucosidase Activity by Tea and Grape Seed Extracts and their Constituent Catechins. *J. Agric. Food Chem.* **2012**, *60*, 8924–8929. [CrossRef]
21. Wasai, M.; Fujimura, Y.; Nonaka, H.; Kitamura, R.; Murata, M.; Tachibana, H. Postprandial glycaemia-lowering effect of a green tea cultivar Sunrouge and cultivar-specific metabolic profiling for determining bioactivity-related ingredients. *Sci. Rep.* **2018**, *8*, 16041. [CrossRef]
22. Mrabti, H.N.; Jaradat, N.; Fichtali, I.; Ouedrhiri, W.; Jodeh, S.; Ayesh, S.; Cherrah, Y.; Faouzi, M E.A. Separation, Identification, and Antidiabetic Activity of Catechin Isolated from *Arbutus unedo* L. Plant Roots. *Plants* **2018**, *7*, 31. [CrossRef]
23. Bräunlich, M.; Slimestad, R.; Wangensteen, H.; Brede, C.; Malterud, K.E.; Barsett, H. Extracts, Anthocyanins and Procyanidins from Aronia melanocarpa as Radical Scavengers and Enzyme Inhibitors. *Nutrients* **2013**, *5*, 663–678. [CrossRef] [PubMed]
24. Tong, T.; Ren, N.; Soomi, P.; Wu, J.; Guo, N.; Kang, H.; Kim, E.; Wu, Y.; He, P.; Tu, Y.; et al. Theaflavins Improve Insulin Sensitivity through Regulating Mitochondrial Biosynthesis in Palmitic Acid-Induced HepG2 Cells. *Molecules* **2018**, *23*, 3382. [CrossRef] [PubMed]
25. Ojelabi, O.A.; Lloyd, K.P.; De Zutter, J.K.; Carruthers, A. Red wine and green tea flavonoids are cis-allosteric activators and competitive inhibitors of glucose transporter 1 (GLUT1)-mediated sugar uptake. *J. Biol. Chem.* **2018**, *293*, 19823–19834. [CrossRef] [PubMed]
26. Yan, J.; Zhao, Y.; Suo, S.; Liu, Y.; Zhao, B. Green tea catechins ameliorate adipose insulin resistance by improving oxidative stress. *Free. Rad. Biol. Med.* **2012**, *52*, 1648–1657. [CrossRef]

27. Takagaki, A.; Yoshioka, Y.; Yamashita, Y.; Nagano, T.; Ikeda, M.; Hara-Terawaki, A.; Seto, R.; Ashida, H. Effects of Microbial Metabolites of (-)-Epigallocatechin Gallate on Glucose Uptake in L6 Skeletal Muscle Cell and Glucose Tolerance in ICR Mice. *Biol. Pharm. Bull.* **2019**, *42*, 212–221. [CrossRef]
28. Scazzocchio, B.; Varì, R.; Filesi, C.; D'Archivio, M.; Santangelo, C.; Giovannini, C.; Iacovelli, A.; Silecchia, G.; Li Volti, G.; Galvano, F.; et al. Cyanidin-3-O-β-glucoside and protocatechuic acid exert insulin-like effects by upregulating PPARγ activity in human omental adipocytes. *Diabetes* **2011**, *60*, 2234–2244. [CrossRef]
29. Álvarez-Cilleros, D.; Martín, M.Á.; Ramos, S. (−)-Epicatechin and the Colonic 2,3-Dihydroxybenzoic Acid Metabolite Regulate Glucose Uptake, Glucose Production, and Improve Insulin Signaling in Renal NRK-52E Cells. *Mol. Nutr. Food Res.* **2018**, *62*, 1700470. [CrossRef]
30. Álvarez-Cilleros, D.; Martín, M.Á.; Ramos, S. Protective effects of (−)-epicatechin and the colonic metabolite 3,4-dihydroxyphenylacetic acid against glucotoxicity-induced insulin signalling blockade and altered glucose uptake and production in renal tubular NRK-52E cells. *Food Chem. Toxicol.* **2018**, *120*, 119–128. [CrossRef]
31. Kaneko, Y.K.; Takii, M.; Kojima, Y.; Yokosawa, H.; Ishikawa, T. Structure-Dependent Inhibitory Effects of Green Tea Catechins on Insulin Secretion from Pancreatic β-Cells. *Biol. Pharm. Bull.* **2015**, *38*, 476–481. [CrossRef]
32. Yang, K.; Chan, C. Epicatechin potentiation of glucose-stimulated insulin secretion in INS-1 cells is not dependent on its antioxidant activity. *Acta Pharmacol. Sin.* **2018**, *39*, 893–902. [CrossRef]
33. Koonyosying, P.; Uthaipibull, C.; Fucharoen, S.; Koumoutsea, E.V.; Porter, J.B.; Srichairatanakool, S. Decrement in Cellular Iron and Reactive Oxygen Species, and Improvement of Insulin Secretion in a Pancreatic Cell Line Using Green Tea Extract. *Pancreas* **2019**, *48*, 636–643. [CrossRef] [PubMed]
34. Sun, P.; Wang, T.; Chen, L.; Yu, B.; Jia, Q.; Chen, K.; Fan, H.; Li, Y.; Wang, H. Trimer procyanidin oligomers contribute to the protective effects of cinnamon extracts on pancreatic β-cells in vitro. *Acta Pharmacol. Sin.* **2016**, *37*, 1083–1090. [CrossRef]
35. Mo, Y.; Lei, J.; Sun, Y.; Zhang, Q.; Wei, G. Conformational Ensemble of hIAPP Dimer: Insight into the Molecular Mechanism by which a Green Tea Extract inhibits hIAPP Aggregation. *Sci. Rep.* **2016**, *6*, 33076. [CrossRef] [PubMed]
36. Meng, F.; Abedini, A.; Plesner, A.; Verchere, C.B.; Raleigh, D.P. The flavanol (-)-epigallocatechin 3-gallate inhibits amyloid formation by islet amyloid polypeptide, disaggregates amyloid fibrils, and protects cultured cells against IAPP-induced toxicity. *Biochemistry* **2010**, *49*, 8127–8133. [CrossRef] [PubMed]
37. Xu, Z.X.; Zhang, Q.; Ma, G.L.; Chen, C.H.; He, Y.M.; Xu, L.H.; Zhang, Y.; Zhou, G.R.; Li, Z.H.; Yang, H.J.; et al. Influence of Aluminium and EGCG on Fibrillation and Aggregation of Human Islet Amyloid Polypeptide. *J. Diabetes Res.* **2016**, *2016*, 1–14. [CrossRef]
38. Fernández-Millán, E.; Ramos, S.; Alvarez, C.; Bravo, L.; Goya, L.; Martín, M.Á. Microbial phenolic metabolites improve glucose-stimulated insulin secretion and protect pancreatic beta cells against tert-butyl hydroperoxide-induced toxicity via ERKs and PKC pathways. *Food Chem. Toxicol.* **2014**, *66*, 245–253. [CrossRef]
39. Carrasco-Pozo, C.; Gotteland, M.; Castillo, R.L.; Chen, C. 3,4-Dihydroxyphenylacetic acid, a microbiota-derived metabolite of quercetin, protects against pancreatic β-cells dysfunction induced by high cholesterol. *Exp. Cell Res.* **2015**, *334*, 270–282. [CrossRef]
40. Bitner, B.F.; Ray, J.D.; Kener, K.B.; Herring, J.A.; Tueller, J.A.; Johnson, D.K.; Tellez Freitas, C.M.; Fausnacht, D.W.; Allen, M.E.; Thomson, A.H.; et al. Common gut microbial metabolites of dietary flavonoids exert potent protective activities in β-cells and skeletal muscle cells. *J. Nutr. Biochem.* **2018**, *62*, 95–107. [CrossRef]
41. Waltner-Law, M.E.; Wang, X.L.; Law, B.K.; Hall, R.K.; Nawano, M.; Granner, D.K. Epigallocatechin Gallate, a Constituent of Green Tea, Represses Hepatic Glucose Production. *J. Biol. Chem.* **2002**, *277*, 34933–34940. [CrossRef]
42. Collins, Q.F.; Liu, H.Y.; Pi, J.; Liu, Z.; Quon, M.J.; Cao, W. Epigallocatechin-3-gallate (EGCG), a green tea polyphenol, suppresses hepatic gluconeogenesis through 5′-AMP-activated protein kinase. *J. Boil. Chem.* **2007**, *282*, 30143–30149. [CrossRef]
43. Yadollah, S.; Kazemipour, N.; Bakhtiyari, S.; Nazifi, S. Palmitate-induced insulin resistance is attenuated by Pioglitazone and EGCG through reducing the gluconeogenic key enzymes expression in HepG2 cells. *J. Med. Life* **2017**, *10*, 244–249. [PubMed]

44. González-Abuín, N.; Martínez-Micaelo, N.; Blay, M.; Green, B.D.; Pinent, M.; Ardévol, A. Grape-seed procyanidins modulate cellular membrane potential and nutrient-induced GLP-1 secretion in STC-1 cells. *Am. J. Physiol. Cell Physiol.* **2013**, *306*, C485–C492. [CrossRef]
45. Kim, J.J.; Tan, Y.; Xiao, L.; Sun, Y.L.; Qu, X. Green tea polyphenol epigallocatechin-3-gallate enhance glycogen synthesis and inhibit lipogenesis in hepatocytes. *BioMed. Res. Int.* **2013**, *2013*, 1–8. [CrossRef]
46. Vazquez-Prieto, M.A.; Bettaieb, A.; Haj, F.G.; Fraga, C.G.; Oteiza, P.I. (−)-Epicatechin prevents TNFα-induced activation of signaling cascades involved in inflammation and insulin sensitivity in 3T3-L1 adipocytes. *Arch. Bioch. Biophys.* **2012**, *527*, 113–118. [CrossRef] [PubMed]
47. Najmanová, I.; Pourová, J.; Vopršalová, M.; Pilarˇová, V.; Semecký, V.; Nováková, L.; Mladěnka, P. Flavonoid metabolite 3-(3-hydroxyphenyl) propionic acid formed by human microflora decreases arterial blood pressure in rats. *Mol. Nutr. Food Res.* **2016**, *60*, 981–991. [CrossRef]
48. Qian, Y.; Babu, P.V.A.; Symons, J.D.; Jalili, T. Metabolites of flavonoid compounds preserve indices of endothelial cell nitric oxide bioavailability under glucotoxic conditions. *Nutr. Diabetes* **2017**, *7*, e286. [CrossRef]
49. Álvarez-Cilleros, D.; Ramos, S.; Goya, L.; Martín, M.Á. Colonic metabolites from flavanols stimulate nitric oxide production in human endothelial cells and protect against oxidative stress-induced toxicity and endothelial dysfunction. *Food Chem. Toxicol.* **2018**, *115*, 88–97. [CrossRef]
50. Verzelloni, E.; Pellacani, C.; Tagliazucchi, D.; Tagliaferri, S.; Calani, L.; Costa, L.G.; Brighenti, F.; Borges, G.; Crozier, A.; Conte, A.; et al. Antiglycative and neuroprotective activity of colon-derived polyphenol catabolites. *Mol. Nutr. Food Res.* **2011**, *55*, S35–S43. [CrossRef]
51. Giménez-Bastida, J.A.; Zielinski, H.; Piskula, M.; Zielinska, D.; Szawara-Nowak, D. Buckwheat bioactive compounds, their derived phenolic metabolites and their health benefits. *Mol. Nutr. Food Res.* **2017**, *61*, 1600475. [CrossRef] [PubMed]
52. Zhong, H.; Xue, Y.; Lu, X.; Shao, Q.; Cao, Y.; Wu, Z.; Chen, G. The Effects of Different Degrees of Procyanidin Polymerization on the Nutrient Absorption and Digestive Enzyme Activity in Mice. *Molecules* **2018**, *23*, 2916. [CrossRef]
53. Yamashita, Y.; Okabe, M.; Natsume, M.; Ashida, H. Cacao liquor procyanidin extract improves glucose tolerance by enhancing GLUT4 translocation and glucose uptake in skeletal muscle. *J. Nutr. Sci.* **2012**, *1*, E2. [CrossRef] [PubMed]
54. Yamashita, Y.; Okabe, M.; Natsume, M.; Ashida, H. Cacao liquor procyanidins prevent postprandial hyperglycaemia by increasing glucagon-like peptide-1 activity and AMP-activated protein kinase in mice. *J. Nutr. Sci.* **2019**, *8*, E2. [CrossRef] [PubMed]
55. Yamashita, Y.; Wang, L.; Nanba, F.; Ito, C.; Toda, T.; Ashida, H. Procyanidin Promotes Translocation of Glucose Transporter 4 in Muscle of Mice through Activation of Insulin and AMPK Signaling Pathways. *PLoS ONE* **2016**, *11*, e0161704. [CrossRef]
56. Ueda-Wakagi, M.; Nagayasu, H.; Yamashita, Y.; Ashida, H. Green Tea Ameliorates Hyperglycemia by Promoting the Translocation of Glucose Transporter 4 in the Skeletal Muscle of Diabetic Rodents. *Int. J. Mol. Sci.* **2019**, *20*, 2436. [CrossRef] [PubMed]
57. Cremonini, E.; Bettaieb, A.; Haj, F.G.; Fraga, C.G.; Oteiza, P. (−)-Epicatechin improves insulin sensitivity in high fat diet-fed mice. *Arch. Biochem. Biophys.* **2016**, *599*, 13–21. [CrossRef] [PubMed]
58. Bettaieb, A.; Vazquez Prieto, M.A.; Rodriguez Lanzi, C.; Miatello, R.M.; Haj, F.G.; Fraga, C.G.; Oteiza, P.I. (−)-Epicatechin mitigates high-fructose-associated insulin resistance by modulating redox signaling and endoplasmic reticulum stress. *Free Radic. Biol. Med.* **2014**, *72*, 247–256. [CrossRef] [PubMed]
59. Othman, A.I.; El-Sawi, M.R.; El-Missiry, M.A.; Abukhalil, M.H. Epigallocatechin-3-gallate protects against diabetic cardiomyopathy through modulating the cardiometabolic risk factors, oxidative stress, inflammation, cell death and fibrosis in streptozotocin-nicotinamide-induced diabetic rats. *Biomed. Pharmacother.* **2017**, *94*, 362–373. [CrossRef]
60. Cedó, L.; Castell-Auví, A.; Pallarès, V.; Blay, M.; Ardévol, A.; Pinent, M. Grape Seed Procyanidin Extract Improves Insulin Production but Enhances Bax Protein Expression in Cafeteria-Treated Male Rats. *Int. J. Food Sci.* **2013**, *2013*, 875314. [CrossRef]
61. Gan, L.; Meng, Z.; Xiong, R.; Guo, J.; Lu, X.; Zheng, Z.; Deng, Y.; Luo, B.; Zou, F.; Li, H. Green tea polyphenol epigallocatechin-3-gallate ameliorates insulin resistance in non-alcoholic fatty liver disease mice. *Acta Pharmacol. Sin.* **2015**, *36*, 597–605. [CrossRef]

62. Ortsäter, H.; Grankvist, N.; Wolfram, S.; Kuehn, N.; Sjöholm, A. Diet supplementation with green tea extract epigallocatechin gallate prevents progression to glucose intolerance in db/db mice. *Nutr. Metab.* **2012**, *9*, 11. [CrossRef]
63. Franko, A.; Rodriguez Camargo, D.C.; Böddrich, A.; Garg, D.; Rodríguez Camargo, A.; Rathkolb, B.; Janik, D.; Aichler, M.; Feuchtinger, A.; Neff, F.; et al. Epigallocatechin gallate (EGCG) reduces the intensity of pancreatic amyloid fibrils in human islet amyloid polypeptide (hIAPP) transgenic mice. *Sci. Rep.* **2018**, *8*, 1116. [CrossRef] [PubMed]
64. Fu, Z.; Zhen, W.; Yuskavage, J.; Liu, D. Epigallocatechin gallate delays the onset of type 1 diabetes in spontaneous non-obese diabetic mice. *Br. J. Nutr.* **2011**, *105*, 1218–1225. [CrossRef] [PubMed]
65. Fu, Z.; Yuskavage, J.; Liu, D. Dietary flavonol epicatechin prevents the onset of type 1 diabetes in nonobese diabetic mice. *J. Agric. Food Chem.* **2013**, *61*, 4303–4309. [CrossRef]
66. Yamashita, Y.; Okabe, M.; Nasume, M.; Ashida, H. Cinnamtannin A2, a Tetrameric Procyanidin, Increases GLP-1 and Insulin Secretion in Mice. *Biosc. Biotech. Biochem.* **2013**, *77*, 888–891. [CrossRef] [PubMed]
67. Samarghandian, S.; Azimi-Nezhad, M.; Farkhondeh, T. Catechin Treatment Ameliorates Diabetes and Its Complications in Streptozotocin-Induced Diabetic Rats. *Dose-Response* **2017**, *15*, 1–7. [CrossRef] [PubMed]
68. Haidari, F.; Omidian, K.; Rafiei, H.; Zarei, M.; Mohamad Shahi, M. Green Tea (Camellia sinensis) Supplementation to Diabetic Rats Improves Serum and Hepatic Oxidative Stress Markers. *IJPR* **2013**, *12*, 109–114. [PubMed]
69. De Sandoval-Muñiz, R.J.; Vargas-Guerrero, B.; Flores-Alvarado, L.J.; Gurrola-Díaz, C.M. Glucotransporters: Clinical, molecular and genetic aspects. *Gac. Med. Mex.* **2016**, *152*, 547–557.
70. Hajiaghaalipour, F.; Khalilpourfarshbafi, M.; Arya, A. Modulation of Glucose Transporter Protein by Dietary Flavonoids in Type 2 Diabetes Mellitus. *Int. J. Biol. Sci.* **2015**, *11*, 508–524. [CrossRef] [PubMed]
71. Chen, C.; Cohrs, C.M.; Stertmann, J.; Bozsak, R.; Speier, S. Human beta cell mass and function in diabetes: Recent advances in knowledge and technologies to understand disease pathogenesis. *Mol. Metab.* **2017**, *6*, 943–957. [CrossRef]
72. Haataja, L.; Gurlo, T.; Huang, C.J.; Butler, P.C. Islet amyloid in type 2 diabetes, and the toxic oligomer hypothesis. *Endocr. Rev.* **2008**, *29*, 303–316.
73. Del Prato, S. Role of glucotoxicity and lipotoxicity in the pathophysiology of Type 2 diabetes mellitus and emerging treatment strategies. *Diab. Med.* **2009**, *26*, 1185–1192. [CrossRef] [PubMed]
74. Cersosimo, E.; Solis-Herrera, C.; Trautmann, M.E.; Malloy, J.; Triplitt, C.L. Assessment of pancreatic β-cell function: Review of methods and clinical applications. *Curr. Diabetes Rev.* **2014**, *10*, 2–42. [CrossRef] [PubMed]
75. Hatting, M.; Tavares, C.D.; Sharabi, K.; Rines, A.K.; Puigserver, P. Insulin regulation of gluconeogenesis. *Ann. N. Y. Acad. Sci.* **2018**, *1411*, 21–35. [CrossRef] [PubMed]
76. Nauck, M.A.; Meier, J.J. Incretin hormones: Their role in health and disease. *Diabetes Obes. Metab.* **2018**, *1*, 5–21. [CrossRef]
77. Strat, K.M.; Rowley, T.J.; Smithson, A.T.; Tessem, J.S.; Hulver, M.W.; Liu, D.; Davy, B.M.; Davy, K.P.; Neilson, A.P. Mechanisms by which cocoa flavanols improve metabolic syndrome and related disorders. *J. Nutr. Biochem.* **2016**, *35*, 1–21. [CrossRef]
78. Kohlgruber, A.; Lynch, L. Adipose tissue inflammation in the pathogenesis of type 2 diabetes. *Curr. Diabetes Rep.* **2015**, *15*, 92. [CrossRef]
79. Petrie, J.R.; Guzik, T.J.; Touyz, R.M. Diabetes, Hypertension, and Cardiovascular Disease: Clinical Insights and Vascular Mechanisms. *Can. J. Cardiol.* **2018**, *34*, 575–584. [CrossRef]
80. Vlassara, H.; Uribarri, J. Advanced glycation end products (AGE) and diabetes: Cause, effect, or both? *Curr. Diabetes Rep.* **2014**, *14*, 453. [CrossRef]
81. Zhang, H.; Su, S.; Yu, X.; Li, Y. Dietary epigallocatechin 3-gallate supplement improves maternal and neonatal treatment outcome of gestational diabetes mellitus: A double-blind randomised controlled trial. *J. Hum. Nutr. Diet.* **2017**, *30*, 753–758. [CrossRef]
82. Grassi, D.; Desideri, G.; Necozione, S.; Lippi, C.; Casale, R.; Properzi, G.; Blumberg, J.B.; Ferri, C. Blood pressure is reduced and insulin sensitivity increased in glucose-intolerant, hypertensive subjects after 15 days of consuming high-polyphenol dark chocolate. *J. Nutr.* **2008**, *138*, 1671–1676. [CrossRef]

83. Curtis, P.J.; Sampson, M.; Potter, J.; Dhatariya, K.; Kroon, P.A.; Cassidy, A. Chronic ingestion of flavan-3-ols and isoflavones improves insulin sensitivity and lipoprotein status and attenuates estimated 10-year CVD risk in medicated postmenopausal women with type 2 diabetes: A 1-year, double-blind, randomized, controlled trial. *Diabetes Care* **2012**, *35*, 226–232. [CrossRef] [PubMed]
84. Hsu, C.-H.; Liao, Y.-L.; Lin, S.-C.; Tsai, T.-H.; Huang, C.-J.; Chou, P. Does supplementation with green tea extract improve insulin resistance in obese type 2 diabetics? A randomized, double-blind, and placebo-controlled clinical trial. *Altern. Med. Rev.* **2011**, *16*, 157–163. [CrossRef] [PubMed]
85. Nagao, T.; Meguro, S.; Hase, T.; Otsuka, K.; Komikado, M.; Tokimitsu, I.; Yamamoto, T.; Yamamoto, K. A catechin-rich beverage improves obesity and blood glucose control in patients with type 2 diabetes. *Obesity* **2008**, *17*, 310–317. [CrossRef] [PubMed]
86. Fukino, Y.; Ikeda, A.; Maruyama, K.; Aoki, N.; Okubo, T.; Iso, H. Randomized controlled trial for an effect of green tea-extract powder supplementation on glucose abnormalities. *Eur. J. Clin. Nutr.* **2008**, *62*, 953–960. [CrossRef] [PubMed]
87. Fukino, Y.; Shimbo, M.; Aoki, N.; Okubo, T.; Iso, H. Randomized controlled trial for an effect of green tea consumption on insulin resistance and inflammation markers. *J. Nutr. Sci. Vitaminol.* **2005**, *51*, 335–342. [CrossRef] [PubMed]
88. Ryu, O.H.; Lee, J.; Lee, K.W.; Kim, H.Y.; Seo, J.A.; Kim, S.G.; Kim, N.H.; Baik, S.-H.; Choi, D.S.; Choi, K.M. Effects of green tea consumption on inflammation, insulin resistance and pulse wave velocity in type 2 diabetes patients. *Diabetes Res. Clin. Pract.* **2006**, *71*, 356–358. [CrossRef]
89. Kar, P.; Laight, D.; Rooprai, H.K.; Shaw, K.M.; Cummings, M. Effects of grape seed extract in Type 2 diabetic subjects at high cardiovascular risk: A double blind randomized placebo controlled trial examining metabolic markers, vascular tone, inflammation, oxidative stress and insulin sensitivity. *Diabet. Med.* **2009**, *26*, 526–531. [CrossRef]
90. Dicks, L.; Kirch, N.; Gronwald, D.; Wernken, K.; Zimmermann, B.F.; Helfrich, H.P.; Ellinger, S. Regular Intake of a Usual Serving Size of Flavanol-Rich Cocoa Powder Does Not Affect Cardiometabolic Parameters in Stably Treated Patients with Type 2 Diabetes and Hypertension-A Double-Blinded, Randomized, Placebo-Controlled Trial. *Nutrients* **2018**, *10*, 1435. [CrossRef]
91. Stote, K.S.; Clevidence, B.A.; Novotny, J.A.; Henderson, T.; Radecki, S.V.; Baer, D.J. Effect of cocoa and green tea on biomarkers of glucose regulation, oxidative stress, inflammation and hemostasis in obese adults at risk for insulin resistance. *Eur. J. Clin. Nutr.* **2012**, *66*, 1153–1159. [CrossRef] [PubMed]
92. Basu, A.; Betts, N.M.; Leyva, M.J.; Fu, D.; Aston, C.E.; Lyons, T.J. Acute Cocoa Supplementation Increases Postprandial HDL Cholesterol and Insulin in Obese Adults with Type 2 Diabetes after Consumption of a High-Fat Breakfast. *J. Nutr.* **2015**, *145*, 2325–2332. [CrossRef]
93. Rynarzewski, J.; Dicks, L.; Zimmermann, B.F.; Stoffel-Wagner, B.; Ludwig, N.; Helfrich, H.P.; Ellinger, S. Impact of a Usual Serving Size of Flavanol-Rich Cocoa Powder Ingested with a Diabetic-Suitable Meal on Postprandial Cardiometabolic Parameters in Type 2 Diabetics-A Randomized, Placebo-Controlled, Double-Blind Crossover Study. *Nutrients* **2019**, *11*, 417. [CrossRef]
94. Del Rio, D.; Calani, L.; Cordero, C.; Salvatore, S.; Pellegrini, N.; Brighenti, F. Bioavailability and catabolism of green tea flavan-3-ols in humans. *Nutrition* **2010**, *26*, 1110–1116. [CrossRef] [PubMed]
95. Ottaviani, J.I.; Borges, G.; Momma, T.Y.; Spencer, J.P.E.; Keen, C.L.; Crozier, A.; Schroeter, H. The metabolome of [2-(14) C] (-)-epicatechin in humans: Implications for the assessment of efficacy, safety, and mechanisms of action of polyphenolic bioactives. *Sci. Rep.* **2016**, *6*, 29034. [CrossRef] [PubMed]
96. Urpi-Sarda, M.; Monagas, M.; Khan, N.; Llorach, R.; Lamuela-Raventós, R.M.; Jáuregui, O.; Estruch, R.; Izquierdo-Pulido, M.; Andrés-Lacueva, C. Targeted metabolic profiling of phenolics in urine and plasma after regular consumption of cocoa by liquid chromatography–tandem mass spectrometry. *J. Chromatogr. A* **2009**, *1216*, 7258–7267. [CrossRef] [PubMed]
97. Wiese, S.; Esatbeyoglu, T.; Winterhalter, P.; Kruse, H.-P.; Winkler, S.; Bub, A.; Kulling, S.E. Comparative biokinetics and metabolism of pure monomeric, dimeric, and polymeric flavan-3-ols: A randomized cross-over study in humans. *Mol. Nutr. Food Res.* **2015**, *59*, 610–621. [PubMed]
98. Rodriguez-Mateos, A.; Feliciano, R.P.; Boeres, A.; Weber, T.; Dos Santos, C.N.; Ventura, M.R.; Heiss, C. Cranberry (poly)phenol metabolites correlate with improvements in vascular function: A double-blind, randomized, controlled, dose-response, crossover study. *Mol. Nutr. Food Res.* **2016**, *60*, 2130–2140. [CrossRef]

99. Castello, F.; Costabile, G.; Bresciani, L.; Tassotti, M.; Naviglio, D.; Luongo, D.; Ciciola, P.; Vitale, M.; Vetrani, C.; Galaverna, G.; et al. Bioavailability and pharmacokinetic profile of grape pomace phenolic compounds in humans. *Arch. Biochem. Biophys.* **2018**, *646*, 1–9.
100. Feliciano, R.P.; Boeres, A.; Massacessi, L.; Istas, G.; Ventura, M.R.; Nunes dos Santos, C.; Heiss, C.; Rodriguez-Mateos, A. Identification and quantification of novel cranberry-derived plasma and urinary (poly) phenols. *Arch. Biochem. Biophys.* **2016**, *599*, 31–41. [CrossRef]
101. Tagliazucchi, D.; Martini, S.; Conte, A. Protocatechuic and 3,4-Dihydroxyphenylacetic Acids Inhibit Protein Glycation by Binding Lysine through a Metal-Catalyzed Oxidative Mechanism. *J. Agric. Food Chem.* **2019**, *67*, 7821–7831. [CrossRef]
102. Pourová, J.; Najmanová, I.; Vopršalová, M.; Migkos, T.; Pilařová, V.; Applová, L.; Nováková, L.; Mladěnka, P. Two flavonoid metabolites, 3,4-dihydroxyphenylacetic acid and 4-methylcatechol, relax arteries ex vivo and decrease blood pressure in vivo. *Vascul. Pharmacol.* **2018**, *111*, 36–43. [CrossRef]

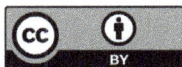

© 2020 by the authors. Licensee MDPI, Basel, Switzerland. This article is an open access article distributed under the terms and conditions of the Creative Commons Attribution (CC BY) license (http://creativecommons.org/licenses/by/4.0/).

MDPI
St. Alban-Anlage 66
4052 Basel
Switzerland
Tel. –41 61 683 77 34
Fax –41 61 302 89 18
www.mdpi.com

Nutrients Editorial Office
E-mail: nutrients@mdpi.com
www.mdpi.com/journal/nutrients

www.ingramcontent.com/pod-product-compliance
Lightning Source LLC
LaVergne TN
LVHW070438100526
838202LV00014B/1621